Guidebook for Support Programs in Aural Rehabilitation

Guidebook for Support Programs in Aural Rehabilitation

Carole E. Johnson, Ph.D.
Associate Professor
Department of Communication Disorders
Auburn University
Auburn, Alabama

Jeffrey L. Danhauer, Ph.D.
Professor
Department of Speech and Hearing Sciences
University of California at Santa Barbara
Santa Barbara, California

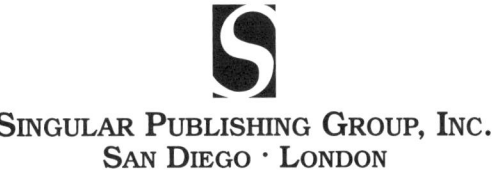

SINGULAR PUBLISHING GROUP, INC.
SAN DIEGO · LONDON

Singular Publishing Group, Inc.
401 West A Street, Suite 325
San Diego, California 92101-7904

Singular Publishing Ltd.
19 Compton Terrace
London N1 2UN, UK

Singular Publishing Group, Inc., publishes textbooks, clinical manuals, clinical reference books, journals, videos, and multimedia materials on speech-language pathology, audiology, otorhinolaryngology, special education, early childhood, aging, occupational therapy, physical therapy, rehabilitation, counseling, mental health, and voice. For your convenience, our entire catalog can be accessed on our website at **http//www.singpub.com**. Our mission to provide you with materials to meet the daily challenges of the everchanging health care/educational environment will remain on course if we are in touch with you. In that spirit, we welcome your feedback on our products. Please telephone (**1-800-521-8545**), fax (**1-800-774-8398**), or e-mail (**singpub@singpub.com**) your comments and requests to us.

© 1999 by Singular Publishing Group, Inc.

Typeset in 10/12 Bookman by So Cal Graphics
Printed in the United States of America by McNaughton & Gunn

All rights, including that of translation, reserved. No part of this publication may be reproduced, stored in a retrieval system or transmitted in any form or by any means, electronic, mechanical, recording, or otherwise, without the prior written permission of the publisher.

Library of Congress Cataloging-in-Publication Data

Johnson, Carole E.
   Guidebook For support programs in aural rehabilitation / by Carole
E. Johnson, Jeffrey L. Danhauer
      p.   cm.
   Includes bibliographical references and index.
   ISBN 1-565-93-905-0 (softcover : alk. paper)
   1. Hearing disorders—Patients—Rehabilitation—Social aspects.
2. Hearing impaired—Rehabilitation—Social aspects.   3. Managed
care plans (Medical care) I. Danhauer, Jeffrey L. II. Title.
   [DNLM: 1. Rehabilitation of Hearing Impaired. 2. Managed Care
Programs. 3. Marketing of Hearing Health Services.   WV 276 J66g 1999]
RF291.J617   1999
362.4'68—dc21
DNLM/DLC
for Library of Congress   99-10767
                                                                                                              CIP

CONTENTS

Foreword by Nancy Tye-Murray	ix
Preface	xi
CD-ROM	xv
Chapter 1 Current Climate of Health Care	**1**
Introduction	1
Learning Objectives	2
Managed Care: An Overview	2
Advantages and Disadvantages of Managed Care	3
Trends in Managed Care	5
Managed Care and the Practice of Audiology	5
A Proactive Approach to Managed Care	7
Summary	9
Learning Activities	10
References	10
Appendix	12
Chapter 2 Multiskilling and the Use of Support Personnel: An Overview	**15**
Introduction	15
Learning Objectives	16
Team Concepts in Aural Rehabilitation	16
Multiskilling	17
Use of Support Personnel	19
A Model	21
Summary	23
Learning Activities	24
References	24
Appendices	26

Chapter 3 Defining and Marketing Support Programs — 33

Introduction — 33
Learning Objectives — 34
Impact of Support Programs on Private Practices — 34
Defining Support Programs — 34
Marketing Support Programs — 37
Summary — 43
Learning Activities — 43
References — 44
Appendices — 45

Chapter 4 Funding Sources for Support Programs — 51

Introduction — 51
Learning Objectives — 52
Strategic Philanthropy — 52
Factors Related to Funding Support Programs — 53
Funding Sources for Support Programs — 55
Summary — 59
Learning Activities — 59
References — 59
Appendices — 60

Chapter 5 Creating Effective Inservice Programs — 65

Introduction — 65
Learning Objectives — 66
Preparedness of Related Professionals to Serve as Audiologic
   Support Personnel — 66
Selection of the Appropriate Model of Multiskilling — 68
Components of Complete Inservice Programs — 69
Types of Inservice Formats — 70
Creating Meaningful Adult Learning Experiences — 74
Summary — 76
Learning Activities — 76
References — 76
Appendices — 78

Chapter 6 Establishing Support Programs in Educational Settings — 147

Introduction — 148
Learning Objectives — 148

The Law	148
Current Realities in Educational Settings	150
Informal Support Programs	152
Amplification Device Support Programs	154
Support Programs in Central Auditory Processing Disorders (CAPD) Service Delivery	161
Counseling Support Programs	167
Support Programs in Postsecondary Educational Institutions	172
Summary	176
Learning Activities	176
References	176
Appendices	180

Chapter 7 Establishing Support Programs in Rehabilitation Hospitals — 207

Introduction	207
Learning Objectives	208
The Rehabilitation Industry for the Next Millenium: The HealthSouth Model	208
Typical Audiologic Service-Delivery Model in a Rehabilitation Hospital	209
Effects of Disability and Hearing Loss	210
Support Programs for Rehabilitation-Hospital Patients with Hearing Impairment	213
Summary	222
References	222
Appendices	225

Chapter 8 Establishing Support Programs in Long-Term Residential Care Facilities for the Elderly — 263

Introduction	263
Learning Objectives	265
Aspects of Aging: Myths Versus Reality	265
Why Should Audiologists Care?	267
Continuum of Housing for the Elderly: Important Considerations	269
Establishing Support Programs in Residential Facilities for the Elderly	270
Patient Services	273
Facility Services	293
Special Services	296
Summary	296
Learning Activities	297

References	297
Appendices	301

Chapter 9   Sustaining Stellar Support Programs: Outcome Measures   331

Introduction	331
Learning Objectives	332
Terminology in Outcomes Measurement	332
Critical Areas of Outcomes Measurement for Support Programs	334
Outcomes Measurement Across Service-Delivery Sites	336
Outcome Measures for Fiscal Responsibility	338
Summary	339
Learning Activities	339
References	339
Appendices	341

Chapter 10   Aural Rehabilitation Programming in the Future   345

Introduction	345
Learning Objectives	346
Research Needs in Aural Rehabilitation	346
Aural Rehabilitation Needs in Training Programs	350
Audiologists' Promotion of Aural Rehabilitation	352
Summary	353
Learning Activities	353
References	354

Index   **355**

Foreword

Students of audiology leave their training programs with an arsenal of knowledge about how to diagnose and habilitate hearing loss. They have spent several years taking courses about how to detect and measure hearing loss, how to fit listening aids, and how to counsel patients and their communication partners. They may have learned fundamental principles of auditory training and communication-strategies training.

Filled with enthusiasm and good will, they charge into the market place. Unfortunately, many new graduates find themselves unprepared to deal with the realities of the U.S. health-care system. Their professors may have had little experience with operating a successful audiological practice, and may have conveyed to them primarily "book knowledge." As a result, students may have learned little about managed care: how managed care operates, the types of managed care organizations that exist in the United States today, and the implications of managed care for the provision of audiological services. Morever, they may not know how to market their services in a competitive marketplace or how to make their services cost effective with the use of multiskilling and support personnel. Students may find that a second stage of their education begins on completion of their formal instruction. They must learn to provide aural rehabilitation to patients through service-delivery models that are appropriate for today's health-care system, and all too often, they do so by the seat of their pants.

The publication of this textbook represents an epochal event in the discipline of aural rehabilitation. This is the first such text I know of that includes a comprehensive overview of managed care, a consideration of marketing principles in the context of hearing health care, and a detailed look at realistic outcome measures. This is the kind of information that is so critical for the successful execution of aural rehabilitation in the real world, yet is so lacking in coverage in most current textbooks.

In addition to important information, this text also includes ready-to-use materials and provides a myriad of resources to the practicing audiologist. For example, materials from the appendices can be made directly into overheads and used for providing inservice training to other professionals. Sample letters can be modified for marketing and fundraising purposes. The materials will greatly simplify and streamline the preparation of aural rehabilitation services.

In sum, many students, whether they are in graduate training or seeking continuing education, will find this textbook to be an invaluable resource. My hunch is that it will have an influence on subsequent textbooks in our discipline, so they too will likely begin to include information about the nuts-and-bolts of private practice and managed care. This book is indeed an important first.

Nancy Tye-Murray

Preface

The hearing health-care profession is a rapidly growing force bolstered in particular by two recent events. First, advances in technology related to the early identification of hearing loss and the amplification systems to remedy it have done much to change the public's opinion about hearing loss. Second, the aging population and its accompanying hearing difficulties can no longer ignore the importance of hearing health care. Today, audiologists must acknowledge the current realities of the hearing health-care arena as it relates to their broadened scope of practice. Probably more than ever before, participation in this arena encompasses aural rehabilitation programs across several service-delivery sites in addition to the traditional office setting.

The future looks bright for the audiology profession because the number of patients is steadily increasing and now exceeds the number of audiologists available to provide services. Audiologists must devise ways to maximize the effectiveness of their efforts to meet all patients' needs, while also containing costs in light of reductions in funds available for health-related services. One way to meet these requirements is through the establishment of support programs for patients with hearing impairment across service-delivery sites. These programs should be designed using multiskilled audiologic support personnel so that patients' hearing health-care needs are met in service delivery sites in which managing audiologists are not present on a day-to-day basis.

Presently, only about one-fifth the necessary number of audiologists are available to treat children with hearing impairment in U.S. public schools. Many of the hearing aids used by this population are frequently nonfunctional, and less than 50% of public agencies have adequate provisions to maintain children's hearing aids and personal FM systems. Similarly, rehabilitation hospitals and long-term residential care facilities for the elderly rarely employ audiologists to meet the hearing health-care needs of their patients. Such patients are often elderly individuals with hearing loss who may not be able to benefit from any type of rehabilitation efforts because of their inability to communicate with therapists. Also, few, if any, hearing health-insurance plans offered through corporate audiology networks have provisions for aural rehabilitation beyond the purchase of hearing aids.

Consequently, most audiologists are left with the reality that although aural rehabilitation principles are worthy of consideration, they are rarely implemented. There are a variety of reasons. First, audiologists do not have the time or financial resources to provide the services. Second, patients often are unwilling to commit the necessary time, effort, or money to attend aural rehabilitation classes. Finally, some audiologists may not have the training or expertise to provide aural rehabilitation (Tye-Murray, Witt, Schum, Kelsay, & Schum, 1994). Thus, audiologists must try to "bridge the gap" by providing hearing health-care services to vast numbers of unserved and underserved individuals with hearing impairment in various service delivery sites. The task is complicated by the current trends and perspectives in health care mandated by managed care.

We wanted to write a textbook for students and for those professionals (audiologists, speech-language pathologists, and administrators) who are challenged to meet patients' hearing health-care needs under less than optimal circumstances. At first we envisioned a handbook that would cover all aspects of aural rehabilitation necessary to accomplish this goal. That task was overwhelming for a single text, however, because each service-delivery site and each patient have unique challenges and needs. What we have done instead is to provide a guidebook to assist professionals in establishing support programs for patients with hearing impairment in service-delivery sites where patients' hearing health-care needs are either unserved or underserved.

Support programs can help ensure the communication accessibility of patients with hearing impairment so that they can meet the demands of their environments. Support programs are necessary when traditional audiologic service delivery is either difficult or impossible to achieve. These programs require the coordination and cooperation of other multiskilled (cross-trained) professionals. These colleagues may serve as audiologic support personnel to meet patients' communication needs in service-delivery sites where the managing audiologist is not available on a day-to-day basis (e.g., public schools, rehabilitation hospitals, and long-term residential care facilities for the elderly). For each of these sites, clinical-management concepts, managed-care principles, preferred practice patterns, position statements, and practice guidelines are discussed and integrated for contextual relevance and for direct application. Numerous useful suggestions and materials are provided regarding the use of multiskilling and audiologic support personnel to establish innovative aural rehabilitation support programs that augment traditional audiologic service-delivery models. The accompanying CD-ROM provides useful forms that can be downloaded and adapted for clinicians' use.

The first four chapters of this book lay the foundation for establishing these support programs. Chapter 1 discusses the current climate of health care with an introduction to managed care, including its definition and primary principles, advantages and disadvantages for health-care providers and patients, current trends, and implications for aural rehabilitation. Most important, this chapter emphasizes the fact that audiologists must assume a proactive approach to managed care. Chapter 2 provides an overview of multiskilling, which refers to training one professional to perform tasks that are typically conducted by professionals in other disciplines. This chapter places the use of multiskilling and audiologic support personnel within the context of a team approach to aural rehabilitation. In addition, multiskilling is discussed in terms of its various models; advantages and disadvantages for health-care providers, patients, manangement, and third-party payers; the American Speech-Language-Hearing Association's Position Statement: Multiskilled Personnel (1997); the history of using support personnel in the profession; and the Position Statement and Guidelines of the Consensus Panel on Support Personnel in Audiology (AAA, 1997).

Chapter 3 defines support programs and methods of marketing them. Audiologists must effectively market clearly defined support programs in order to obtain the necessary start-up resources for their initiation. With the knowledge that audiologists could not implement these support programs unless there was a way to pay for them, a chapter on funding has been included in this text. Thus, Chapter 4 is devoted to means by which audiologists can practice "strategic philanthropy" in raising funds to provide aural rehabilitation services to deserving patients through support programs.

Chapters 5 through 8 are the "nuts and bolts" of the book. Chapter 5 explains how to create effective inservice programs for training participants to serve competently in support programs for patients with hearing impairment. Numerous inservice protocols (i.e., formats, handouts, instructors' overheads, and quizzes) are provided for readers' use. Chapters 6, 7, and 8 provide specifics about how to establish these support programs in educational settings, rehabilitation hospitals, and long-term residential care facilities for the elderly, respectively. Chapters 5 through 8 provide audiologists with essential information and useful materials to implement state-of-the-art aural rehabilitation support programs in each of these service-delivery sites.

Chapter 9 discusses sustaining stellar support programs through outcomes measurement, which is extremely important because third-party payers expect health-care providers to be accountable and demonstrate quality (Hicks, 1998). In addition, readers are provided with the following information regarding outcomes measurement: terminology, requirements of accrediting bodies, and measures specific to service-delivery sites. Finally, Chapter 10 ties the book together, highlighting the important points by discussing future research and training program needs in aural rehabilitation. In addition, this chapter discusses how audiologists can promote aural rehabilitation in audiologic service delivery.

We have attempted to provide cost-efficient ways to provide aural rehabilitation services to patients with hearing impairment in traditionally unserved or underserved service-delivery sites. The development of efficient support programs may help to reduce the amount of direct involvement required of managing audiologists. At the same time, such programs should be beneficial, demonstrating the hearing healthcare professional's sensitivity and ability to meet patients' communication needs. We are aware that some aspects of aural rehabilitation in these service-delivery sites may have been overlooked. Nevertheless, we believe that our approach is timely, innovative, and consistent with many principles of managed care. We hope that this text stimulates more audiologists to provide aural rehabilitation services in these and other service-delivery sites. Furthermore, we hope that this textbook changes the way that aural rehabilitation services are provided to patients. Aural rehabilitation can change not only the lives of patients' with hearing impairment, but the lives of their family, friends, and associates as well.

We would like to acknowledge our families, friends, colleagues, and our students for their support in the completion of this project. We would like to thank Nancy Tye-Murray for writing the foreword to this book. We would also like to thank the staff at Singular Publishing Group (Candice Janco, Kristin Banach, Sandy Doyle, Brad Bielawski, and Angie Singh) for their input and expertise throughout all phases of this project. In addition, we would like to thank Sue Abel, Traci Miller, Jill Mize, Alese Morgan, and other student assistants who assisted with proofreading the text and compiling the references. The first author would also like to thank Sandra Clark-Lewis and Donna Griffin for the wonderful opportunity to participate in and observe the innovative audiologic service-delivery model developed at HealthSouth Rehabilitation Hospital in Montgomery, AL, and Dr. William O. Haynes who was always available to answer my questions. Last, but not least, we would like to thank our patients who have taught us the most.

REFERENCES

American Academy of Audiology. (1997). Position statement and guidelines of the consensus panel on support personnel in audiology. *Audiology Today, 9*(3), 27–28.

American Speech-Language-Hearing Association. (1997, Spring). Position statement: Multiskilled personnel. *Asha 39*(Suppl. 17), 13.

Hicks, P. L. (1998). Outcomes measurement requirements. In C. M. Frattali (Ed.), *Measuring outcomes in speech-language pathology* (pp. 28–54). New York: Thieme.

Tye-Murray, N., Witt, S., Schum, L., Kelsay, D., & Schum, D. J. (1994). Feasible aural rehabilitation services for busy clinical settings. *American Journal of Audiology: A Journal of Clinical Practice, 3*(3), 33–37.

CD-ROM

A special feature of this Guidebook is an accompanying CD-ROM that contains forms and handouts from the text appendices in Microsoft Word 7.0 (PC-based format). Some of these materials contain images that have been scanned directly into the documents. Therefore, users should always choose the "Enable Macros" option when opening the text file. The CD-ROM feature allows the user the advantage of printing of original copywork as well as the ability to adapt the materials to include new information or to modify for relevance to specific service-delivery sites. Users are asked to retain the book title, authors, and publisher printed at the bottom of each page to maintain the identity with the Guidebook. Materials that have been authored by others should not be adapted unless permission of the original authors is obtained. Prior to using the CD-ROM, copy the documents to a separate disk to use as a working file. The contents of the CD-ROM are listed below and the file names correspond to the appropriate appendices.

CONTENTS

Chapter 3   Defining and Marketing Programs
Appendix III-D: Marketing Effectiveness Log

Chapter 5   Creating Effective Inservice Programs
Appendix V-B: Staff Inservice Participation Documentation Form
Appendix V-C: Inservice Participant Evaluation Form
Appendix V-D: Inservice for the Americans with Disabilities Act (1990)
Appendix V-E: Inservice on Hearing Loss and its Effect on Communication
Appendix V-F: Inservice on, "How Do You Communicate with Someone with a Hearing Loss?"
Appendix V-G: Inservice on Hearing Aids, Their Care and Their Use
Appendix V-H: Inservice on Cochlear Implants, Their Care and Their Use

Chapter 6   Establishing Support Programs in Educational Settings
Appendix VI-B: Classroom Amplification Device Inventory Sheet
Appendix VI-D: Hearing Aid Check Sheet
Appendix VI-E: Cochlear Implant Check Sheet
Appendix VI-F: Personal FM System Check Sheet
Appendix VI-G: Sound-Field FM Amplification System Check Sheet

Chapter 7 Establishing Support Programs in Rehabilitation Hospitals

- Appendix VII-A: Informed Consent for Participation in Hearing Support Program
- Appendix VII-B: Notification of Patient Participation in Hearing Support Program
- Appendix VII-C: Otoacoustic Emissions Fact Sheet
- Appendix VII-E: Inservice on Otoacoustic Emissions (OAEs) for Audiologic Support Personnel
- Appendix VII-F: Hearing Screening Form
- Appendix VII-G: Hearing Handicap Inventory for the Elderly—Screening
- Appendix VII-H: Hearing Handicap Inventory for Adults—Screening
- Appendix VII-K: Handouts for the Hearing Aid Delivery
- Appendix VII-L: Motor Skills and Sequencing for Hearing Aid Use and Manipulation
- Appendix VII-M: Visualization and Imagery Task for CIC Insertion
- Appendix VII-P: Hearing Aid Check Sheet
- Appendix VII-Q: Daily Log of Hearing Aid Use for Patients Requiring Assistance
- Appendix VII-R: Facility Communication Accessibility Checklist
- Appendix VII-S: Listening Questionnaire
- Appendix VII-U: Handout on "Clear Speech"
- Appendix VII-V: Speechreading Materials

Chapter 8 Establishing Support Programs in Long-Term Residential Care Facilities for the Elderly

- Appendix VIII-B: Facility Checklists
- Appendix VIII-D: Sample Audiologic Case-History Intake Form
- Appendix VIII-E: Communication/Environment Assessment and Planning Guide
- Appendix VIII-G: Checklist of Holistic Factors in Planning Aural Rehabilitation
- Appendix VIII-K: Hearing Aid Skills Checklist
- Appendix VIII-L: Group Interaction Checklist
- Appendix VIII-N: Documentation of ALD Selection Protocol
- Appendix VIII-O: ALD Fitting and Orientation Checklist

Chapter 9 Sustaining Stellar Support Programs: Outcomes Measures

- Appendix IX-A: Customer-Satisfaction Questionnaire for Educational Support Programs
- Appendix IX-B: Customer-Satisfaction Questionnaire for Rehabilitation Hospital Support Programs
- Appendix IX-C: Customer-Satisfaction Questionnaire for Support Programs in Nursing Homes

CHAPTER 1

Current Climate of Health Care

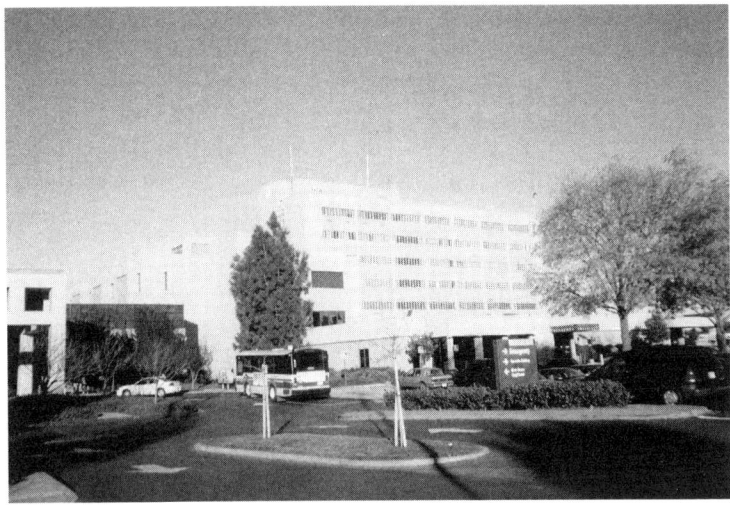

Figure 1-1. New health-care policies affect service delivery in most facilities.

INTRODUCTION

Since the end of World War II, the American health-care system has generally operated under the traditional fee-for-service reimbursement model that provides little incentive for service care providers to cut costs (ASHA, 1996). A disadvantage of fee-for-service reimbursement models is that they can monetarily reward unethical health-care providers who prescribe unnecessary treatment (Seppala, 1995). High volumes of unnecessary care have driven the cost of health care to higher and higher levels. Health-care costs account for one out of every six to seven dollars or 14% of the gross domestic product (GDP) (ASHA, 1996). Estimates suggest that the cost of health care could increase to nearly 20% of the GDP by the year 2000 if changes are not made to the system and its financing mechanisms (Hattie Larlham Bulletin, 1996).

At present, our unfocused, inefficient health-care system consists of millions of independent profit centers (e.g., solo practices, clinics, hospitals, nursing homes, and so on) that have few, if any, financial or operational linkages (Seppala, 1995). *Managed care has been offered as one way to reduce the costs of health care by combining financing, clinical services, and management under a single system.* Managed care changes the role of the "customer" from the patient to the third-party payer. The first party is the patient, the second party is the health-care provider, and the third party is the insurer (ASHA, 1996). The second party, usually the primary-care physician, is the gatekeeper who is rewarded by the managed-care organization (MCO) for treating its members while also reducing health-care costs.

Managed care is becoming increasingly popular. For example, more than 50% of the Fortune 500 companies have their employees enrolled in managed-care programs; 30% of those programs offer hearing aid benefits and 82% offer hearing assessment benefits (Berkowitz, 1996). More than 53% of dispensing audiologists now provide hearing care under managed-care contracts and receive 19% of their revenues for these services (Skafte, 1997). Also, public schools are now billing third-party payers for services provided by audiologists. Thus, *audiologists must be familiar with the principles of managed care in order to compete in today's health-care arena.*

Unfortunately, managed-care organizations do not reimburse for aural rehabilitation services except in some cases, for the purchase and fitting of hearing aids. In the near future, audiologists will struggle to balance the aural rehabilitation needs of patients and the pressures of managed care through innovative service-delivery models. *The focus of this book is to be a guide for clinicians in establishing cost-efficient, stellar support programs for persons with hearing impairment across various service delivery sites.* Chapter 1 provides an introduction to managed care and its implications for the practice of audiology, especially aural rehabilitation.

LEARNING OBJECTIVES

This chapter will enable the reader to:

- Define managed care
- Describe the primary principles of managed care
- Describe the different types of managed-care organizations
- Discuss the advantages and disadvantages of managed care for health-care providers and patients
- Discuss current trends in managed care
- Discuss implications of managed care on aural rehabilitation
- Understand the importance of a proactive approach to managed care for the practice of audiology

---

MANAGED CARE: AN OVERVIEW

Principles of Managed Care

There are eight basic principles to managed care (ASHA, 1996). First, health-care services are provided by a specific group of health-care professionals grouped under one organization for a covered population (i.e., enrollees) under the terms of a contract. Second, capitation is the most common and fastest growing managed-care payment system. Payment is completely unrelated to services rendered. A fixed amount of money is prospectively paid on a "per-member-per-month" (PMPM) unit basis based on: (1) plan enrollment, (2) plan experience, and (3) health-risk factors. Third, the health-care providers are paid by the managed-care plan either on a salary or through a contract. The MCO provides incentives for the primary-care physician to act as gatekeeper (i.e., controls enrollees' access to health-care services) to reduce costs. Fourth, the gatekeeper must authorize health-care services provided by specialists. Fifth, the MCO offers a continuum of health services emphasizing preventative care (e.g., health education), primary care, acute care, subacute care, and long-term care (Deloitte & Touche, 1996). Sixth, the focus of health care is shifting away from hospitalization toward medical-care processes that can be provided in community clinics closer to patients' homes (Hattie Larlham Bulletin, 1996). Seventh, resource management is the key to cutting costs. Table 1–1 lists the components of resource management (ASHA, 1996). Eighth, managed care strongly emphasizes information systems to monitor costs, processes of care, and outcomes.

Table 1-1. Components of resource management.

- Admission planning
- Utilization management
- Productivity standards
- Quality assessment and improvement activities
- Use of practice guidelines, clinical paths, and treatment protocols
- Risk management
- Infection control
- Discharge planning

Source: From *Curriculum Guide to Managed Care*, 1996, p. 32. Rockville, MD: American Speech-Language Hearing Association. Reprinted with permission.

Types of Managed-Care Organizations (MCOs)

There are several different types of managed-care organizations. The three most common types of MCOs are the following (Griffin & Fazen, 1993):

- ***Managed indemnity insurance programs*** are traditional fee-for-service plans that reimburse providers based on their billed charges for medical-care services in return for payment of a monthly premium by the enrollee.
- ***Preferred Provider Organizations (PPOs)*** are organized by either insurers or providers themselves who contract with either networks or providers who have agreed to provide health-care services on a negotiated fee schedule. With PPOs, enrollees can seek health-care services from nonaffiliated providers, but they have to pay a higher fee.
- ***Health Maintenance Organizations (HMOs)*** provide a defined, comprehensive set of health services to a group of enrollees. There are four types of HMOs (ASHA, 1996):
  ⇒ *Staff Model:* requires that all health-care providers are employees of the HMO and work at the same facility.
  ⇒ *Group Model:* involves health-care provider groups contracted with the HMO to provide services either in their own offices or in company facilities.
  ⇒ *Individual Practice Association (IPA):* involves a group of health-care practitioners with whom an HMO has contracted to provide services in their own offices.
  ⇒ *Networks:* contract with HMOs and are multispecialty groups of individual practitioners in a wide geographic area who serve a large population of enrollees.

The most common HMO arrangement for audiologists is the network. There are two types of networks: (1) vertically integrated networks and (2) horizontally integrated networks (Klontz, 1997). Vertically integrated networks involve different types of associated providers (e.g., physical therapists, speech-language pathologists) who offer a continuum of care (Klontz, 1997). Horizontally integrated networks are formed when providers in the same profession combine over a geographic area (Klontz, 1997). Audiologists most often affiliate with horizontally integrated networks. Some successful horizontally integrated networks include the National Ear Care Plan, Sonus, and Integrated Audiology Network (Minnesota).

ADVANTAGES AND DISADVANTAGES OF MANAGED CARE

There are advantages and disadvantages of managed care to health-care providers and patients. Tables 1-2 and 1-3 illustrate the pros and cons of managed care for health-care providers and patients.

For health-care providers, the positive aspects of managed care are numerous (ASHA, 1996; Casey & Grimes, 1997). Managed-care organizations often will advertise health-care providers' practices, give a guaranteed referral base, provide a steady cash flow, and stimulate business (Casey & Grimes, 1997). Affiliating with an MCO enables practitioners to gain new patients, as well as keep their current ones (Casey & Grimes, 1997). As part of a managed-care system, the practitioner becomes involved in outcomes measurement and is part of a management system (ASHA, 1996). These processes can help practitioners provide quality care and unify practice patterns. The term "quality managed care" is not an oxymoron (Northern, 1997). Managed-care organizations must prove that they are meeting or even exceeding rigorous accredi-

Table 1-2. Advantages and disadvantages of managed care for health-care providers.

ADVANTAGES

- Advertises professional practices to consumers
- Brings in business
- Enables practitioners to keep current patients
- Guarantees referral base
- Maintains revenue flow
- Provides new patients
- Provides opportunity for participation in outcomes measurement and management systems
- Unifies practice patterns

DISADVANTAGES

- Demands data and documentation
- Forces participation for viability
- Limits opportunities for price negotiation
- Limits visits to specialists
- Restricts autonomy
- Restricts coverage

Sources: Adapted from *Curriculum Guide to Managed Care*, 1996. Rockville, MD: American Speech-Language-Hearing Association and *Enhancing Your Audiologic Practice*, by P. Casey and A. M. Grimes, 1997. A preconvention workshop at the Ninth Annual Convention of the American Academy of Audiology, Ft. Lauderdale, FL.

Table 1-3. Advantages and disadvantages of managed care for patients.

ADVANTAGES

- Offers case management for complex solutions
- Offers coordinated health care
- Offers low-cost treatment options
- Promotes wellness
- Provides full coverage for diagnostic care and hospitalization
- Requires minimal or no deductibles
- Requires no screening for pre-existing conditions
- Requires only small copayment for office visit
- Stresses preventative care

DISADVANTAGES

- Complicates process to obtain referral to specialist
- Disenrolls members who are out of the area for 90 days or more
- Discourages expensive care
- Eliminates freedom to choose one's health-care provider
- Limits coverage to patients with special needs
- Limits referral to specialists
- May alter treatment options
- Provides limited care for travelers

Sources: Adapted from *Curriculum Guide to Managed Care*, 1996. Rockville, MD: *American Speech-Language-Hearing Association* and *Enhancing Your Audiologic Practice*, by P. Casey and A. M. Grimes, 1997. A preconvention workshop at the Ninth Annual Convention of the American Academy of Audiology, Ft. Lauderdale, FL.

tation standards by groups such as the National Committee on Quality Assurance (NCQA) (Casey, 1997). Unification of practice patterns establishes standards of health care for patients. On the other hand, many health-care providers are threatened by managed care and believe that they must affiliate with an MCO to survive. Furthermore, MCOs often restrict autonomy, coverage for services, and opportunities for price negotiation. They generally demand data and documentation from providers as well (ASHA, 1996). Recently, Danhauer (1998) provided a discussion of issues pertinent to audiologists in private practice and large audiology networks. He suggested that, although many audiologists have already affiliated with large provider networks, there is still room for those who wish to maintain their private practices to do so.

Managed care also has positive and negative aspects for patients (ASHA, 1996; Casey & Grimes, 1997). Managed care can provide a low-cost alternative to traditional fee-for-service reimbursement models (ASHA, 1996). Typically, patients need only to pay a low premium in exchange for small copayments for office visits with little or no annual deductible (ASHA, 1996). In addition, full coverage is provided for diagnostic care and hospitalization (ASHA, 1996). Other advantages include improved patient care through an emphasis on prevention, wellness, and coordinated care (ASHA, 1996). Coordinated care results in an efficient use of resources, communication among practitioners, and a case-management approach for cases that require complex solutions. Unfortunately, managed care limits patients' freedom to choose their healthcare providers (ASHA, 1996). If patients seek treatment from nonaffiliated practitioners, they may have to pay "out of pocket" for services (ASHA, 1996; Casey & Grimes, 1997). Patients may find it complicated to seek authorization for a referral to a specialist or to obtain expensive treatments (ASHA, 1996). Managed-care organizations are often local and may disenroll members who are out of the area for 90 days or more with no provisions for those who travel (Casey & Grimes, 1997). Managed care may also limit coverage to patients with special needs. In "Principles for Health Care Reform from a Disability Perspective," however, the Consortium for Citizens with Disabilities (CCD) Health Task Force advocates that any health-care reform must be based on the following principles: nondiscrimination, comprehensiveness, appropriateness, choice, equity, and efficiency (ASHA, 1996; Hattie Larlham Bulletin, 1996). For patients having disabilities, MCOs must: (1) not discriminate, (2) make available a full range of health and health-related services in an efficient manner based on individual needs and choices, and (3) not burden these individuals with inequitable and disproportionate costs (Hattie-Larlham Bulletin, 1996).

TRENDS IN MANAGED CARE

Griffin and Fazen (1993) charted six future trends in managed care. They contend that managed care will:

- continue to increase in importance and scope;
- move rapidly toward shared risk, or capitated, arrangements rather than discount for fees-for-service;
- undergo mergers and consolidations among plans, resulting in fewer—but larger—players;
- base gatekeeping functions and payment strategies on severity-adjusted clinical outcomes and clinical protocols;
- develop more specialty managed-care organizations to provide segmented care to self-insured employers and to subcontract with managed-care plans for that segment of health care; and
- urge acute-care and rehabilitation hospitals to form lower cost alternatives for longer stay patients (e.g., outpatient rehabilitation and subacute rehabilitation centers).

MANAGED CARE AND THE PRACTICE OF AUDIOLOGY

Hearing Plans

Physicians were introduced to managed care nearly 20 years ago (Casey, 1995). Dental plans and vision plans have been included as benefits by HMOs to entice individuals to enroll in their organizations for some time (Casey, 1995). Health maintenance organizations are applying to the Health Care Finance Administration (HCFA) to provide Medicare services to the elderly population, as well as providing benefits such as "hearing plans," through subcontracting with networks of audiologists who provide an array of managed products and services (Casey & Grimes, 1997). Besides HMOs, other organizations that purchase hearing plans include: (1) employers, (2) multiemployer trust funds, (3) group-purchasing coalitions, and (4) consumer-discount organizations (Casey & Grimes, 1997). Audiology networks are sweeping the nation. Hearing networks work with benefit administrators to design hearing plans that: (1) contain overall program costs, (2) provide allowance for testing and hearing aids, (3) reduce patients' out-of-pocket expenses, (4) minimize patient costs for network development and administration, and (5) assure that audiologists deliver quality services (Charles D. Spencer & Associates, 1997).

Benefit administrators ask the following questions when evaluating hearing plans (Charles D. Spencer & Associates, 1997):

- Are providers readily available, even in remote locations?
- Are there any geographical restrictions on where the plan applies?
- Are benefits for employees and retirees the same regardless of where they are provided?
- Are plan costs measurable and predictable?
- What are the plans' reporting capabilities with respect to claims utilization?
- Is claims-dispute resolution handled promptly and consistently?

Casey (1995) outlined the characteristics of hearing plans that ensure high quality professional care and products, as well as those plans that may be questionable. High quality hearing plans provide:

- a credentialed provider network;
- reimbursements for hearing assessments only when performed by licensed and/or certified audiologists;
- a reasonable allowance toward the purchase of hearing aids;
- flexible hearing aid pricing to account for differing technologies while still providing significant discounts; and
- freedom for enrollees and audiologists to select appropriate technologies, regardless of brand.

Questionable hearing plans may include:

- "free" hearing testing by individuals whose qualification may vary widely,
- use of "mail order" hearing aid companies,
- use of single-brand dispensers,
- little or no allowance for purchasing hearing aids,
- managing hearing aid costs through discounts from overly inflated "suggested retail" prices, and
- limiting patients to the least expensive hearing aid circuitry and features.

Implications for Aural Rehabilitation

Increasingly, managed care is having an impact on private-practice audiologists. As a result, many audiologists view managed care with caution, suspicion, and fear (Casey, 1995). Private-practice audiologists face the dilemma of either affiliating with a network or remaining independent practitioners. Affiliated audiologists should expect to discount their products and services, to face restrictions on testing (e.g., billable codes), and to deal with lots of paperwork (Casey & Grimes, 1997). On the other hand, they should not have to tolerate unethical practices, an inability to do basic testing, being asked to provide services "for free," or the placement of severe restrictions on hearing aid technology (Casey & Grimes, 1997). Ormsby, Sawyer, and Benziger (1997) state that good networks will allow audiologists certain freedoms as outlined in Table 1–4.

Many HMOs want audiologic testing to be capitated under the primary-care physician and to contract only for the purchase of hearing aids. Furthermore, few hearing plans have provisions for aural rehabilitation services beyond the fitting of hearing aids. This restriction can be a disadvantage for patients because many affiliated audiologists who have already discounted the cost of hearing aids will not want to provide aural rehabilitation for free. In addition, many states have enacted "Any Willing Provider" laws requiring HMOs and similar health plans to accept into their network any licensed professional (not necessarily audiologists) to dispense hearing aids (Seppala, 1995). These laws prohibit otolaryngologists from restricting networks to audiologists, and also keep audiologists from restricting the network to hearing aid dispensers. Thus, private-practice audiologists are not just competing with other audiologists, but also with high-volume, retail-authorized dispensers, manufacturers, and corporations (e.g., Kmart, Wal-Mart, Price Club, and so on) who know little about the rehabilitative aspects of hearing care (Casey & Grimes, 1997). To compete, audiologists must take a proactive approach to managed care to ensure the fiscal viability of their

Table 1-4. Allowances afforded audiologists by good networks.

AUDIOLOGIST ALLOWANCES

- Negotiation for professional fees
- Education of the MCO regarding audiology as a profession
- Recognition of the importance of patient satisfaction
- Explanation of laws and MCO requirements
- Automation of systems necessary for efficient outcomes reporting, utilization of information, standardization of services, and diagnostic capabilities
- Automation of third-party administrative services
- Freedom to take risks
- Involvement in the process of change

Source: Adapted from "Managed Care: Open the Window of Opportunity," by M. Ormsby, D. Sawyer, and L. Benziger, 1997, p. 44. *The Hearing Journal, 50*(6), 42, 43–44. Reprinted with permission.

practices and the continued availability of employment for our graduates.

A PROACTIVE APPROACH TO MANAGED CARE

A proactive approach to managed care requires audiologists to take action on at least three levels: personal, professional, and clinical practice. Figure 1–2 depicts the necessary steps in each area that contribute to a proactive approach to managed care.

Personal Level

On a personal level, audiologists should make a commitment to provide the highest quality of care possible to consumers regardless of the cost-cutting trends in managed care. By establishing high ethical standards for professional practice, audiologists should be able to withstand the pressures of third-party payers and still preserve their autonomy. Nevertheless, simply being the best clinical audiologist one can be and ignoring the status of managed care probably will not suffice to sustain private practices in the millenium. In addition, audiologists should educate themselves about and keep up-to-date with managed-care issues and the current directions of health care through a variety of resources. Professional organizations can be excellent resources for audiologists. The American Speech-Language-Hearing Association and the American Academy of Audiology also provide timely information about managed care as it applies to the profession. Relevant ASHA publications and instructions for receiving "FAX on Demand" information also appear in Appendix I-A. In addition, provider-relations personnel or case-management personnel from local MCOs can provide valuable information to audiologists about the managed-care scene in their local areas (Griffin & Fazen, 1993). Many public libraries have books on managed care, as well as access to useful Web sites on the Internet. Several useful managed-care books and Web site addresses are also listed in Appendix I-A.

Professional Level

On a professional level, audiologists should request that their professional organizations include managed care in their continuing-education programs (Griffin & Fazen, 1993). Audiologists should check to see if their states have "Any Willing Provider" laws and determine how they are enforced by local MCOs (Seppala, 1995). After care- ful study, audiologists can consider affiliating with a provider network. Well-informed affiliated audiologists can make positive changes from within the managed-care system. As part of a net- work, audiologists should learn contract negotiation as early as possible to avoid costly mistakes (Griffin & Fazen, 1993). In addition, audiologists should know about the costs involved in maintaining their practices so that they can evaluate their fiscal soundness with the network (Casey & Grimes, 1997). Hosford-Dunn,

PERSONAL REALM
- Learn about managed care from:
  ⇒ books
  ⇒ Internet resources
  ⇒ local MCOs
  ⇒ professional organizations
- Commit to ethical/high-quality care
- Understand current directions in health care

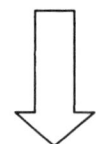

PROFESSIONAL REALM
- Consider affiliating with a provider network
- Check state "Any Willing Provider" legislation
- Evaluate fiscal soundness with MCOs
- Learn about contract negotiation
- Learn about the operational costs of private practice
- Market services to physicians and MCOs
- Request managed-care topics for continuing education through professional organizations
- Work with MCOs in formulating hearing plans
- Consider forming your own network

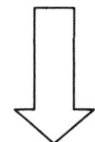

CLINICAL PRACTICE
- Define operational clinical protocols
- Develop an outcome-oriented quality improvement system
- Give MCOs what they want:
  ⇒ communicate/follow-up with referring physicians
  ⇒ cover a broad geographic area
  ⇒ establish protocols for care
  ⇒ offer comprehensive services
  ⇒ report outcomes of quality services
  ⇒ take a risk with cost sharing
- Strive for excellence in patient satisfaction

Figure 1-2. Steps to a proactive approach to managed care. (Adapted from Griffin and Fazen (1993), Casey (1995), Seppala (1995), Casey (1997), Casey and Grimes (1997), and Klontz (1997).)

Dunn, and Harford (1995) have provided excellent information and materials (e.g., worksheets) regarding how to determine business costs and the worth of a private practice. Successful network-affiliated audiologists can eventually be involved with benefits administrators in creating viable hearing packages for MCOs that incorporate a full range of hearing health-care services according to the highest standards of professional practice (Casey, 1995). In particular, benefit administrators must be educated about what constitutes a "routine hearing examination" and what type of hearing aids can be purchased for $400 (Casey, 1997).

Audiologists should seek every opportunity to market audiologic services to MCOs, physicians, and patients. They might find ways to be included on MCO's health-education calendars to discuss new technology in hearing diagnostics, hearing instruments (Seppala, 1995), and aural rehabilitation services. The use of otoacoustic emissions (OAEs) (Danhauer, 1997) is a relatively new development in diagnostic audiology. Although OAE testing has become the standard of practice in audiology, many audiologists have not yet incorporated it into their test protocols. Use of OAEs can assist audiologists in establishing a strong position with MCOs due to their low cost, noninvasiveness, and clinical utility with patients of all ages. Emphasizing OAEs in a practice at this time is an ideal way to distinguish one's business from the many others who do not offer them. Similarly, keeping abreast of the newest technology in hearing instruments (e.g., completely-in-the-canal (CIC), programmable, and digital hearing aids) and offering it to patients can help distinguish one's practice to MCOs. The key is finding ways to make the use of such technology accountable and cost-effective for MCO patients so that they will see the benefits and request it. Furthermore, establishing cost-effective stellar aural rehabilitation support programs for patients with hearing impairment across service-delivery sites can also be attractive to MCOs and other third-party payers. Defining and marketing these support programs is covered in Chapter 3.

Obviously, involvement in MCO activities takes time away from other clinical and professional opportunities, but it is becoming a necessary part of operating a successful private practice. Training programs must begin including this type of information in their curricula to prepare students for the challenges of managed care. Unfortunately, many university faculty members are often inexperienced in the basics of managing a successful private practice in today's health-care arena. Few audiologists in clinical practice were given any business acumen in their graduate preparation. Instead, they have had to develop a practice the hard way through the "college of hard knocks," a series of mistakes, or both. This type of informal, trial-and-error education has been the downfall of many audiology practices over the years, even those that were run by well-qualified audiologists. Simply being a "good audiologist" and the "best one can be" is not enough. Students in training need a business background, knowledge of managed-care principles, and a certain mindset to develop and maintain successful audiology practices. Audiologists in private practice must be fearless risk takers who realize that success or failure is in their own hands. Most audiologists are unwilling to take that risk and would rather work for someone else on a salary. However, even audiologists who are employed by practices and clinics have to be more knowledgeable about business and managed-care concerns, especially if their employer chooses to affiliate with an audiologist network.

Audiologists who choose not to affiliate with an existing network might consider forming their own. In forming one's own network, Klontz (1997) suggested that audiologists:

- evaluate their goals;
- evaluate market demographics;
- know their capabilities;
- know their limitations;
- allow sufficient time to form a network (i.e., 6 to 18 months);
- get assistance from accountants, consultants, and attorneys;
- assess information technology up front; and
- establish a common terminology.

Clinical Practice

Affiliated audiologists should implement managed-care principles in their clinical practices. Managed-care organizations want audiologists to: (1) take a risk with cost sharing, (2) have a broad geographic coverage, (3) offer comprehensive services, (4) establish protocols for care, (5) report outcomes of quality services, and (6) communicate and follow up with referring physicians (Seppala, 1995). Affiliated audiologists take a risk by discounting products and services in exchange for a steady source of referrals. Networks ensure a referral base from a wide geographic area that can give certain underserved populations access to comprehensive audiologic services. In addition, managed-care companies want to use facilities and providers that produce documented positive outcomes in the most cost-effective manner possible (Frattali, 1991; Goldberg, 1996). Thus, audiologists should define operational clinical protocols that result in documented positive patient outcomes at the lowest cost. Services provided without documentation may be excluded from future coverage (Frattali, 1991; Goldberg, 1996). Audiologists should report their findings to ASHA's National Outcome Measurement System (NOMS), which collects information for the national outcomes data base managed by ASHA's National Center for Treatment Effectiveness in Communication Disorders (Frattali, 1991; Goldberg, 1996). With this data bank, audiologists can compare their data to national averages, a process called benchmarking. Benchmarking allows standards for comparison for continual improvement (Frattali, 1991; Goldberg, 1996). Audiologists must be patient, however, because it can take a long time to collect sufficient data to determine one's performance (Casey, 1997). At the same time, audiologists should strive for excellence in patient satisfaction, communication, and follow-up with referring physicians (Seppala, 1995). Patients must be encouraged to tell MCOs if they are not receiving adequate care (Casey, 1997) and also to provide positive feedback for quality services. For example, Seppala (1995) suggested sending patient satisfaction questionnaires to their referrals and then reporting the results back to the referring physicians. In summary, using managed-care principles in audiologic practices can result in optimal patient care, fiscal success, and satisfied third-party payers, ensuring viability of the profession.

SUMMARY

The challenge for audiologists is to provide quality clinical services across service-delivery settings in spite of the changing health-care climate, personnel shortages, public-policy initiatives, economic considerations, and reductions in provider reimbursements (ASHA, 1997). Audiologists must be aware of the need for strategic advocacy with legislators and for marketing services to health-care providers. This will ensure that persons with hearing impairment have access to quality management of their disorders (Hallowell, 1996). Audiologists should support local, state, and national lobbying groups in these efforts. The application of managed-care principles throughout the scope of audiology practice will be a long and complicated process.

This text focuses on developing cost-efficient, stellar support programs for persons with hearing impairment across several service-delivery sites. Effective support programs require the use of trained support personnel, which is a relatively new concept to most audiologists. Therefore, this text will serve as a guidebook for students and practicing audiologists in managing multiskilled professionals and audiologic support personnel in aural-rehabilitation support programs. For each service-delivery site, clinical management and managed-care principles are integrated for contextual relevance and for the direct application of knowledge. This first chapter presented the basics of managed care, as well as its implications for the profession.

LEARNING ACTIVITIES

- Interview local audiologists about the impact of managed care on their private practices.
- Evaluate how managed care differentially affects audiologists in a variety of work settings.
- Determine if the local MCOs in your regional area offer hearing plans and evaluate their soundness with the criteria presented in the chapter (Casey, 1995).
- Explore the Internet for managed-care Web sites and download useful information to create a reference notebook.
- Investigate the "Any Willing Provider" laws in your state and determine how they are enforced.

REFERENCES

American Speech-Language-Hearing Association. (1996). *Curriculum guide to managed care*. Rockville, MD: American Speech-Language-Hearing Association.

American Speech-Language-Hearing Association. (1997, Spring). Guidelines for audiology service delivery in nursing homes. *Asha, 39*(Suppl. 17), 15–19.

Berkowitz, A. O. (1996). Piloting the managed care highway. *The Hearing Review, 3*(5), 8–9, 46.

Casey, P. (1995). Viewpoint: Managed care and dispensing audiology . . . To play or not to play? *Audiology Today, 7*(3), 17–18.

Casey, P. (1996). Ask the experts: Have you heard the news about hearing benefits? *Employee Benefits News: Strategies and Solutions for the Business of Employment. 10*(6), Reprint.

Casey, P. (1997). Meeting the challenges of managed care. *The Hearing Journal, 50*(6), 32–34.

Casey, P., & Grimes, A. M. (1997). Enhancing your audiologic practice. A preconvention workshop of the Ninth Annual Convention of the American Academy of Audiology, Ft. Lauderdale, FL.

Charles D. Spencer & Associates, Inc. (1997, January). Managed hearing care plan offers employers low-cost way of enhancing health benefits. *Employee Benefit Plan Review*, January 1997.

Danhauer, J. L. (1997). How otoacoustic emissions testing can change your audiology practice. *The Hearing Journal, 50*(4), 62, 64, 66, 68–69.

Danhauer, J. L. (1998). Who are those major multi-office audiology groups moving in on us, and—Is this town big enough for the both of us? *Audiology Today, 10*(2), 47–51.

Deloitte & Touche, L.L.P. (1996, May/June). New roles, new responsibilities for health: Responding to imperatives for change. Cited in *Hattie Larlham Bulletin* [On-line], *1*(3). Available Internet: www.larlham.org/hlbul.html.

Frattali, C. (1991). From quality assurance to total quality management. *American Journal of Audiology: A Journal of Clinical Practice, 1*(1), 41–47.

Goldberg, B. (1996). Imagining tomorrow: What's ahead for our professions? *Asha, 38*(3), 22–23, 25–28.

Griffin, K. M., & Fazen, M. (1993). A managed care strategy for practitioners. In C. M. Frattali (Ed.) *Quality improvement digest: Current information on issues related to quality evaluation and improvement* (pp. 1–7). Rockville, MD: American Speech-Language-Hearing Association.

Hallowell, B. (1996). *Measuring educational outcomes*. Paper presented at the Annual Conference of the Council of Graduate Programs in Communication Sciences and Disorders, San Diego, CA.

Hosford-Dunn, H., Dunn, D. R., & Harford, E. R. (1995). *Audiology business and practice management*. San Diego, CA: Singular Publishing Group.

How will managed care fit into the lives of people with disabilities? (1996, May-June). *Hattie Larlham Bulletin* [On-line], 1(3). Available Internet: www.larlham.org/hlbul.html.

Klontz, H. (1997). Managed care 101: A primer on whats, whys, and hows. *The Hearing Journal, 50*(6), 26, 28–29.

Northern, J. L. (1997). Quality managed care: It's not an oxymoron. *The Hearing Journal, 50*(6), 35, 38, 40.

Ormsby, M., Sawyer, D., & Benziger, L. (1997). Managed care: Open the window of opportunity! *The Hearing Journal, 50*(6), 42, 43–44.

Seppala, T. (1995). Viewpoint: Health care reform: Issues for audiologists. *Audiology Today, 7*(3), 19–20.

Skafte, M. D. (1997). The 1996 hearing instrument market: The dispensers' perspective. *The Hearing Review, 4*(3), 8, 12, 22–42.

APPENDIX I-A

Resources On Managed Care and Related Professional Issues

Useful Web Sites on Managed Care

- *http://www.ncqa.org/* National Committee for Quality Assurance (NCQA): The NCQA is an independent, not-for-profit organization dedicated to assessing and reporting on the quality of managed-care plans, including HMOs. More than one-half of the nation's 650 HMOs have been reviewed, have a decision pending, or are scheduled for review as part of the NCQA's accreditation process for managed care. This Web site has separate pages pertaining to government issues, health-care organizations, employers and unions, consumers, health-care providers, NCQA teams, researchers, and a useful index.
- *http://www.asha.org/* American Speech-Language-Hearing Association: This Web site is for the national professional organization for speech-language pathologists and audiologists. Users can access up-to-date information on managed care by using the "Search Site" feature and typing in "managed care." Users will find numerous references to managed care ranging from ASHA publications on the topic to current news for practitioners.

Relevant Publications from the American Speech-Language-Hearing Association

- A Practical Guide to Applying Treatment Outcomes and Efficacy Resources
- ASHA Audiology Campaign: The Marketing Kit
- ASHA Desk Reference: Audiology
- ASHA-QA Consumer Satisfaction Measure: Audiology/Rehabilitation
- Business Practices: Laying the Foundation for Successful Service Delivery in Communication Disorders
- Communication, Creativity, Collaboration: Current Challenges for School Supervisors and Administrators
- Curriculum Guide to Managed Care
- Development and Management of Audiology Practices
- Enhancing Communication Services for Older Persons in Extended Care Settings
- Ethics: Resources for Professional Preparation and Practice
- How to Establish a Quality Improvement Process: A Ten Step Model
- Managed Care Contracting: An Actuarial Analysis
- Managing Managed Care: A Practical Guide for Audiologists and Speech-Language Pathologists
- Marketing Manual: A Resource Guide
- Medicare Handbook for Speech-Language-Pathology and Audiology Services
- Meeting the Managed Care Challenge: Strategies for Professionals and the Professions
- Private Health Plans Handbook for Speech-Language Pathology and Audiology Services
- Professional Collaboration: A Team Approach to Health Care, Clinical Series 11
- Promoting your Services to Health Plans
- Successful Operations in the Treatment Outcomes Driven World of Managed Care, Clinical Series 13
- Technical Packets: Each packet contains information from the Association for each area, including reports, position statements, guidelines, and related documents. May also include supporting documents.
    ⇒ Professional Autonomy
    ⇒ Audiology Private Practice Packet
    ⇒ Home Health Care Packet
    ⇒ Productivity Information Packet
    ⇒ Quality Assurance Packet
    ⇒ Treatment Outcomes and Managed Care Information Packet

- The Competitive Edge for Audiologists Negotiating with Managed Care Organizations (MCOs)
- Total Quality Management: A Continuous Process for Improvement
- Treatment Outcome Data Collection Instruments

Ordering by phone:
Call (888) 498-6699 and ask for product sales.

Ordering by FAX:
Send order form to: (301) 897-7355

Ordering by mail:
ASHA
10801 Rockville Pike
Rockville, MD 20852-3279

American Speech-Language-Hearing Association's FAX on Demand

A member service providing up-to-date information. Call (703) 531-0866 to order anything on the menu. Just follow the operator's prompts, making sure to enter your FAX number correctly. You will receive the item by FAX within minutes.

CHAPTER 2

Multiskilling and the Use of Support Personnel: An Overview

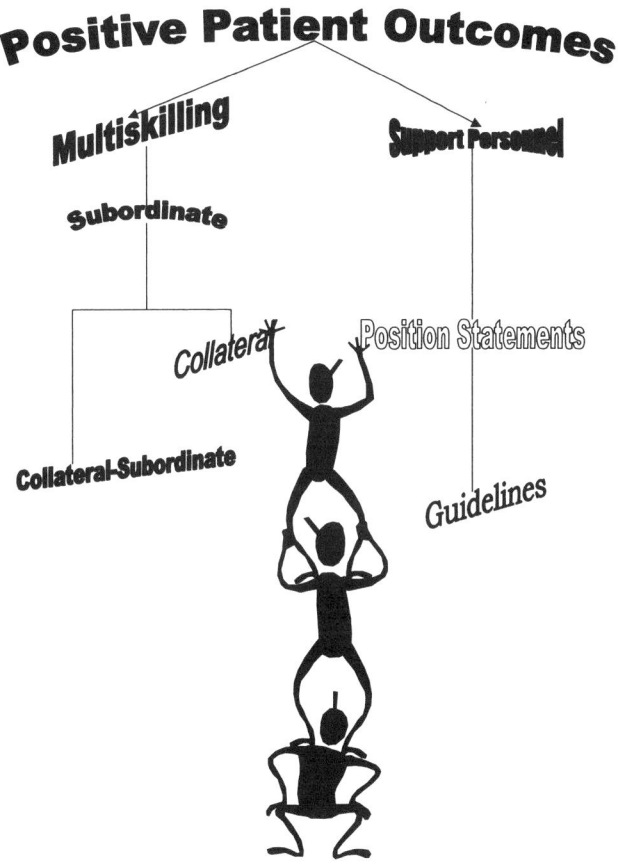

Figure 2-1. Positive patient outcomes can be achieved through the use of multiskilling and support personnel.

INTRODUCTION

The high cost of technology, the budget deficit, the early identification of disorders, and the aging of the population (i.e., more than 30 million over 65 years of age today and 68 million expected by the year 2050) have all contributed to high health-care costs (Goldberg, 1996). In 1960, the cost of health care in the United States totalled $27 billion or about 5.3% of the gross national product (GNP), whereas in 1995, it was $903 billion or 16% of the GNP (Goldberg, 1996). As discussed in Chapter 1, one solution to the problem is managed care. Since World War II, health care has operated under the traditional fee-for-service reimbursement model. Under this model, there was no incentive for cutting costs (ASHA, 1996a). In managed care, the customer is changing from the patient to the employer or the insurer. It is no longer the patient who: (1) chooses the service provider, (2) decides what services will be provided, and (3) determines the length of service (ASHA, 1996a). The advantages and disadvantages of managed care were discussed in Chapter 1.

Multiskilling and the use of support personnel have been proposed as strategies for increasing the effectiveness, efficiency, and coordination of health-care services. *Multiskilling* refers to training one professional to perform tasks that are typically performed by other professionals (Foto, 1996). The application of multiskilling can be found in a broad spectrum of health-related jobs ranging in complexity from the nonprofessional to the professional, including clinical, nonclinical, and management functions (Bamberg, Blayney, Vaughn, & Wilson, 1989). The American Speech-Language-Hearing Association (ASHA) has considered the use of support personnel for the past 30 years. Like multiskilling, use of support personnel has been considered as a way to limit health-care costs. *Support personnel* are people who, after appropriate training, perform tasks that are prescribed, directed, and supervised by a professional, such as a certified and licensed audiologist (AAA, 1997). The use of multiskilling and support personnel evoke strong and diverse responses from audiologists and speech-language pathologists (Pietranton & Lynch, 1995). Audiologists and speech-language pathologists must: (1) consider the diverse issues regarding multiskilling and the use of support personnel, (2) identify when the use of multiskilled personnel is or is not in their patients' best interests, and (3) determine how multiskilling and the use of support personnel may or may not apply to the professions (ASHA, 1996d).

LEARNING OBJECTIVES

This chapter will enable the reader to:

- Place multiskilling and the use of support personnel within the context of a team approach to rehabilitation

- Define multiskilling; differentiate models of multiskilling; understand the pros and cons of multiskilling to health-care providers, patients, and management/third-party payers; and know the position of the American Speech-Language-Hearing Association on multiskilling

- Define the use of support personnel, trace the use of support personnel within the professions, and know the position of the Consensus Panel on Support Personnel in Audiology

- Apply the guidelines of the Consensus Panel on Support Personnel in Audiology

- Understand the proposed model of the regulatory influences on the practice of audiology

---

TEAM CONCEPTS IN AURAL REHABILITATION

In the past, teams of professionals have provided health services in rehabilitative medicine. Rehabilitation teams have been traditionally thought of as "multidisciplinary" or "interdisciplinary" (ASHA, 1996a). *Multidisciplinary teams* utilize discipline-specific skills and view rehabilitation efforts as the combined efforts of each discipline involved (ASHA, 1996a). *Interdisciplinary teams*, on the other hand, involve professionals from different disciplines who possess discipline-specific skills, plus the ability to contribute to a team effort in accomplishing goals (ASHA, 1996a). An innovative new approach, *transdisciplinary teams*, involves breaking down boundaries between professional disciplines and has the promise of being a more cost-efficient method of providing rehabilitative care (ASHA, 1996a). The concept of transdisciplinary teams has advocated the use of other cost-efficient staffing strategies including: (1) multiskilling and (2) support personnel.

MULTISKILLING

Multiskilling has had two models at the professional level of practice involving either (1) replacing allied-health professionals with generalists or (2) maintaining traditional discipline-specific knowledge and skills, as well as developing cross-disciplinary skills (ASHA, 1996a). Multiskilling has been applied in various health-care disciplines such as (1) dietetics (American Dietetic Association, 1995), (2) nursing (American Nurses Association, 1994), (3) occupational therapy (American Occupational Therapy Association, 1995), and (4) physical therapy (American Physical Therapy Association, 1995). *Multiskilling is not new to the practice of audiology.* Audiologists have used multiskilling for years. Audiologists have cross-trained public-school nurses to perform hearing screenings and/or visual and listening checks on children's hearing aids, for example (Johnson, Stein, & Lass, 1992). Currently, guidelines are being drafted for the use of support personnel for newborn hearing screening (AAA Committee on Infant Hearing, 1998).

Three variations of these models are appropriate for the practice of audiology. The first model is *subordinate multiskilling* in which support personnel are prescribed, directed, and supervised by a licensed and/or certified audiologist (AAA, 1997) such as in using an audiology assistant to perform a variety of audiologic tasks at the nonprofessional level of practice. Another model is *collateral multiskilling* in which health-care professionals from other disciplines are cross-trained in nonprofessional audiology skills. A rehabilitation-hospital nurse instructed to perform a visual and listening check on patients' hearing aids is an example of a professional who has discipline-specific skills but has been cross-trained in basic patient-care skills that are typically performed by an audiologist. A third model is *collateral-subordinate multiskilling* in which support personnel from other professions are cross-trained to perform nonprofessional audiology tasks, such as instructing physical-therapy assistants to teach patients who have had strokes to insert and remove their hearing aids.

The model of multiskilling used depends on the setting (e.g., acute care, subacute care, outpatient clinic, long-term care facility, home-health agency, preschool programs, elementary schools, secondary schools, residential programs, special-education facilities, and so on), patient population (e.g., age, prevalent etiologies, disorders exhibited, and so on), and geographic location (e.g., remote, rural, suburban, urban, metropolitan, and so on) (ASHA, 1996d). Audiologists may use one model or a combination of the three. Selection of the appropriate model of multiskilling should be the result of a systematic analysis of the service-delivery site to ensure cost-efficiency, accessibility of services, and quality of care. Specific system analysis strategies for various service-delivery sites will be covered in later chapters of this book.

Multiskilling offers numerous advantages and disadvantages for health-care professionals and patients, as well as management and third-party payers as depicted in Tables 2–1 and 2–2.

On a positive note, multiskilling allows some professional disciplines opportunities for salary equity (ASHA, 1996a). If important tasks are to be shared across health-care professions, so should higher salary benefits. Furthermore, cross-disciplinary assignment of tasks alleviates professional shortages (ASHA, 1996a). Rural areas often experience personnel shortages in certain critical health-care positions. Cross-training support personnel or other professionals to perform routine, frequently provided, easily trainable, low-risk procedures allow key health-care professionals to focus on more clinically challenging issues (ASHA, 1996a). Multiskilled health-care professionals benefit from professional growth, expanding scopes of practice, employability, and job security (ASHA, 1996d). Many health-care professionals have a negative view of multiskilling, however. Some believe that it erodes the scope of clinical practice, reduces professional autonomy, and may encourage management to hire lower paid "technicians" to perform tasks usually assigned to higher paid health-care professionals (ASHA, 1996d). In ad-

Table 2-1. Advantages of multiskilling.

ADVANTAGES

FOR HEALTH-CARE PROFESSIONALS

- Achieves salary parity among disciplines
- Alleviates discipline-specific shortages
- Enhances opportunities for professional growth and development
- Ensures employability and job security
- Expands the career ladder
- Expands scope of practice
- Focuses attention on clinically challenging issues
- Greater flexibility in justifying staff increases

FOR PATIENT CARE

- Accessibility to services
- Contributes to better and quicker treatment outcomes
- Improved efficiency in and coordination of clinical services

FOR MANAGEMENT AND THIRD-PARTY PAYERS

- Contributes to patient satisfaction
- Contributes to service provider satisfaction
- Enhances cost-efficiency

Sources: Adapted from *Curriculum Guide to Managed Care*, 1996. Rockville, MD: American Speech-Language-Hearing Association and "Technical Report of the Ad Hoc Committee on Multiskilling," 1996. *Asha, 38*(Suppl. 16), 53–61. Rockville, MD: American Speech-Language-Hearing Association.

Table 2-2. Disadvantages of multiskilling.

DISADVANTAGES

FOR HEALTH-CARE PROFESSIONALS

- Erodes the scope of practice
- Reduces likelihood of reimbursement from third-party payers
- Reduces professional autonomy
- Reduces revenue
- Reduces the number of positions for some clinical disciplines

FOR PATIENT CARE

- Compromises quality of care through the elimination of clinical specialties
- Limits accessibility to specialized clinical services

FOR MANAGEMENT AND THIRD-PARTY PAYERS

- Requires a large investment in cross-training
- Compromises trust of health-care providers
- Compromises trust of patients

Sources: Adapted from *Curriculum Guide to Managed Care*, 1996. Rockville, MD: American Speech-Language-Hearing Association and "Technical Report of the Ad Hoc Committee on Multiskilling," 1996. *Asha, 38*(Suppl. 16), 52–61. Rockville, MD: American Speech-Language-Hearing Association.

dition, many reimbursement and regulatory guidelines have no provisions for services provided by multiskilled personnel, resulting in a denial of payment (ASHA, 1996d).

Multiskilling has advantages and disadvantages for patients as well. Multiskilling provides patients greater access to certain services. Basic problems with residents' hearing aids can be circumvented by the use of nurse's assistants trained to perform visual and listening checks in a long-term residential care facility for the elderly that has contracted with an audiologist to provide services only one day a month or on an "as-needed basis." In addition, multiskilling can contribute to better and quicker treatment outcomes (ASHA, 1996a). Rehabilitation-hospital patients with hearing impairment whose communication is facilitated through a multiskilled staff may be sent home sooner than if their hearing needs were not met. Multiskilling can ultimately result in improved efficiency in and coordination of clinical services for patients with hearing impairment (ASHA, 1996d). On the other hand, multiskilling can compromise the quality of care and limit patients' access to specialized clinical services if management tries to replace professionals with lower paid, multiskilled support personnel (ASHA, 1996d).

Multiskilling has both positive and negative aspects for management and third-party payers. The most obvious benefit of multiskilling is cost-efficiency (ASHA, 1996a, 1996d). Operational costs can be reduced through reorganization and streamlining of staff assignments. Successful multiskilling can result in job satisfaction for health-care providers and happy, well-cared for patients. While some administrators dread the cost of cross-training, others generously support inservice training because they believe that support personnel can be more efficient, have less "down time," and be more effective than professionals traditionally trained to perform discipline-specific tasks (ASHA, 1996a). Successful multiskilling and use of support personnel require: (1) commitment of supervising personnel; (2) cooperation and support of administrators; (3) consistent implementation of state, facility, and professional-organization guidelines; and (4) ongoing review of the effects on patients and staff (Runnels, 1994; Werven, 1993). Multiskilling and use of support personnel have been viewed with skepticism by audiologists and speech-language pathologists. Many are threatened by administrators' attempts to implement multiskilling. In addition, administrators may find that patients will not have confidence in services provided in a facility that uses support personnel.

The American Speech-Language-Hearing Association recently published the technical report of their Ad-Hoc Committee on Multiskilling that: (1) identified the issues related to the concept of multiskilling, (2) provided definitions, (3) discussed implications for patient care, (4) explored the potential impact on speech-language pathologists, and (5) served as the basis for the development of a position statement about multiskilled personnel (ASHA, 1996d). In the spring of 1997, ASHA published its position paper on the use of multiskilled personnel stating that multiskilling is not a unidimensional concept, and it cannot be applied across a diverse clinical work force. The position paper conveyed that multiskilling can involve cross-training the following: (1) clinical skills (e.g., training practitioners in one discipline to perform services traditionally regarded as within the scope of practice of another discipline), (2) basic patient-care skills (e.g., routine, frequently provided, easily trainable, low-risk procedures), (3) professional, nonclinical skills (e.g., skills and services including patient education, technical writing, team dynamics/communication/leadership, and so on), and (4) administrative skills (e.g., programmatic activities such as quality improvement, case management, systems design, and the management of clinical services). The American Speech-Language-Hearing Association strongly stated that the cross-training of clinical skills at the professional level of practice is not appropriate, but that cross-training of basic patient-care skills, professional nonclinical skills, and administrative skills is a viable option (ASHA, 1997a). The American Speech-Language-Hearing Association's "Position Statement on Multiskilled Personnel" appears in Appendix II-A.

USE OF SUPPORT PERSONNEL

History

The use of support personnel in speech-language pathology and audiology is not a new concept. In 1967, John P. Moncur, chair of the first Committee on Support Personnel appointed by the American Speech-Language-Hearing Association, concluded that the use of support personnel was not an issue to be left for the future and needed immediate attention (O'Brien, 1997). ASHA attempted to clarify the use of support personnel in 1969 when its Legislative Council adopted the first guidelines (Moncur, 1967). The ASHA Ethical Practices Board published an Issues in Ethics Statement, which went into effect in June 1979, that highlighted the professional and ethical responsibilities of the supervising professional while de-emphasizing the role of support personnel. In 1981, the second Committee on Supportive Personnel published "Guidelines for the Employment and Utilization of Supportive Personnel" (ASHA, 1981). Over the next few years, various ASHA committees debated and evaluated the use of support personnel in the professions. In 1992, ASHA published a policy statement on support personnel in the professions. In 1994, the most current ASHA Task Force on Support Personnel prepared "Guidelines for the Training, Credentialing, Use, and Supervision of Speech-Language Pathology Assistants," which were not implemented until 1996 (ASHA, 1996c).

The implementation of support personnel in speech-language pathology has been successful in the public-school systems of several states (O'Brien, 1997). Freilinger (1992) reported the successful use of support personnel in Iowa. Support personnel have had various titles, such as associate, communication assistant, paraprofessional, speech/audiology assistant, audiometrist, audiometric technician, communication helper, and so on (ASHA, 1992). In 1995, Larson and Lynch found that in the 45 states that regulate one or both professions of audiology and speech-language pathology, 30 recognize support personnel; 22 of those have published rules regarding the use of support personnel, and five states were in the process of defining them. We can expect to see these numbers increase as we enter the next millenium.

Use of Support Personnel in Audiology

The use of support personnel in speech-language pathology has been well-defined (ASHA, 1996c), but not in audiology. To resolve this, a Consensus Panel on Support Personnel in Audiology was formed consisting of members from organizations representing audiologists: Academy of Dispensing Audiologists (ADA), American Academy of Audiology (AAA), American Speech-Language-Hearing Association (ASHA), Educational Audiology Association (EAA), Military Audiology Association (MAA), and the National Hearing Conservation Association (NHCA). The panel developed the "Position Statement and Guidelines of the Consensus Panel on Support Personnel in Audiology" (AAA, 1997). The document does not supersede federal legislation and regulation requirements or any existing state licensure laws, and its does not affect the interpretation or implementation of such laws. It may, however, serve as a guide for the development of new laws or, at the appropriate time, for the revision of existing licensure laws (AAA, 1997).

The document consists of two parts: (1) the Position Statement and (2) Guidelines. The position statement states that the professional organizations represented on the Consensus Panel on Support Personnel in Audiology agree that support personnel may assist audiologists in the delivery of services under the following conditions:

- The roles and tasks of audiology support personnel will be assigned only by supervising audiologists.
- Supervising audiologists will provide appropriate training that is competency-based and specific to job performance.
- Supervision will be comprehensive, periodic, and documented.
- The supervising audiologists maintain the legal and ethical responsibilities for all assigned audiology activities provided by support personnel.
- The needs of the consumer of audiology services and the protection of that consumer will always be paramount (ASHA, 1994; NHCA, 1995; AAA, 1996; ASHA, 1996c; AAA, 1997).

The guidelines for the use of support personnel appear in Appendix II-B. They provide definitions, qualifications for support personnel, their training, and supervision. The document serves as a starting point for audiologists contemplating using multiskilling and support personnel in their practices. Although helpful, the document is not very specific and leaves much to the discretion of the audiologist.

A MODEL

The use of multiskilling and/or support personnel depends on the professional setting, patient population, and geographic location. Many external rules and regulations may affect the implementation of new programs. Thus, audiologists need to consider the following dynamic, multidimensional model of regulatory influences on the practice of audiology that is depicted in Figure 2–2.

Practicing audiologists should consider the code of ethics of their professional organization(s) prior to implementation of multiskilling and the use of support personnel. The ASHA Code of Ethics (ASHA, 1996b) provides guidelines for ethical practice in the professions. The situation is complicated for audiologists, as most belong to two or more professional organizations. The two main professional organizations for audiologists, ASHA and the AAA, each have their own code of ethics. In addition, other professional organizations related to the practice of audiology, such as the National Hearing Conservation Association (NHCA), may also have a code of ethics. Professional issues can be quite complicated for audiologists who belong to two or more of these organizations. Audiologists who belong to all three organizations, for example, and who use support personnel in hearing conservation programs should consult the code of ethics for each professional organization.

At the next level, audiologists should be aware of federal and state laws affecting their practice. Federal legislation pertinent to the practice of audiology includes the Individuals with Disabilities Education Act (IDEA) (1990), the Americans with Disabilities Act (ADA) (1990), and so on. As discussed in later chapters of this book, audiologists can use these federal laws to justify the use of multiskilling and support personnel in the creation of support programs for persons with hearing impairment. A staff audiologist at an acute-care hospital can explain to administrators that a multiskilled staff trained in managing assistive listening devices could help ensure that patients with hearing impairment have equal access to hospital services as required by the ADA (1990). At the state level, licensure laws regulate the practice of audiology. Many state licensure boards have passed regulations regarding the use of support personnel. Audiologists should contact state licensure boards prior to implementing any program involving the use of multiskilling and support personnel.

At the next level, accrediting bodies of health-care organizations, such as the Joint Commission on the Accreditation of Healthcare Organizations (JCAHO), regulate the performance of health-care providers working in many medical facilities. In their Accreditation Manual for Hospitals, this body specifies dimensions of performance with regard to: efficacy, appropriateness, availability, timeliness, effectiveness, continuity, safety, efficiency, respect, and caring. The Professional Service Board (PSB) of ASHA accredits speech and hearing centers that operate according to specific regulations ensuring quality of care. Each health-care facility will have its own operating procedures that will influence the implementation of the use multiskilling and support personnel by audiologists.

At the next level, the Scope of Practice in Audiology (ASHA, 1996b) (1) describes the services provided by audiologists as primary service providers, case managers, and/or members of multidisciplinary teams and interdisciplinary teams; (2) serves as a reference for health-care, education, and other professionals, as well as for consumers, members of the general public, and policy makers concerned with legislation, regulation, licensure, and third-party reimbursement; and (3) informs members of ASHA, certificate holders, and students of the activities for which certification is required in accordance with the ASHA Code of Ethics (ASHA, 1996b). The Scope of Practice in Audiology includes "administration and supervision of professional and technical personnel who provide support functions to the practice of audiology" (ASHA, 1996b). The Scope of Practice in Audiology can also assist audiologists in determining the appropriateness of requests made by their employers to cross-train and perform tasks typically assigned to other disciplines.

Because the Scope of Practice in Audiology is rather broad, audiologists within ASHA have published preferred practice patterns, position statements, and guidelines. Preferred practice patterns are statements that define universally applicable characteristics of specific clinical activities including definitions, which professionals perform the procedures, expected outcomes,

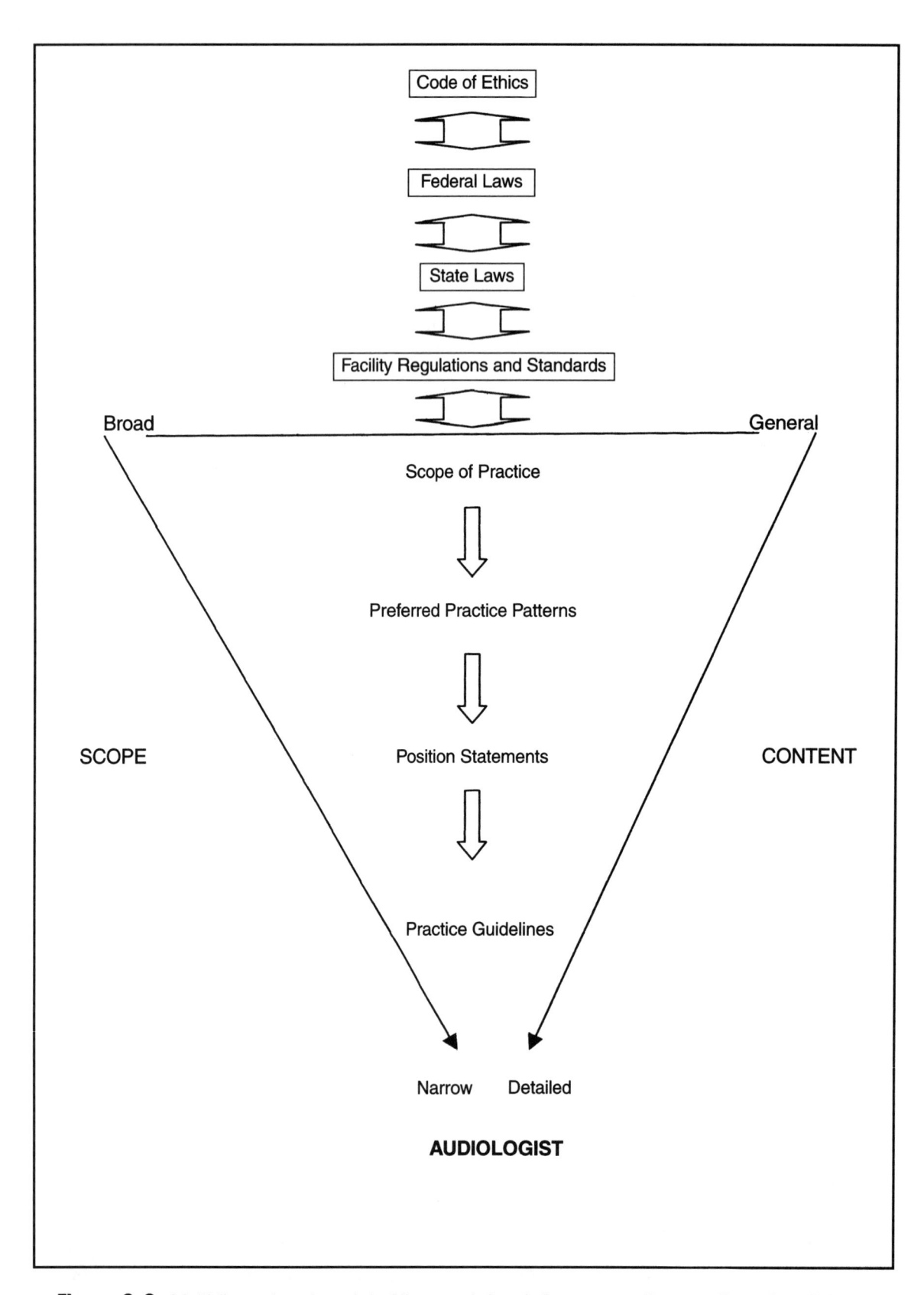

Figure 2-2. Multidimensional model of the regulatory influences on the practice of audiology.

clinical indications, clinical processes, setting and equipment specifications, and documentation (ASHA, 1997b). Preferred Practice Patterns for Audiology and Speech-Language Pathology are not official standards, but they serve as guidelines for enhancing the quality of professional services to consumers (Grantham, 1996). Preferred practice patterns have been developed for audiology on the following topics: speech-language-hearing screenings, follow-up procedures, consultation, prevention, occupational and environmental hearing conservation, audiologic assessment (basic, pediatric, and advanced), external ear procedures (examination and cerumen management), electrodiagnostic test procedures, auditory evoked response evaluation, neurophysiologic intraoperative monitoring, audiologic (aural) rehabilitation (assessment and management), assessment/treatment of central auditory processing disorders (adults and children), counseling, balance system assessment, hearing aid fitting, product dispensing, product repair/modification, assistive listening system/device selection, and sensory aids assessment. The preferred practice patterns must be revised and updated as needed due to expanding technology, a broadening scope of practice in audiology, and so on. A preferred practice pattern for the use of multiskilling and support personnel in the professions should be developed. Until then, the earlier reviewed technical reports and position statements are the only resources on this topic available to audiologists and to other outside agencies. These documents are rather generic and must be applied individually to specific areas of practice. In this case, practice guidelines (recommended sets of procedures for specific areas of practice) can be used to assist audiologists in determining how, or if, the use of multiskilling and support personnel is appropriate across various service-delivery sites.

Throughout this textbook, we will refer to this model in applying the concept of multiskilling and the use of support personnel in the establishment of support programs for persons with hearing impairment across various service-delivery sites. The model will assist practitioners in designing programs that operate according to regulatory constraints at every level. Unfortunately, the use of multiskilling and support personnel may be warranted but not possible due to regulatory contraindications at some level of the system. In this case, *it is important to realize that audiologists can change regulations through advocacy*. The purposes of advocacy are to: (1) keep policy and decision-makers informed about important issues and (2) build public support for audiologists and audiologic services (ASHA, 1996a). Audiologists can have an impact on federal legislation by getting involved in ASHA's grass roots networks of Ed-Net (i.e., issues related to education) and Health-Net (i.e., issues related to health), as well as their Political Action Committee (ASHA-PAC). The purposes of ASHA-PAC are to (1) influence election of individuals supportive of the professions, (2) raise funds, (3) encourage understanding, (4) promote interests of the professions, and (5) promote public policy. The American Academy of Audiology (AAA) also has a political action committee called AAA-PAC, which functions in much the same way and for the same purposes as ASHA-PAC. Appendix II-C contains pertinent resources including (1) important ASHA/AAA publications related to the topic of multiskilling and the use of support personnel, (2) useful Web sites, and (3) specific ASHA e-mail addresses for inquiries concerning regulatory policies that may be related to this topic at various levels of the model.

SUMMARY

This chapter has provided readers with basic concepts for the use of multiskilling and support personnel in audiology. By being able to define, differentiate various models, and understand the pros and cons of multiskilling, audiologists can cross-train competent support personnel to participate in stellar support programs for persons with hearing impairment. Furthermore, audiologists' knowledge of the "Position Statement and Guidelines of the Consensus Panel on Support Personnel in Audiology" (AAA, 1997) and understanding of the model defining the regulatory influences on the profession assist them in appropriately using multiskilling in their own practices or places of employment. Other chapters in this textbook will show readers how to define, market, develop, and maintain aural rehabilitation support programs in specific service-delivery sites.

> **LEARNING ACTIVITIES**
>
> - List as many examples as possible in which multiskilling and support personnel are currently being used in the practice of audiology across service-delivery settings. For each example, classify each as subordinate, collateral, or collateral-subordinate multiskilling. Determine if each example complies with the Consensus Panel's "Statement and Guidelines on Support Personnel in Audiology."
>
> - Compare and contrast the Consensus Panel's "Statement and Guidelines on Support Personnel in Audiology" (AAA, 1997) and ASHA's "Guidelines for Training, Credentialing, Use, and Supervision of Speech-Language Pathology Assistants" (ASHA, 1996c) and discuss the following: How do the two professions differ in their approach to the use of support personnel with regard to training, credentialing, use, and supervision of support personnel? In what areas are the documents vague? In what areas are the documents controversial?
>
> - Using the model proposed in the chapter, trace the regulatory influences on the possible implementation of multiskilling and the use of support personnel in various students' clinical externship sites or in various service-delivery sites in your practice.
>
> - Debate the use of multiskilling and support personnel in the profession.

REFERENCES

American Academy of Audiology. (1993). Audiology: Scope of practice. *Audiology Today, 5*(1), 16–17.

American Academy of Audiology. (1996). Code of ethics. McLean, VA: Author.

American Academy of Audiology. (1997). Position statement and guidelines of the consensus panel on support personnel in audiology. *Audiology Today, 9*(3), 27–28.

American Dietetic Association. (1995). Multiskilling dietetics students for the future. Chicago: Author.

American Nurses Association. (1994). Unlicensed assistive personnel in community settings. (Policy/Position #11.42). Washington, DC: Author.

American Occupational Therapy Association. (1995, January). White Paper: Occupational therapy and cross-training initiatives. *OT Week, 9*, 31.

American Physical Therapy Association. (1995). Position on multiskilled personnel (HOD 06–95–27–17, Program 32). Alexandria, VA: Author.

American Speech-Language-Hearing Association. (1981, March) Employment and utilization of supportive personnel in audiology and speech-language pathology. *Asha, 23*, 165–169.

American Speech-Language-Hearing Association. (1992). ASHA policy regarding support personnel. *Asha, 34*(Suppl. 5), 51–58.

American Speech-Language-Hearing Association. (1994, March). Code of ethics. *Asha, 36*(Suppl. 13), 1–2.

American Speech-Language-Hearing Association. (1995, March). Position statement of the training, credentialing, use and supervision of support personnel in speech-language pathology. *Asha, 37*(Suppl. 14), 21.

American Speech-Language-Hearing Association. (1996a). *Curriculum guide to managed care*. Rockville, MD: Author.

American Speech-Language-Hearing Association. (1996b, Spring). Scope of practice in audiology. *Asha, 38*(Suppl. 16), 12–14.

American Speech-Language-Hearing Association. (1996c, Spring). Guidelines for the training, credentialing, use, and supervision of speech-language pathology assistants. *Asha, 38*(Suppl. 16), 21–34.

American Speech-Language-Hearing Association. (1996d, Spring). Technical report of the ad hoc committee on multiskilling. *Asha, 38*(Suppl. 16), 53–61.

American Speech-Language-Hearing Association. (1997a, Spring). Position statement: Multiskillied personnel. *Asha, 39*(Suppl. 17), 13.

American Speech-Language-Hearing Association. (1997b, November). Preferred practice patterns for the profession of audiology. Rockville, MD: Author.

Americans with Disabilities Act of 1990, Public Law 101-336, 42, U.S.C. 12101 *et seq. U.S. Statutes at Large, 104*, 327–378 (1991).

Bamberg, R., Blayney, K. D., Vaughn, D. G., & Wilson, B. R. (1989). *Multiskilled health practitioner education: A national perspective*. Birmingham, AL: University of Alabama at Birmingham, School of Health Related Professions, National Multiskilled Health Practitioner Clearinghouse.

Educational Testing Service. (1995). *The practice of audiology—A study of clinical activities and knowledge areas for the certified audiologist*. Rockville, MD: American Speech-Language-Hearing Association.

Foto, M. (1996). Multiskilling: Who, how, when, and why? *The American Journal of Occupational Therapy, 50,* 1.

Freilinger, J. (1992). Support personnel. *Asha, 34*(10), 51–53.

Goldberg, B. (1996). Imagining tomorrow: What's ahead for our professions. *Asha 38*(3), 22–23, 25–28.

Grantham, R. B. (1997). ASHA and the schools. In P. F. O'Connell (Ed.), *Speech, language, and hearing programs in the schools: A guide for students and practitioners* (pp. 24–65). Gaithersburg, MD: Aspen Publishers, Inc.

Griffin, K. M., & Fazen, M. (1993). A managed care strategy for practitioners. In C.M. Frattali (Ed.) *Quality improvement digest: Current information on issues related to quality evaluation and improvement* (pp. 1–7). Rockville, MD: American Speech-Language-Hearing Association.

Individuals with Disabilities Education Act of 1990 (IDEA), Public Law 101-476, 20, U.S.C. 1400 *et seq.: U.S. Statutes at Large, 104,* 1103–1151 (1990).

Johnson, C. E., Stein, R. L, & Lass, N. J. (1992). Public school nurses' preparedness for a hearing aid monitoring program. *Language Speech, and Hearing Services in the Schools, 23,* 141–144.

Joint Commission on the Accreditation of Health-Care Organizations. (1996). *Comprehensive accreditation manual for hospitals.* Oakbrook, IL: Author.

Larson, S., & Lynch, D. (1995). *Report: State regulation of audiology and speech-language pathology support personnel.* Rockville, MD: American Speech-Language- Hearing Association. Unpublished manuscript.

Moncur, J. P. (1967). *Institute on the utilization of support personnel in school speech and hearing programs.* Washington, DC: American Speech and Hearing Association.

National Hearing Conservation Association. (1995). Code of ethics. Milwaukee, WI: Author.

O'Brien, M. A. (1997). Third party payments, supervision, and support personnel. In P. F. O'Connell, (Ed.), *Speech, language, and hearing programs in the schools: A guide for students and practitioners* (pp. 305–344). Gaithersburg, MD: Aspen Publishers, Inc.

Pietranton, A., & Lynch, C. (1995). Multiskilling: A renaissance or dark age. *Asha, 37*(6–7), 37–40.

Runnels, C. A. (1994). Support personnel. In C. Peters-Johnson, S. Karr, & J. Langsam (Eds.), *Reference manual: Communication, creativity, collaboration: Current challenges for school supervisors and administrators* (pp. 75–78). Rockville, MD: American Speech-Language-Hearing Association.

Werven, G. (1993). Support personnel: An issue for our times. *American Journal of Speech-Language Pathology: A Journal of Clinical Practice, 2*(2), 9–12.

APPENDIX II-A

American Speech-Language-Hearing Association's Position Statement on Multiskilled Personnel

It is the position of the American Speech-Language-Hearing Association that multiskilling is not a unidimensional concept and that it cannot be evenly applied across the diverse clinical workforce. Specifically, cross-training of clinical skills is not appropriate at the professional level of practice (i.e., audiologists or speech-language pathologists). Cross-training of basic patient-care skills, professional nonclinical skills, and/or administrative skills is a reasonable option that clinical practitioners at all levels of practice may need to consider depending on the service delivery setting, geographic location, patient/client population, and clinical workforce resources. (See glossary for definition of terms used in this position statement. For further clarification, please refer to the American Speech-Language-Hearing Association. [1996, Spring]. Technical report of the ad hoc committee on multiskilling. Asha, 38 [Suppl. 16,] pp. 53–61.)

Glossary of Terms

- **Cross-training of clinical skills**—involves training practitioners in one discipline to perform services traditionally regarded as within the purview or scope of practice of another discipline in an attempt to more efficiently deploy the clinical workforce to meet the needs of the patient caseload as it fluctuates at any particular point in time. Examples include training respiratory therapists to perform EEGs (electroencephalograms), or medical technologists to perform certain radiological procedures.
- **Cross-training of basic patient care skills**—includes routine, frequently provided, easily trainable, low-risk procedures such as suctioning patients, monitoring vital signs, and transferring and positioning patients. Identifying a facility/agency/program-specific set of patient-care skills that can be performed by various practitioners in that particular setting may lead to less fragmented and less costly patient care (e.g., bedside treatment sessions do not have to be delayed waiting for another practitioner to suction the patient; home care patients' compliance with prescribed medications can be verified by clinicians already coming to the home on a regular basis; diabetic preschoolers' blood sugar levels can be monitored by on-site clinicians).
- **Cross-training of professional nonclinical skills**—includes skills and services such as patient education, technical writing, team dynamics/communication/leadership, and such. Establishing competency standards for such skills across the workforce may enhance the overall quality, efficiency, and coordination of service delivery.
- **Cross-training of administrative skills**—includes programmatic activities such as quality improvement, case management, systems design, and the management of clinical services. Increasingly, as organizations downsize, such responsibilities are moving from centralization in one or more "administrative positions" to distribution among clinical practitioners. Doing so may result in more efficient use of staff and better integration of these functions with clinical service delivery.

APPENDIX II-B

Position Statement and Guidelines of the Consensus Panel on Support Personnel in Audiology

This policy paper was developed by the Consensus Panel on Support Personnel in Audiology whose members come from the following professional organizations that represent audiologists: Academy of Dispensing Audiologists (ADA), American Academy of Audiology (AAA), American Speech-Language-Hearing Association (ASHA), Educational Audiology Association (EAA), Military Audiology Association (MAA), and the National Hearing Conservation Association (NHCA). Audiologists who served as organizational representatives to the panel included Donald Bender (AAA) and Evelyn Cherow (ASHA), co-chairs; James McDonald and Meredy Hase (ADA); Albert deChiccis and Cheryl DeConde Johnson (AAA); Chris Halpin and Deborah Price (ASHA); Peggy Benson (EAA); James Jerome (MAA); and Lloyd Bowling and Richard Danielson (NHCA).

I. Introduction

The consensus panel recognizes that federal and state health care and education reform Initiatives, changing U.S. demographics, and the broadening scope of practice of audiologists (ASHA, 1996; Educational Testing Service, 1995; AAA, 1993) have affected the delivery of audiology services. Audiologists are using support personnel in audiology service delivery systems to ensure both the accessibility and the highest quality of audiology care while addressing productivity and cost-benefit concerns. In an analysis of state licensure laws (Larson & Lynch, 1995), ASHA found that in the 45 states that regulate one or both professions of audiology and speech-language pathology, 30 recognize support personnel. Not all of these states actually regulate support personnel; 22 states have promulgated rules regulating support personnel in all work settings and five were in the process of creating these rules. This position statement and guidelines do not supersede federal legislation and regulation requirements, any exisiting state licensure laws, or affect interpretation or implementation of such laws. The document may serve, however, as a guide for the development of new laws or, at the appropriate time, for revising existing licensure laws.

II. Position Statement

It is the position of the following organizations represented on the Consensus Panel on Support Personnel in Audiology (Academy of Dispensing Audiologists, American Academy of Audiology, Educational Audiology Association, Military Audiology Association, and National Hearing Conservation Association) that support personnel may assist audiologists in delivery of services.

The roles and tasks of audiology support personnel will be assigned only by supervising audiologists. Supervising audiologists will provide appropriate training that is competency-based and specific to job performance. Supervision will be comprehensive, periodic, and documented. The supervising audiologist maintains the legal and ethical responsibilities for all assigned audiology activities provided by support personnel. The needs of the consumer of audiology services and protection of that consumer will always be paramount (ASHA, 1996; ASHA, 1994; AAA, 1996-97; NHCA, 1995). Audiologists are uniquely educated and specialize in the diagnosis and rehabilitation of hearing and related disorders. As such, audiologists are the appropriate, qualified professionals to hire, supervise, and train audiology support personnel.

III. Guidelines

A. Definitions
SUPPORT PERSONNEL: People who, after appropriate training, perform tasks that are prescribed, directed, and supervised by an audiologist.

SUPERVISING AUDIOLOGIST: An audiologist who has attained license (where applicable) or certification credentials and who has been practicing for at least one year after meeting these requirements.

B. Qualifications for Support Personnel
1. Have a high school degree or equivalent.
2. Have communication and interpersonal skills necessary for the tasks assigned.
3. Have a basic understanding of the needs of the population being served.
4. Have met training requirements and have competency-based skills necessary to the performance of specific assigned tasks.
5. Have any additional qualifications established by the supervising audiologist to meet the specific needs of the audiology program and the population being served.

C. Training

Training for support personnel should be well-defined and specific to the assigned task(s). The supervising audiologist will ensure that the scope and intensity of training encompass all of the activities assigned to the support personnel. Training should be competency-based and provided through a variety of formal and informal instructional methods. Audiologists should provide support personnel with information on roles and functions. Continuing opportunities should be provided to ensure that practices are current and that skills are maintained. The supervising audiologist will maintain written documentation of training activities.

D. Role

Audiology support personnel may engage in only those tasks that are planned, delegated, and supervised by the audiologist. The specific roles of audiology support personnel will be influenced by the particular needs of the audiologist and must be determined by the audiologist responsible for the support personnel's training and supervision.

Audiology support personnel **will not engage independently** in the following activities. **This list provides examples and is not intended to be all-inclusive.**

- Interpreting observations or data into diagnostic statements of clinical management strategies or procedures.
- Determining case selection.
- Perform habilitative or rehabilitative tasks that require in process clinical judgements.
- Transmitting clinical information, either verbally or in writing, to anyone without the approval of the supervising audiologist.
- Composing clinical reports except for progress notes to be reviewed by the audiologist and held in the patient's/client's records.
- Referring a patient/client to other professionals or agencies.
- Referring him- or herself either orally or in writing with a title other than one determined by the supervising audiologist.
- Signing any formal documents (e.g., treatment plans, reimbursement forms, or reports).
- Discharging a patient/client from services.
- Communicating with the patient/client, family, or others regarding any aspect of patient/client status or service without the specific consent of the supervising audiologist.

E. Supervision

Supervising audiologists will have the primary role in all administrative actions related to audiology support personnel, such as hiring, training, determining competency, and conducting performance evaluations. In addition, the supervising audiologist maintains final approval of all directives given by administrators and other professionals regarding audiology tasks.

Supervising audiologists will assign specific tasks to the support person. Such tasks **must not**: 1) require the exercise of professional judgment, 2) entail of interpretation of results (with the exception of hearing screening), or 3) encompass the development or modification of treatment plans.

The amount and type of supervision required should be based on skills and experience of the support person, the needs of patients/clients served, the service delivery setting, the tasks assigned, and other factors. For example, more intense supervision will be required during orientation of a new support person; initiation of a new program task, or equipment; or a change in patient/client status.

The number of support personnel supervised by a given audiologist must be consistent with the delivery of appropriate, quality service. It is the responsibility of the individual supervisor to protect the interests of patients/clients in a manner consistent with state licensure requirements, where applicable, and the Code of Ethics of that audiologist's respective professional organization.

APPENDIX II-C

Resources on the Use of Multiskilling and Support Personnel

Useful E-mail Addresses at the ASHA National Office for Issues Related to the Use of Multiskilling and Support Personnel

- **Consumer Information:** *actioncenter@asha.org*
- **Audiology:** *audiology@asha.org*
  Provides general information about the practice of audiology.
- **Educational Programs:** *ashaeducation@asha.org*
  Provides information on continuing-education programs developed by ASHA.
- **Ethics:** *ethics@asha.org*
  Provides information about the ASHA Code of Ethics.
- **Governance:** *governance@asha.org*
  Provides information about boards, committees, task forces, legislative council, etc.
- **Governmental Affairs, Federal:** *federal@asha.org*
  Provides information on federal appropriations, budget, legislation; the ASHA PAC (Political Action Committee); its grassroots networks (HealthNet and EdNet); members of and candidates for Congress; federal advocacy coalitions; federal legislation related to speech pathology, audiology, and speech and hearing science.
- **Governmental Affairs, Federal Education and Regulatory Policy:** *regs@asha.org*
  Provides information on federal education rules, regulations, policy, legislation; Improving American Schools Act; Higher Education Act; Deaf Education Act; federal officials; IDEA legislation; OSHA; FDA regulations/legislation; qualified provider/school settings; special-education legislation and funding for infants and toddlers.
- **Governmental Affairs, States:** *states@asha.org*
  Provides information on state legislation and regulations related to professionals, services and consumers, state advocacy, and taking action.
- **Health Services:** *healthservices@asha.org*
  Provides information on admission/discharge reports, American Board of Disability Analysts (ABDA), Competencies (JCAHO), efficacy, and ASHA-FACs (information on important topics).
- **Professional Services Board (PSB):** *psb@asha.org*
  Provides information about PSB accreditation, including applications and annual reports of PSB accredited programs.
- **Reimbursement:** *reimbursement@asha.org*
  Provides information about managed-care insurance appeals, insurance codes, CHAMPUS (health insurance for military personnel), qualified provider (health settings), private health insurance, salary equivalency for health-care insurance reimbursement, Medicare, and Medicaid.
- **Schools:** *schools@asha.org*
  Provides information on practicing in schools.
- **Special Interest Divisions:** *sidivisions@asha.org*
  Provides information on ASHA's Special Interest Divisions.
- **State Agencies:** *actioncenter@asha.org*
  Provides contacts and addresses for state departments of education and health.

Important Professional Publications about Multiskilling and the Use of Support Personnel

American Academy of Audiology Committee on Infant Hearing. (1998). Use of support personnel for newborn hearing screening (proposed guidelines). *Audiology Today, 10*(6), 21–23.

American Speech-Language-Hearing Association. (1992). ASHA policy regarding support personnel. *Asha, 34*(Suppl. 5), 51–58.

American Speech-Language-Hearing Association. (1997, November). Preferred practice patterns for the profession of audiology. Rockville, MD: Author.

American Speech-Language-Hearing Association. (1994, March). Code of ethics. *Asha, 36*(Suppl. 13), 1-2.

American Speech-Language-Hearing Association. (1995, March). Position statement of the training, credentialing, use and supervision of support personnel in speech-language pathology. *Asha, 37*(Suppl. 14), 21.

American Speech-Language-Hearing Association. (1996). *Curriculum guide to managed care.* Rockville, MD: American Speech-Language-Hearing Association.

American Speech-Language-Hearing Association. (1996, Spring). Scope of practice in audiology. *Asha, 38*(Suppl. 16), 12-14.

American Speech-Language-Hearing Association. (1996, Spring). Guidelines for the training, credentialing, use, and supervision of speech-language pathology assistants. *Asha, 38*(Suppl. 16), 21-34.

American Speech-Language-Hearing Association. (1996, Spring). Technical report of the ad hoc committee on multiskilling. *Asha, 38*(Suppl. 16), 53–61.

American Speech-Language-Hearing Association. (1997, Spring). Position statement: Multiskillied personnel. *Asha, 39*(Suppl. 17), 13.

CHAPTER 3

Defining and Marketing Support Programs

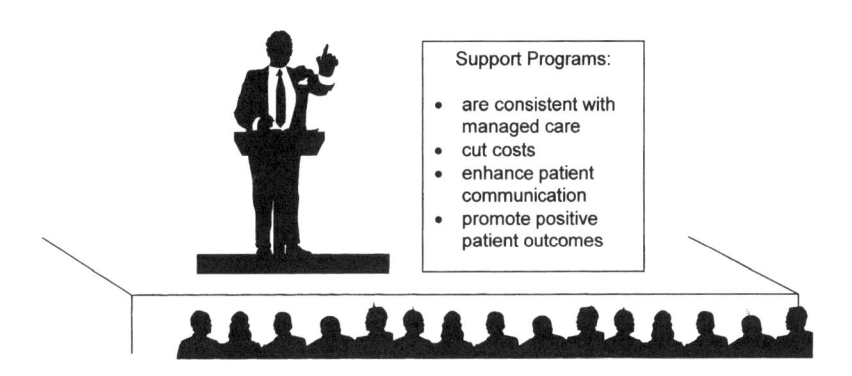

Figure 3-1. Defining and marketing support programs are critical to success.

INTRODUCTION

Chapter 1 highlighted the effects of managed care on the practice of audiology. In recent years, many audiologists believe they are being forced to consider either joining provider networks or maintaining their positions as private practitioners (Danhauer, 1998). Audiology networks claim both to increase the volume of patients audiologists will see and to handle the considerable problems associated with managed hearing health care. In exchange, they require participants to discount hearing aids and audiology services. In some cases, audiologic evaluations are capitated or even expected to be provided at no cost. In addition, audiologists are not likely to receive compensation for aural rehabilitation services in any of the managed-care programs now in existence. All audiologists must adopt a proactive approach toward not only surviving, but flourishing in today's competitive health-care arena. Audiologists in private practice need to find their own niches by defining their business direction and creating innovations for improving their practices (Danhauer, 1998). Private-practice audiologists may find that providing services via comprehensive stellar support programs for patients with hearing impairment in various service-delivery sites will help increase the number of patients seen. For example, providing services through support programs in rehabilitation hospitals to recuperating patients who have had cerebral vascular accidents may increase audiologists' patient-care load once those patients resume their normal day-to-day activities and need ongoing audiologic care. The first step toward success is the audiologists' ability to identify the impact of support programs on their practices, as well as to define and market them. The purpose of this chapter is to provide theoretical frameworks for defining and marketing such programs.

> **LEARNING OBJECTIVES**
>
> **This chapter will enable the reader to:**
>
> - Understand the impact of support programs on private practices
> - Define support programs for persons with hearing impairment
> - Implement strategies for marketing support programs

IMPACT OF SUPPORT PROGRAMS ON PRIVATE PRACTICES

Incorporating support programs across service-delivery sites into audiologists' private practices may increase their number of patients seen. This may expand audiologists' practices to include multiple offices and increase the number of employees. Nonetheless, audiologists must carefully consider the possibility that while they will see "more" patients and be "busier than ever," they may fail to see corresponding increases in income. In some cases, being the "boss" and having several persons on the payroll can cause far more headaches, as well as loss of income and free time, than simply focusing audiologists' energies on a quality, single-office, sole-proprietor practice. Audiologists often have a difficult time grasping this concept when success is often equated with having several offices and employees. Too often, audiologists become preoccupied with this misconception and have to learn the hard way, approaching financial disaster before realizing that smaller may be better. Our goal here is to increase awareness of these issues and offer ways to deal with them. The development of support programs for patients with hearing impairment across service-delivery sites may expand a practice but, for the above stated reasons, should be controlled and monitored for quality. Audiologists should always be "taking the pulse" of these endeavors to ensure that they are not dragging down the practice in terms of resources used and income generated. Audiologists must be vigilant and protective of their resources. They also must take notice when their practices are being pushed to their limits. Constant monitoring can save an audiologist from having to make decisions in a crisis or after it is too late.

DEFINING SUPPORT PROGRAMS

Support programs for persons with hearing impairment can be defined by differentiating between what these programs are and what they are not. Table 3–1 lists characteristics of such programs.

Support programs are specific to the service-delivery site, although they all share the same goal. For example, Chapters 6, 7, and 8 discuss the implementation of support programs in educational settings, rehabilitation hospitals, and long-term care residential facilities for the elderly. Although specific program components

Table 3–1. Characteristics of support programs.

CHARACTERISTICS OF SUPPORT PROGRAMS

- Adhere to managed-care principles
- Undergo a continuous cycle of development, planning, and evaluation
- Require the leadership of audiologists with special skills
- Are not a substitute for comprehensive audiologic care
- Augment ongoing comprehensive diagnostic and rehabilitative audiologic programming
- Are not provided "for free"
- Are not self-sustaining
- Are an excellent marketing tool

may vary according to service-delivery site, all share the same goal of addressing the immediate auditory needs of persons with hearing impairment so that they can meet the communication demands of their environments.

Regardless of service-delivery site, efficient support programs should adhere to the basic principles of managed care (ASHA, 1996). Although managed care may have some disadvantages, its principles have a lot to offer audiologists attempting to market their programs to cost-conscious health-care facilities, school systems, or both. Support programs should: (1) coordinate among practitioners, (2) be applied at the appropriate consistency, (3) adhere to practice guidelines, (4) cost the least amount possible, (5) achieve desired patient outcomes, and (6) be monitored under resource management (ASHA, 1996).

As described in Chapters 7 and 8, the implementation of support programs in rehabilitation hospitals and nursing homes requires a coordinated approach among staff members in order to manage patients' communication needs successfully. Staff members should be consistent in performing daily visual/listening checks of patients' hearing aids. Similarly, support programs for both short- and long-term residential care facilities should conform to practice guidelines (e.g., ASHA, 1997a) and federal laws (e.g., the Americans with Disabilities Act, 1990), when applicable, while still being cost-efficient.

Cost-efficiency must be considered from the perspectives of both health administrators and audiologists. Health administrators want to know how much a program will cost. They want to know who will pay for the services and who will handle the billing and paperwork. Generally, they will be more supportive if required resources for the support program are kept at a minimum. They also want to know if the program contributes to positive patient outcomes and enhanced recovery, or quality of life. Audiologists, on the other hand, are concerned with whether they will receive a profitable return on their investment of time and resources, and whether the services can be maintained once set in place. Assessment of cost versus benefits of support programs requires skilled resource management (e.g., allocation of human and financial resources) and implementation of productivity standards, quality assessment, and improvement activities (e.g., performance management, outcomes assessment, and program evaluation). Adequate resource management of support programs requires a continuous cycle of development, planning, and evaluation (Johnson, Benson, & Seaton, 1997) in order to be successful. Figure 3–2 shows the continual process that should be completed annually and then updated every 3 to 5 years thereafter (Johnson et al., 1997).

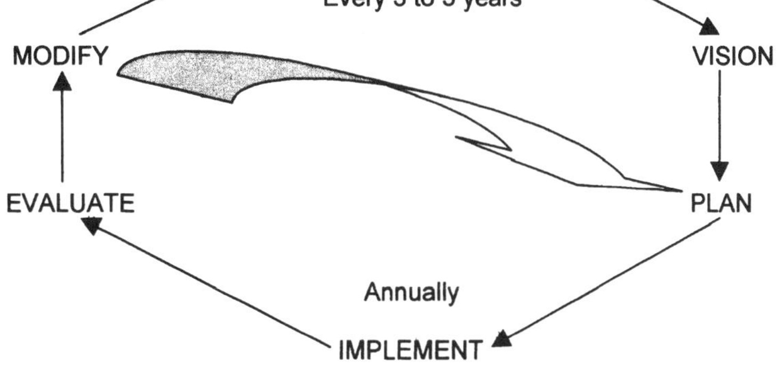

Figure 3-2. Continuous cycle of development, planning, and evaluation of support programs. (Adapted from the *Educational Audiology Handbook*, by C. D. Johnson, P. V. Benson, & J. B. Seaton, 1997. San Diego, CA: Singular Publishing Group, Inc.)

Support program development adapted from Johnson et al. (1997) includes: (1) lining up funding sources; (2) laying the foundation by providing standards and guidelines for audiology services according to specific service-delivery site; (3) enlisting the support of key individuals and administrators; (4) conducting a needs survey to determine critical program components to meet standards of care; (5) establishing a program vision with specific goals based on the results of the needs assessment; (6) performing a systematic analysis (e.g., feasibility, cost containment, and administrative approval) of possible program scenarios to achieve identified goals; (7) selecting a scenario, obtaining necessary materials (e.g., hearing aid check kits and ALDs), and training appropriate support personnel; (8) developing a long-range plan that identifies activities in each of the program component areas; (9) determining budget requirements and other possible limitations to carry out identified activities; (10) prioritizing activities for resource allocation; (11) planning for annual evaluations; and (12) making necessary modifications.

Successful support programs are managed by audiologists who possess certain unique technical, human-relation, and conceptual skills. Table 3–2 displays the requisite skills in each area as adapted from Bodenhemier (1994).

First, audiologists must possess technical skills requiring familiarity with the preferred practices (ASHA, 1997b), guidelines, applicable state and federal laws, and knowledge of administrative issues, including budgeting across service-delivery sites. For example, in establishing support programs for children with hearing impairment in public schools, audiologists must be knowledgeable about preferred practices and guidelines for educational audiology. They must also be familiar with the Individuals with Disabilities Education Act (IDEA) (1990), the Americans with Disabilities Act (ADA) (1990), and the administrative policies of the local school system. Second, audiologists must have excellent human-relation skills to work effectively with administrators, colleagues, audiologic support personnel, patients and their families, and others. This often requires certain personality traits that include the ability to obtain respect, flexibility, communication skills, leadership, and support-personnel policy development skills. Third, conceptual skills are needed not only to establish support programs, but to sustain them

Table 3–2. Requisite skills for managing support programs.

TECHNICAL SKILLS

- Knowledge of preferred practices and guidelines for care across service-delivery sites
- Knowledge of state and federal laws mandating communication accessibility
- Knowledge of administrative issues specific to service-delivery site including budgeting
- Clinical expertise in effective service-delivery across settings

HUMAN-RELATIONS SKILLS

- "Personality skills" needed to work effectively with administrators, other professionals, and support personnel to execute short- and long-term objectives
- Leadership skills
- Support-personnel policy development skills
- Ability to gain respect of support personnel
- Good communication skills (written, oral, and listening)
- Flexibility

CONCEPTUAL SKILLS

- Ability to perform a systematic analysis of service-delivery site to specify program needs
- Ability to understand the importance of all support program components so that priorities about future directions can be made
- Ability to predict future program needs (i.e., visioning)
- Ability to stress the importance of support programs to administrators, other professionals, and support personnel
- Ability to market support programs

Source: Adapted from "Managing a Hearing Conservation Service," by W. G. Bodenhemier, 1994. In D. M. Lipscomb (Ed.), *Hearing Conservation* (pp. 273–286). San Diego: Singular Publishing Group, Inc.

as well. The managing audiologist, for example, must be able to market and convince administrators, other professionals, audiologic support personnel, and so on as to the value of the program and their participation in optimizing patient outcomes. Achieving positive patient outcomes depends on the ability of the audiologist to analyze the service-delivery site systematically and then logistically design a cost-efficient program that supports the communication needs of all patients with hearing impairment and the persons who come into contact with them. In addition, program development and continuation requires that the audiologist establishes program priorities, charts future directions, and projects ongoing needs. Thus, audiologists who possess the necessary technical, human-relation, and conceptual skills can create stellar support programs for patients with hearing impairment, regardless of service-delivery site. Furthermore, *successful programming requires that the managing audiologist understands both the characteristics and the limitations of these programs.*

Support programs for patients with hearing impairment have several limitations. First, support programs using multiskilling and support personnel should not be a substitute for quality hearing health care provided by a licensed and certified audiologist. The managing audiologist should be assisted by other professionals and audiologic support personnel in order to meet the communication needs of as many patients as possible, while also establishing a continuum of hearing health care. Second, audiologic support programs are not complete within themselves, but should augment ongoing comprehensive diagnostic and rehabilitation programming. Third, support programs should not be expected to be self-sustaining, nor provided "free-of-charge." They will need constant monitoring by audiologists. This takes time, and time is money. As a profession, audiologists must vigorously market aural rehabilitation by presenting support programs in cost-efficient packages that are appealing to hospital administrators, third-party payers, MCOs, and others. *Audiologists must clearly state the necessary support needed, charge for services provided, and document program efficacy.* Once successfully established, stellar support programs can be excellent marketing tools. Satisfied patients and their families will seek follow-up, diagnostic, and rehabilitation services from managing audiologists' practices. In addition, satisfied patients and their families will refer their friends to those practices.

MARKETING SUPPORT PROGRAMS

Marketing can be an exciting endeavor, incorporating sociology, psychology, education, human engineering, product and public relations, cost analysis, and management (Hosford-Dunn, Dunn, & Harford, 1995). Simply stated, *marketing* means getting into the minds of a target audience and then making a connection by creating an image, developing messages to communicate the image, and finally disseminating those messages (Smith, 1992). Marketing support programs for persons with hearing impairment is similar to marketing other aspects of audiologic practice.

Although most audiologists are quite confident about their knowledge and their clinical skills, many are frightened at the prospect of having to market their practices. Many audiologists spend their entire careers in "protected environments" (e.g., academic or hospital settings) where they work for someone else and never have to market themselves, their products, or their services. Even for those whose primary income is produced through the sale of hearing aids, it is usually the hearing instrument manufacturers who market the devices in national and local promotions. The increase in the number of practicing audiologists who work at least part-time in a private practice (presently about 40% of all audiologists, Stach, 1998) reflects the need for an enhanced awareness and development of marketing skills for the profession. Those in private practice will either have to acquire marketing skills rapidly, affiliate with one of the many emerging corporate audiology networks active in marketing, or suffer the consequences of not promoting their practices. Like it or not, audiologists must become involved with marketing, be it for their own private practices or as an employee of someone else, in order to survive in today's hearing health-care arena. As Danhauer (1998) suggested, these skills have not been taught as part of our academic preparation in the past but should be in the future, especially in the new Au.D. curricula.

As depicted in Figure 3–3, developing a successful marketing plan has been described as a four-phase process that combines the principles of marketing theory with the practical realities of one's audiologic practice (Smith, 1992).

PRELIMINARY WORK

- Define marketing goals and objectives.
- Determine marketing audience.
- Execute market research (feasibility study).
  - *Preliminary analysis
  - *Market survey
  - *Planning/financing for practice expansion
  - *Data review/analysis
  - *Decision making
- Identify marketing tools.

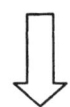

⇩

MARKET POSITION & STRATEGIES

- Determine market position.
- Select marketing tools.
- Develop a timeline.

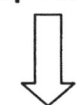

⇩

ASSESSMENT OF MARKETING PLAN

- Assess financial plan.
- Implement strategies.
- Continue evaluation.

⇩

CONTINUOUS QUALITY IMPROVEMENT (CQI)

- Create constancy of quality.
- Adopt the new philosophy.
- Cease dependence on inspection.
- Think beyond profit.
- Improve constantly and forever.
- Institute on-the-job training.
- Institute leadership.
- Drive out fear.
- Breakdown staff barriers.
- Eliminate slogans.
- Eliminate quotas.
- Instill pride of workmanship.
- Institute educational programs.
- Get everyone involved.

Figure 3-3. Marketing plan. (Adapted from Walton, 1986; ASHA, 1991; Reisberg & Frattali, 1990; Smith, 1992; and Hosford-Dunn et al., 1995).

Phase 1: Preliminary Work

The first phase is the preliminary work that involves four steps.

Step 1: Define Marketing Goals and Objectives

First, define goals or marketing objectives. In marketing support programs, audiologists must decide which service-delivery sites to target and what message to convey. (Although this textbook discusses the establishment of programs in educational settings, rehabilitation hospitals, and long-term residential care facilities for the elderly, readers should be able to adapt these procedures to other sites as needed.) An audiologist may, for example, decide to market support programs to nursing homes in the area with the following objectives (adapted from Smith, 1992):

- Explain the effects of hearing impairment on residents' quality of life.
- Discuss the role of the audiologist and support programs in enhancing residents' communication with nursing-home personnel, family members, and peers.
- Educate other professionals about the importance of their participation in these support programs. (The use of regular inservice programs for staff can be very helpful here.)
- Expand the number of residential care facilities for the elderly that are familiar with your services to increase referrals. (Be sure you have the staff and the resources to avoid being spread too thin.)
- Improve working relationships with professional colleagues and possible referral sources.
- Build enthusiasm for support programs within nursing homes that you currently serve.
- Preserve and expand the funding base of your current operations. (This should occur in part as a result of this expanded coverage; if not, you may have a difficult time justifying this new outreach.)
- Retain existing contracts.
- Increase your caseload, keeping in mind the above caviates.

Step 2: Determine Marketing Audience

The second step involves determining the audience, market target, or group of consumers toward which marketing efforts will be directed (Bodenhemier, 1994). Audiologists must consider their relationship to those consumers and the particular service-delivery site. Will marketing efforts be aimed at referral sources, the general public, or current patients? Is the audiologist an employee of the facility, or merely a provider of services to the facility through a contract? Does the audiologist have any current relationship with the facility? Full-time employees may be more successful at marketing within a given facility because administrators and other staff members may be more receptive to ideas from professionals within the organization than from someone who may provide services only once a week or less. Contract-for-service audiologists, for example, may be unsure of how best to market the idea of development of a support program for rehabilitation-hospital patients with hearing impairment without jeopardizing their own relationships with the administration. The audiologist's immediate supervisor or close colleagues (e.g., staff speech-language pathologists or physical therapists) can be invaluable in marketing ideas to hospital administrators. Obtaining the enthusiastic support of directors of the speech-language pathology departments has been shown to be instrumental in successfully marketing hospital-wide support programs to administrators (e.g., Griffin, Clark-Lewis, & Johnson, 1997). Directors of other departments that will be directly impacted by the program also should be included in the marketing campaign. Their early involvement can garner their support, suggestions, and enthusiasm, rather than breeding resentment for leaving them out of the process. In a rehabilitation hospital, directors of the nursing, occupational-therapy, and physical-therapy departments must be supportive for a program to succeed (e.g., Griffin et al., 1997). After identifying the target market, audiologists must conduct research and identify potential marketing tools.

Step 3: Execute Market Research (Feasibility Study)

The third step involves doing market research and completing a feasibility study that involves gathering, analyzing, and evaluating the costs and benefits of initiating a business or adding new programs (ASHA, 1991). Appendix III-B contains a worksheet for completing a five-stage feasibility study on establishment of support programs for persons with hearing impairment.

The first stage of a feasibility study involves a preliminary analysis of marketing potential by determining funding sources:

- Who constitutes your market?
- How many potential customers are there?
- Would support programs serve a currently unserved need?
- Does the need for support programs exceed supply in the market?
- What are some potential payment/funding sources for your market?
- Can the proposed support program compete with already existing services available in the market?
- What are the potential referral sources that apply to your potential market?
- Can establishing support programs be lucrative to your practice without draining human and capital resources?
- Are there any serious contraindications to this business venture?

If the answers to the above questions are favorable, the feasibility study continues to the second stage.

The second stage of a feasibility study includes conducting a market survey that projects a realistic estimate of revenue. The market survey should consist of at least the following five steps as adapted from ASHA (1991):

- Assess geographic influence on the market.
- Review population trends, demographic features, cultural factors, and so on within the community.
- Analyze competitors in the community to assess their strengths and weaknesses (e.g., pricing strategies, product lines, types of services and equipment provided, sources of referral, and so on).
- Determine the total sales volume in the market area and estimate expected market share.
- Estimate the possibilities for market expansion.

If the outcome of the marketing survey is favorable, then the feasibility study progresses to the third stage.

The third stage involves planning and financing operations for practice expansion in sufficient detail to determine the feasibility and costs needed for start-up, fixed investment, and operations (ASHA, 1991). Several questions must be asked. First, what are the costs and the availability of the equipment needed for the support program? What equipment do you need for your practice to manage support programs (e.g., portable audiometers, immittance meters, hearing aid analyzers, video-otoscope, and so on)? What equipment does the facility require for establishing and maintaining a support program for patients with hearing impairment (e.g., assistive listening devices, hearing aid check kits, and so on)? What are the prices for needed equipment?

Second, what merchandising methods will be used for goods and services in establishing support programs? Will you dispense the needed equipment for support programs? Which services will you charge for, and what will be the fee structure? What services could you offer if you had additional training? Third, what are locations of the facilities you will serve? What is their layout and operational structure? What support personnel are needed to accomplish program goals? Usually, audiologists must envision creating the most cost-efficient plan for managing a support program for the facility. Fourth, what is the cost and availability of personnel? Recall that support programs require the use of multiskilling and support personnel. Availability of enthusiastic and cooperative audiologic support personnel within the facility is critical for program success. Furthermore, administrators must be willing to allocate staffs' time for training and program participation. Fifth, what is the availability of supplies for the program (e.g., vendors, pricing schedules, exclusive or franchised products)? Audiologists must design an efficient system for supplying facilities with materials to sustain support programs. Sixth, do you have the personal characteristics to market, develop, maintain, sustain, and, if necessary, terminate support programs successfully? Do you have the necessary reputation, clinical skills, desire, determination, personality, and self-image to expand your practice to include managing support programs across different service-delivery sites? By answering these or similar questions posed in the planning of business organization and operation, audiologists should be prepared for the fourth and fifth stages of the feasibility study.

The fourth and fifth stages of the feasibility study involve reviewing and analyzing data and then decision making. By reviewing and analyzing data from the feasibility study, audiologists can determine the implications of marketing support programs for persons with hearing impairment and their potential impact on the success of their overall practices. If the outcome of the analysis indicates that implementing support programs in various service-delivery sites should result in a return of investment, and at least a moderate profit and growth potential, then a decision to proceed is appropriate at the end of stage five (ASHA, 1991). Additional questions to ask include (ASHA, 1991): Is there a commitment to make the necessary sacrifices in time, effort, and money? Will implementing support programs satisfy long-term aspirations? In summary, if the results of the feasibility study are favorable, audiologists can proceed to the fourth step in the preliminary work of the marketing plan.

Step 4: Identify Marketing Tools

The fourth step is to identify potential marketing tools. Marketing tools are the building blocks of a marketing plan. They should be compatible with the audiologist's message and consistent with the demographic patterns of the target audience (Smith, 1992). At this point, audiologists should list available marketing tools for possible use. Smith recommended the use of the following:

- Market research (e.g., surveys, focus groups, competitor files, patient response cards)
- Handouts for current and prospective patients (e.g., brochures, newsletters, fact sheets)
- Paid advertising, both print and electronic
- Public-service advertising and education, both print and electronic
- Direct mail to referral sources and consumers
- Public speaking
- Community service
- Proactive media relations
- Person-to-person contact with referral sources
- Give-away items

The identification of potential marketing tools concludes the preliminary phase of the marketing plan.

Phase 2: Market Position and Strategies

The second phase of the marketing plan consists of three steps. It is the most detailed phase and entails the most work.

Step 1: Determine Market Position

The first step involves determining your market position, or what you want your target audience to think, know, read, see, and hear about your practice and support programs (Smith, 1992). The three crucial goals in establishing a marketing position involve: (1) knowing where you are going, (2) knowing the business you are in, and (3) deciding on a position strategy (Hosford-Dunn et al., 1995; McKenna, 1986). A position strategy is the steps taken to identify a practice's product and image (Hosford-Dunn et al., 1995).

In accomplishing these three goals, audiologists will find establishing a marketing mission statement helpful (Educational Audiology Association, 1998). Figure 3–4 shows a marketing mission statement for support programs.

Establishing a market position allows audiologists to match consumer needs with product and service offerings. It involves a combination of strategic plans (Bodenhemier, 1994):

- Product strategy deals with specific products and services, package design, trademarks, service development, and so on.

Mission Statement

To increase people's understanding of the role of audiologists in managing support programs for patients with hearing impairment and the types of services provided to patients across service-delivery sites.

⬇

What do you want your target audience to know?

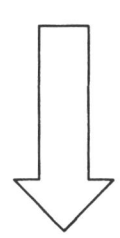

⬇

- My name, where I work, and how I can be reached.
- I did, in fact, go to college and then earned a graduate degree in order to learn my trade.
- My skills are numerous and specialized. My efforts in educating people about hearing impairment improves patients' ability to meet the communication needs of their immediate environments; empowers health-care professionals, educational personnel, and family members; and improves the overall quality of life.
- I chose to provide aural rehabilitation services through managing support programs for persons with hearing impairment across service-delivery sites, and those support programs offer quality services to those patients.
- Because of my efforts through these support programs, many patients are referred for further audiologic evaluation, aural rehabilitation, and possible medical intervention.
- I view the target audience as partners in helping patients with hearing impairment maximize their communication potential.
- I am an information resource.
- I am an advocate for patients with hearing impairment.

Figure 3–4. Mission statement for marketing support programs.

- Pricing strategy involves setting profitable, competitive, and justifiable prices.
- Distribution strategy is the actual delivery of goods and services to the consumer.
- Promotional strategy entails blending personal selling, advertising, and sales promotion for effective communication between the audiologic practice and the marketing audience.

Specifics in developing a marketing position vary with the particular service-delivery site and audiologists' relationship with the facility. Details are covered in the subsequent chapters in the textbook.

Step 2: Select Marketing Tools

The next step in the marketing plan involves selecting the marketing tools needed to implement the plan. Johnson et al. (1997) stated that internal and external marketing require different types of tools. Audiologists use *internal marketing techniques* when they already have an established relationship with a facility and wish to market additional services to include developing support programs. *External marketing* involves communication to target audiences with whom audiologists have no current relationship. Internal marketing often includes inservice presentations and handouts (e.g., brochures, newsletters, fact sheets, and so on). External marketing uses marketing tools such as paid advertising, direct mail, person-to-person phone contacts and so on to establish a preliminary relationship. When the facility shows interest in the goods and services offered by the audiologist, a preliminary relationship has been established. Audiologists can then request an opportunity to make a presentation to administrators and other employees. This presentation should be informative and showcase the benefits of establishing support programs for patients with hearing impairment. Appendix III-C lists some innovative ideas for marketing these support programs to schools, rehabilitation hospitals, and long-term residential care facilities for the elderly.

Marketing materials are a direct representation of audiologists' practices. Johnson et al. (1997) offered some excellent suggestions for written materials and professional presentations. They advised that written materials should:

- be brief and eye-catching, highlighting the primary information to be conveyed;
- contain no more than three bits of information;
- present the most important information in a bold, highlighted font that may be in a different style than less important information; and
- be shown to two or more professionals for evaluation before mass dissemination.

For presentation, they suggested that audiologists:

- determine the primary messages and a few bits of information that the audience should remember,
- gear the content to the interest level of the audience,
- involve the audience by personalizing the information provided,
- supplement oral presentations with visual materials,
- send notice of the presentation to the local news media with an invitation to attend,
- repeat the primary information at the end of the presentation, and
- provide written materials that summarize major points.

Step 3: Develop a Timeline

Once marketing tools have been selected, audiologists must develop a timeline to complete the marketing plan.

Phase 3: Assessment of Marketing Plan

The third phase involves assessment of the marketing plan, which includes three steps (Smith, 1992). First, audiologists must assess the financial impact of the plan. How much is the marketing plan going to cost? If the marketing plan is successful, will the cost of advertising be offset by projected revenue? Second, if the anticipated cost is reasonable, audiologists should then implement their strategies and see what happens. Audiologists must be patient and should allow ample time to receive returns on their investments. Third, audiologists must continually evaluate the effectiveness of their marketing plan. Appendix III-D contains a worksheet adapted from Johnson et al. (1997) that can be used to evaluate marketing strategies. Audiologists should expect to modify their plans as needed. Flexibility is an asset. A good marketing plan is always in response to new market conditions and new information (Hosford-Dunn et al., 1995; Smith, 1992).

Phase 4: Continuous Quality Improvement (CQI)

Initial successful marketing of support programs for persons with hearing impairment is not enough. For continued success, audiologists must focus on continuous quality improvement (CQI), which is the best marketing strategy of all (Hosford-Dunn et al., 1995). Continuous quality improvement requires that support program personnel know what to do and then do their best (Hosford-Dunn et al., 1995). Below are Deming's 14 Points, adapted to apply to sustaining stellar support programs for persons with hearing impairment (Hosford-Dunn et al., 1995; Reisberg & Frattali, 1990; Walton, 1986):

1. *Create a constancy of quality and improvement of product and services.* The marketing goal of providing support programs is not to make money, but to sustain program excellence and meet the needs of patients through innovation, research, constant improvement, and maintenance.
2. *Adopt the new philosophy.* Mistakes and negativism are unacceptable.
3. *Cease dependence on inspection to improve quality.* Quality comes from improving the support program process, not from inspection of what has already been done. Properly instructed support personnel can contribute to this improvement. Manage by good communication and planning, not by crisis.
4. *Think beyond profit.* Judging the success of a support program by the number of hearing aids dispensed to patients has no meaning without the consideration of the overall quality of diagnostic and aural rehabilitation services. Quality of the overall programming is assessed from the perceptions of the managing audiologist and the consumer.
5. *Improve constantly and forever the system of production and service.* Always strive to improve quality and productivity of support programs, thereby reducing costs.
6. *Institute on-the-job training.* Ongoing and effective inservice training is crucial for continuous quality improvement of support programs.
7. *Institute leadership.* Lead by example and instill this philosophy in departmental supervisors. Help support personnel do a better job and identify those who need help.
8. *Drive out fear.* All those involved in support programs need to feel secure in order to do their best and ask the necessary questions to know where they are going, what they are doing, and why they are doing it.
9. *Break down barriers between departments.* Make sure support-program participants from different areas work together as a team.
10. *Eliminate slogans, exhortations, and targets for the work force.* Don't use catchy, vague phrases like, "Be precise." They don't help.
11. *Eliminate quotas.* Do not tell support personnel that they should check all patients' hearing aids within a certain time period. This type of practice is antithetical to the marketing of quality.
12. *Instill pride of workmanship.* Make sure that the support program is well equipped and that all support personnel are encouraged to do their best.
13. *Institute a vigorous program of education and retraining.*
14. *Put everyone to work to accomplish these steps.*

SUMMARY

This chapter has defined and proposed guidelines to market support programs for persons with hearing impairment. With managed care and the streamlining of the U.S. health-care system, audiologists must respond to new demands for cost-efficient, high quality hearing health care. Audiologists must take a proactive approach toward defining and marketing aural rehabilitation according to the trends of the current health-care arena.

LEARNING ACTIVITIES

- Prepare a one-page handout for dissemination regarding the creation of a support program in a local nursing home.
- Write your own mission statement for marketing support programs for persons with hearing impairment for a service-delivery site of your choice.
- Critique local audiologists' marketing efforts using the criteria discussed in the chapter.
- Interview local audiologists concerning the effectiveness of their marketing strategies.
- Explore the Internet for managed-care Web sites and download useful information to create a reference notebook.

REFERENCES

Allen, L. (1998). Easy-to-do marketing ideas. *Educational Audiology Review, 15*(2), 6.

American Speech-Language-Hearing Association. (1991). Consideration for establishing a private practice in audiology and/or speech-language pathology. *Asha, 33*(Suppl. 3), 10–21.

American Speech-Language-Hearing Association. (1996). *Curriculum guide to managed care.* Rockville, MD: Author.

American Speech-Language-Hearing Association. (1997a, Spring). Guidelines for audiology service delivery in nursing homes. *Asha, 39*(Suppl. 17), 15–19.

American Speech-Language-Hearing Association. (1997b, November). *Preferred practice patterns for the profession of audiology.* Rockville, MD: Author.

Americans with Disabilities Act of 1990 (ADA), Public Law 101–336, 42, U.S.C. 12101 et seq.: *U.S. Statutes at Large, 104,* 327–378 (1991).

Bodenhemier, W. G. (1994). Managing a hearing conservation service. In D. M. Lipscomb (Ed.), *Hearing conservation* (pp. 273–286). San Diego, CA: Singular Publishing Group.

Danhauer, J. (1998). Who are those major multi-office audiology groups moving in on us, and—Is this town big enough for the both of us? *Audiology Today, 10*(2), 47–51.

Educational Audiology Association. (1998). Marketing mission statement. *Educational Audiology Review, 15*(2), 3.

Griffin, D. J., Clark-Lewis, S., & Johnson, C. (1997). Hearing can make the difference. *Outcomes: A Publication of HEALTHSOUTH Corporation, 2*(4), 20–21.

Hosford-Dunn, H., Dunn, D. R., & Harford, E. R. (1995). *Audiology business and practice management.* San Diego, CA: Singular Publishing Group.

Individuals with Disabilities Education Act of 1990 (IDEA), Public Law 101–476, 20, U.S.C. 1400 et seq.: *U.S. Statutes at Large, 104,* 1103–1151 (1990).

Johnson, C. D., Benson, P. V., & Seaton, J. B. (1997). *Educational audiology handbook.* San Diego, CA: Singular Publishing Group.

McKenna, R. (1986). *The Regis touch: New marketing strategies for uncertain times.* New York: Addison-Wesley.

Reisberg, M., & Frattali, C. (1990). Toward total quality management. *Quality Assurance Digest,* 1–5.

Smith, T. M. (1992). Marketing and the audiologist. *Asha Reports, 21,* 107–111.

Stach, B. A. (1998). *Clinical audiology: An introduction.* San Diego, CA: Singular Publishing Group.

Walton, M. (1986). *The Deming management method.* New York: Pedigree/Putnam.

APPENDIX III-A

Marketing Resources

Useful Web Sites on Marketing

- *http://www.asha.org/* American Speech-Language-Hearing Association Home Page: Use site "Search" and type in "Marketing" to view a list of current useful marketing links that are available for use.
- *http://www.audiology.org/* American Academy of Audiology Homepage: The Web site has useful information on marketing within the profession of audiology.

Useful Publications on Marketing

- Hiam, A. (1997). *Marketing for Dummies: A Reference for the Rest of Us.* IDG Books Worldwide, $19.99, 366 pages.
- McKeena, R. (1991). *Relationship Marketing: Successful Strategies for the Age of the Customer.* Addison-Wesley Publishing, $16.00, 230 pages.
- Ries, A., & Trout, J. (1993). *The 22 Immutable Laws of Marketing.* HarperCollins Publishers, $13.00, 132 pages.

Relevant Publications from the American Speech-Language-Hearing Association

- Marketing Manual: A Resource Guide
- Audiology Marketing Supplement, Person to Person: Making a Difference (kit)
- ASHA Audiology Campaign: The Marketing Kit: Marketing to Multicultural Audiences Kit (Audiology)

Call (888) 498-6699.

American Speech-Language-Hearing Association FAX on Demand is a member service that provides up-to-date information. Call (703) 531-0866 to order anything on the menu. Just follow the prompts, making sure to enter your FAX number correctly. You will receive the item by FAX within minutes.

APPENDIX III-B

Worksheet for Feasibility Study[1]

MARKET POTENTIAL

- Who will pay for these services?
- How many potential customers are there?
- Would this endeavor serve a currently unserved need?
- Does the need for such programs exceed the current supply in the market?
- What geographical area do you intend to serve?
- What are some potential payment/funding sources for your market?
- Are there competing services that already exist? If so, can your programs compete?
- BE SPECIFIC!

REFERRAL SOURCES

- What are all of the possible referral sources that apply to your potential market?
- Check the Yellow Pages, professional directories, hospital medical staff directories, and clinic directories.
- Determine whether you already have an established referral base for marketing support programs and are willing to make the necessary contacts.

FINANCING

- Prepare a list of ALL equipment and materials, including paper and pencil supplies, that you will need to develop and sustain a support program for each service-delivery site.
- Get actual prices of all equipment and materials. Secure written quotes, prioritize expensive items, and make proposal lists for presentation to potential clients, such as rehabilitation-hospital administration, and so on.
- List equipment you will dispense.
- Decide on merchandising methods.
- Conduct a systematic analysis of known service-delivery sites to determine personnel needs for support programs.
- Budget for advertising and public relations, including Yellow Pages, newspapers, local events, business cards, announcements, open houses, and so on.
- Prepare your business plan to include establishing and sustaining support programs across service-delivery sites.

SERVICES

- List ALL services and products you intend to offer through establishing support programs that fall within your professional expertise.
- Determine fee structure.
- Determine the availability of supplies for your program.
- List services that you could offer with additional training.
- List services that you could provide through the use of multiskilling and support personnel.
- From the above lists, cross out those that seem impractical.
- Go back to the section on market potential to determine if there is still a market for your services.

---

[1] Adapted from "Consideration for Establishing Private Practice in Audiology and/or Speech-Language Pathology," 1991. *Asha, 33*(Suppl. 3) and "Marketing and the Audiologist," by T. M. Smith, 1992. *Asha Reports, 21*, 107–111.

PERSONAL CHARACTERISTICS

- Do you have the necessary experience to develop, maintain, and sustain support programs across service delivery sites?
- Do you have an established reputation in your market community or communities?
- Are you a good clinician with appropriate personal qualities for providing services through a support program?
- Would you like offering support programs?
- Are you willing to work more hours to establish support programs with the possible increase in caseload?
- Are you up for a challenge?
- Are you willing to learn what you don't know?
- Why do you want to do this?
- Can you handle stress and frustration?
- Do you have a strong self-image?
- Are you self-sufficient?
- Are you a good decision-maker?
- Do you have the financial resources to make these programs happen?
- Do you have realistic expectations about the time, money, planning, energy, and so on that will be required to make these programs a success?
- Do you have the proper mind-set to deal with failure and frustration should these endeavors not succeed?
- Are you strong enough to "pull the plug" on these programs if they may jeopardize your primary practice and source of income?

APPENDIX III-C

Innovative, Easy-To-Do Marketing Ideas for Support Programs[1]

- Write up general information articles (i.e., What is hearing loss?) and offer them to schools, rehabilitation hospitals, nursing homes, retirement communities, and local newspapers. Local newspapers are always looking for articles to publish.
- Write letters telling people what you do. Examples include:
    ⇒ describing your services to the local superintendent of schools, administrators in rehabilitation facilities, and nursing homes, or
    ⇒ writing congratulatory letters to new school board members.
- Service-delivery sites are constantly changing. Teachers with whom you work with may become principals, RNs may become directors of nursing, assistant directors of rehabilitation facilities may become directors, and so on. Be sensitive and respectful to the needs of others, and try to work well with everyone.
- If school, rehabilitation-hospital, or nursing-home personnel make special arrangements to accommodate for the support program (e.g., providing a quiet rehabilitation room, optimal inservice environments, and so on), be sure to thank those individuals. They can become your best allies and often make or break a successful support program. You need their support.
- Quietly advertise your services. It may help to wear your audiology T-shirt or sweatshirt on "casual day," or use a tote bag advertising your practice.
- Have a little sign that is visible around your work area summarizing the services provided through the support program during the past year. Example: "During 1999, All-Pro Hearing services identified 20 patients with hearing loss; of those, 12 were fit with hearing aids and/or assistive listening devices."
- Provide fact sheets on the benefits of sound-field amplification and assistive listening devices to school principals, nursing-home directors, and administrators of rehabilitation hospitals to help substantiate the use and cost of these devices.
- Help generate a list of equipment and prices for service-delivery sites that need to make accommodations for patients with hearing loss.
- Generate publications to help schools, rehabilitation hospitals, and nursing homes, as well as the general public, understand more about what you do.
- Offer to teach inservice classes to service-delivery sites about the implications of hearing loss and needs for amplification to reinforce why support programs are important.
- Get involved in state and national organizations.
- Generate a marketing plan for yourself.
- After installing a sound-field FM classroom amplification system or establishing an assistive listening device center, send notes to patients' families and write a short "blurb" for a local newspaper or in-house newsletter.
- Contact local service organizations and offer to give a short presentation about hearing loss (usually 15 to 20 minutes). The Sertoma Club and other groups support persons with speech-language and hearing problems. Solicit their assistance for needy patients and publicize their help.
- Advocate for quieter schools, rehabilitation hospitals, and nursing homes. Provide information and talk with personnel about incorporating acoustical consultation in the design phase of rooms to be used by patients with hearing impairment.
- Make yourself known to the local physicians in the community. Physicians and audiologists can support each other.
- Learn more about giving presentations. Take classes to learn how to use software programs that will make your presentations, newsletters, and publications more attractive to the listener or the reader.
- Respond promptly to the requests of patients, their family members, and service-delivery site personnel.
- Wear a nametag that is easy to read and helps patients understand what you do. Individuals may not understand the word "Audiologist," but inclusion of a statement like, "Support Patients with Hearing Impairment" may help.

[1]Adapted from "Easy-to-Do Marketing Ideas," by L. Allen, 1998. *Educational Audiology Review, 15*(2), 6.

APPENDIX III-D

Marketing Effectiveness Log[1]

ALL-PRO HEARING SERVICES
"So all can hear..."
MARKETING EFFECTIVENESS LOG

Marketing Strategy	Date	Target Audience	Response	Date
XYZ Rehabilitation Hospital introductory letter	6/31/98	Administrators and Department Heads	Scheduled presentation 1	7/5/98

Key to responses: 1 = Referral or request for specific services 2 = Request for information 3 = Request for repeat presentation 4 = Financial or other program support 5 = Other (specify)

[1]Adapted from *Educational Audiology Handbook* by C. D. Johnson, P. V. Benson, and J. B. Seaton, 1997. San Diego: Singular Publishing Group.

CHAPTER 4

Funding Sources for Support Programs

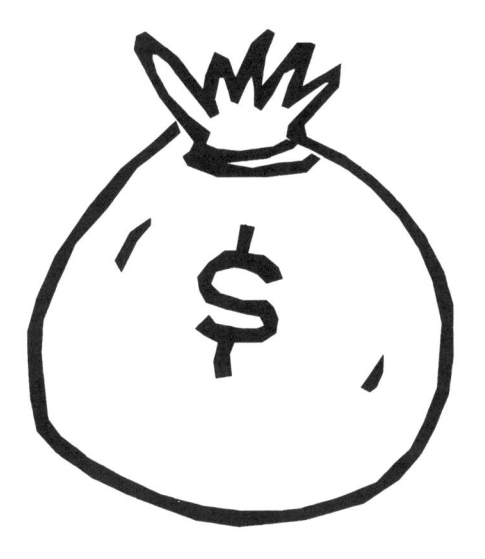

Figure 4-1. Securing funding is the first step in establishing support programs.

INTRODUCTION

"If you build it, they will come." This haunting line that consumed the main character from the movie *Field of Dreams* may be relevant when it comes to establishing support programs for patients with hearing impairment. By now, audiologists reading this textbook should be asking themselves how to fund support programs. With creativity and resourcefulness, audiologists can find funding. As discussed in the previous chapter, marketing plays a big role in acquiring the resources to initiate support programs across service-delivery sites.

Unfortunately, the hearing health-care industry has not maximized market penetration of its services to the segment of the estimated 28 million Americans with hearing loss. According to the National Center for Medical Rehabilitation, poor market penetration results in an estimated annual cost of $56 billion ($216 per capita) to the economy in lost productivity, special education, and medical costs (Chartrand, 1998). Some of the major reasons for poor market penetration include consumers' questioning the value of hearing instruments (Kochkin, 1996), as well as their inability to purchase these devices, aural rehabilitation services, or both (Chartrand, 1998). Thus, *audiologists frequently must play the role of fundraiser for individual patients and for aural rehabilitation programs.* At first glance, fundraising may seem like a drain on the audiologists' time and energy. Audiologists can implement "strategic philanthropy" (Chartrand, 1998) that can enhance their private practices, however.

Audiologists must often use "strategic philanthropy" to locate funding sources for the initiation of support programs for patients with hearing impairment. The support programs described in this text will receive little enthusiasm unless they are funded in their early stages. Audiologists must realize that funding for support programs depends on several factors: (1) status of the support program, (2) service-delivery site, (3) audiologists' relationship with the service-delivery site and its patients, and (4) resources needed. The purpose of this chapter is to discuss factors related to and suggest sources for the funding of support programs.

LEARNING OBJECTIVES

This chapter will enable the reader to:

- Understand the elements of "strategic philanthropy"
- Discuss the factors related to the funding of support programs
- Access possible sources of funding for support programs

STRATEGIC PHILANTHROPY

"Strategic philanthropy" is securing funding for such things as initiation of support programs or meeting the hearing health-care needs of indigent patients through community efforts and national philanthropic hearing health networks (e.g., HEAR NOW) (Chartrand, 1998). By obtaining funding for support programs or the specific needs of particular patients, audiologists can build a bridge of trust, recognition, and acceptance with the largely untapped and distrustful segment of the population with hearing impairment (Chartrand, 1998), as well as with other hearing health-care professionals. Several key elements are critical to the principle of strategic philanthropy (Chartrand, 1998). For example, audiologists must:

- *Lead the way by identifying individuals with hearing impairment who lack adequate resources to purchase the help they need* (e.g., hearing instruments, cochlear implants, assistive listening devices [ALDs], speech therapy, or rehabilitation training).
- *Actively initiate working alliances with local service organizations to help raise funds for support programs and special projects.* Service organizations exist in all communities. As discussed in the previous chapter, marketing plays a big role in acquiring funding to initiate support programs across service-delivery sites. By assisting the truly needy in their communities, audiologists can promote good will, expand their private practices, and reach many other individuals with communication disabilities who may have adequate financial resources to afford treatment.
- *Affiliate with recognized national philanthropic hearing health networks* that may be able to help handle the paperwork to qualify referred individuals. Upon qualification, these organizations can advise during the next steps of the process involving:
  ⇒ the local service organization,
  ⇒ contributing funds to acquire discounted or refurbished devices, and
  ⇒ establishing the audiologist as the liaison and coordinator (and/or provider).
- *Join with other hearing health-care professionals in the community to provide a team approach in meeting the needs of individuals with hearing impairment.* The team could consist of hearing instrument specialists, clinical and educational audiologists, otolaryngologists, cochlear implant teams, speech pathologists, deaf educators, vocational rehabilitation counselors, and other area professionals.

Implementing the principles of "strategic philanthropy" requires an understanding of the many variables affecting the funding of audiologic services. Thus, audiologists must understand these factors when attempting to establish support programs for patients with hearing impairment.

FACTORS RELATED TO FUNDING SUPPORT PROGRAMS

Status of Support Programs

Funding of support programs will likely depend on their status or stage of development. Support program status can be classified as: (1) new programs (process of initiation), (2) developing programs (years one through three), and (3) established programs (beyond three years). New programs may require "start-up funds" to get underway. In many cases, audiologists may only be able to "sell" support programs if funding for the first year has been obtained. First-year funding may be provided by a single sponsor or from multiple sources. For example, a service organization may choose to provide the start-up funds for the first year of a support program for patients with hearing impairment in a local nursing home. If that is not possible, audiologists must be more creative in securing multiple sources of start-up funds.

Securing start-up funds is only the first step in establishing effective support programs. Audiologists may have to convince administrators to provide release time for nursing-home personnel to attend inservices, for example. Most states require staff of long-term residential care facilities for the elderly to attend a minimum number of inservice or continuing-education sessions per year and audiologists should make sure that they are included as speakers in these seminars. In other cases, audiologists may need to convince hearing aid manufacturers to donate "dummy" hearing aid casings illustrating different styles of hearing aids for inservices.

Once start-up funds have been secured, audiologists must tenaciously market new support programs to hospital administrators in order to gain their confidence in and endorsement of the support programs. This can be accomplished by documenting efficacy of services delivered to patients through the collection of appropriate outcome measures. (Appropriate outcome measures are covered in Chapter 9, "Maintaining Stellar Support Programs: Outcome Measures.") Efficacy data demonstrating that support programs result in positive patient outcomes may convince administrators to provide funding for subsequent years of the program. Audiologists must be committed to Continuous Quality Improvement (CQI) (Hosford-Dunn, Dunn, & Harford, 1995; Reisberg & Fratalli, 1990; Walton, 1986) for program initiation, development, and sustenance.

Service-Delivery Site

Funding of support programs can also depend on the service-delivery site. This textbook covers the establishment of support programs for patients with hearing impairment in educational settings, rehabilitation hospitals, and long-term residential care facilities for the elderly. These different settings may have specific requirements for services provision to patients, as well as a variety of funding sources for initiating support programs. School systems, for example, may have funds that are "earmarked" for students with disabilities mandated by the Individuals with Disabilities Education Act (IDEA) (1990) that may be allocated to the development of support programs for children with hearing impairment. If program needs exceed available funding, other support may be obtained from parent-teacher association (PTA) fundraisers, as well as other sources mentioned later in this chapter. Similarly, rehabilitation hospitals and long-term residential care facilities for the elderly are required by the Americans with Disabilities Act (ADA) (1990) to make their facilities communicatively accessible to patients, their families, employees, and visitors with hearing impairment. Administrators should have funds set aside for such purposes that can also be used to initiate support programs. Audiologists' success in obtaining these funds may depend on their relationships with the particular service-delivery sites.

Audiologists' Relationship to Service-Delivery Sites and Patients

Generally, there are two types of relationships audiologists can have with a service-delivery site. Either they are employees of the facility, or they provide services on a contract or fee-for-service basis. Johnson, Benson, and Seaton (1997) described the difference between the two relationships in educational service-delivery sites.

Audiologists who are employees of the service-delivery site will usually have an easier time securing funding for support programs from administrators than will contract-for-service audiologists. Employees are considered permanent members of the staff. They can request materials for support programs in their annual departmental budget with proper justification. On the other hand, administrators and other staff often consider contract-for-service audiologists to be transitory coworkers whose support programs are not a priority given the on-site hierarchy and the limited resources available. Contract-for-service audiologists may have to cover the costs of materials for the program by increasing the budget of their next contract. Administrators may then choose to negotiate with another provider instead. Audiologists' best opportunity for funding is to secure the support of their immediate supervisors in the facility. For example, contract-for-service audiologists providing services to rehabilitation-hospital patients through the speech-language pathology department may be more successful securing funds if the department head is convinced of support program benefits.

In addition to material needs, successful support programs require human resources through the multiskilling or training of other professionals to serve as audiologic support personnel. Again, audiologists who are employees of the service-delivery site will have a much easier time securing the necessary human resources than will contract-for-service audiologists. As in the previous example, a contract-for-service audiologist at a rehabilitation hospital should have the director of the speech-pathology department act as "go-between," enlisting the support of other directors prior to requesting that their staff participate as audiologic support personnel.

Securing the necessary resources for support programs may be difficult, especially for the contract-for-service audiologist. Fee-for-service audiologists often bill Medicare or Medicaid for some of the services provided to patients. Because they obtain funding for these billable services, many audiologists may elect to cover the cost of certain aspects of support programs (e.g., inservices) as a price of doing business.

Funding can also depend on the type of relationship that audiologists have with patients. Obviously, audiologists can lobby for support services to benefit their own patients more easily than they can lobby for strangers. Audiologists who attend their young patients' Individualized Education Plan (IEP) meetings might advocate that someone at the school execute a daily visual and listening check on the children's hearing aids. One dedicated audiologist can make system-wide changes that begin on the behalf of a single child. Similarly, an audiologist can insist that a nursing home adhere to the ADA by providing communication accessibility to all patients, not just their own. In both examples, school systems and long-term residential care facilities for the elderly may seek the professional expertise of audiologists to provide services and establish support programs within those service-delivery sites. In addition, audiologists may be more willing to loan hearing aids to nursing-home residents who are their private patients than to strangers.

Resources Needed

Audiologists cannot secure necessary funding for support programs unless they have determined all of the resources needed to succeed. Expenses are of three types: (1) patient related, (2) human resource, and (3) material.

Patient-related costs include: (1) hearing evaluations, (2) hearing aid evaluations, (3) hearing aids, (4) hearing aid accessories, (5) hearing aid repairs, and (6) aural (re)habilitation. Patient-related costs are highly individualistic depending on the individual health plans and financial status of those involved. In some situations, the particular service-delivery site is required to provide these items free of charge. Audiologists must often play the role of advocate to find alternative sources of funding for patients.

The *human resources* needed for support programs include both the audiologists' time investment and the participation of audiologic support personnel. In most situations collateral or collateral-subordinate multiskilling models are used in support programs for patients with hearing impairment. Recall that with collateral multiskilling, other professionals (e.g., nurses, occupational therapists, physical therapists, and so on) serve as audiologic support personnel. In collateral-subordinate multiskilling, however, assistants from other professional disciplines (e.g., nurse's assistants, occupational-therapy assistants, and physical-therapy assistants) serve in the same capacity. Obtaining funding for the necessary human resources for support programs involves convincing administrators and departmental supervisors to commit the necessary time for staff training and participation. Particular strategies are discussed later in this chapter.

The *material resources* needed for support programs for patients with hearing impairment depend on the service-delivery site. The materials needed in educational settings are different than those needed for rehabilitation hospitals or long-term residential care facilities for the elderly. Examples of materials needed for particular inservices are provided for each topic in Chapter 5. Most of these materials do not need to be purchased by the particular service-delivery site but are owned by the managing audiologist who uses them for presentations in numerous contexts. Although the materials used to maintain a support program are the responsibility of the service-delivery site, they are relatively inexpensive. Hearing aid check kits, for example, can be assembled for less than $50. Most facilities need only one kit per floor, department, or station. Expenses can be higher for school systems that may need to purchase a kit for each public-school nurse, but their budgets may more easily absorb such costs. The most expensive material costs of support programs are assistive listening devices. Audiologists can fund support programs if they are resourceful and consider the suggestions provided below.

FUNDING SOURCES FOR SUPPORT PROGRAMS

Funding sources for support programs differ depending on whether they are for: (1) patient-related costs, (2) human resources, or (3) materials.

Patient-Related Costs

Funding sources for patient-related costs vary according to service-delivery site. In the public schools, hearing evaluations, hearing aid accessories, and aural rehabilitation services are provided by the public agency as mandated by the IDEA. The purchase of children's personal hearing aids by the public agency technically is not required, but this has been challenged by parents in some states who maintain that personal hearing aids are necessary for a free and appropriate education (FAPE) in the least restrictive environment (LRE). Thus, the major part of the budget for audiology services (i.e., medical equipment) should already be covered in the schools.

The type of service-delivery model under which services are provided can severely restrict audiologists' ability to secure funding for a child's hearing aids. An example is contract-for-service audiologists who frequently are hired to perform very specific services (e.g., hearing screenings, hearing evaluations, and hearing aid monitoring). This leaves little time to serve as an advocate for children with hearing impairment. By contrast, it is the school-based audiologists' responsibility to serve as advocates for these children, and thus, these audiologists must find the time to investigate different funding sources for hearing aids.

Generally, audiologists should investigate the policies of the individual school district toward the purchasing of hearing aids for children. Most school systems do not provide this funding. If a child's family cannot afford hearing aids, they may qualify for Medicaid. The purpose of Medicaid, a combined state and federal program, is to assist states in furnishing healthcare services to families who are on welfare programs or categorically eligible (Mueller & Hall, 1998). In addition, the federal government allows state Medicaid agencies to contract with various entities, such as health maintenance organizations (HMOs) and other prepaid health plans (Mueller & Hall, 1998). Most state Medicaid programs cover the cost of hearing aids and their repair for children. Audiologists should consult state and local rules and regulations regarding all potential sources of funding. Collaboration with the school system's social worker can assist with a family's determination of eligibility. Many families who have qualified for Medicaid in the past may become ineligible if there is a lapse in enrollment or change in family income. The social worker can assist otherwise needy families in filing the necessary paperwork to re-establish eligibility. Ineligible families must purchase their children's hearing aids with their personal funds, or request assistance from charitable groups.

Obtaining funds for the repair of children's hearing aids and securing loaners while the devices are being repaired can also be problematic for both the school-based and the contract-for-service audiologist. Obtaining the necessary funding requires the consideration of three factors: (1) Does the child already have a personal audiologist? (2) Is the hearing aid currently under warranty? and (3) Does the family currently qualify for Medicaid or state child-rehabilitation-services (CRS) funding? At the beginning of each school year, audiologists should take inventory of which children have hearing aids, which hearing aids are currently under warranty, and which children qualify for Medicaid services. As a matter of professional courtesy, the child's personal audiologist should be notified and asked to handle hearing aid repairs when needed, including completing all paperwork, and providing the child with a loaner hearing aid. These procedures are covered in detail in Chapter 6, "Establishing Support Programs in Educational Settings."

For rehabilitation-hospital patients and elderly residents of long-term residential care facilities, securing funds for hearing evaluations, hearing aid evaluations, hearing aids, and aural rehabilitation can be challenging. Prior to the delivery of other services, each service-delivery site should have a hearing screening program in place to identify individuals who need further testing. Details of these programs are provided in Chapters 7 and 8. Shultz and Mowry (1995) stated that the elderly in long-term residential care facilities can be subdivided into two groups, private-pay patients and Medicaid or Medicare patients. Private-pay patients are those residents who have their own resources to pay "out-of-pocket" for audiologic services and hearing aids. The problem may be to convince them, their families, or their conservators that audiologic services warrant the use of precious limited funds. Anyone familiar with patients in long-term residential care facilities for the elderly knows how quickly funds can be used up by the needs of daily care. Even a healthy "nest egg" can be depleted in very little time. Once all private funds are gone, most patients must turn to Medicaid or Medicare for assistance.

Medicare patients may have extremely limited private funds for audiologic services. Because individual state laws differ, audiologists should investigate local rules and regulations (Shultz & Mowry, 1995). Medicare was established in 1965 to provide certain health-care services for all individuals over the age of 65 years (Mueller & Hall, 1998). In addition, federally qualified HMOs or other prepaid health plans that obtain competitive medical plan status (CMP) according to the guidelines from the Department of Health and Human Services can be approved to enroll Medicare beneficiaries (Mueller & Hall, 1998). Many of those prepaid health plans and HMOs offer hearing plans by contracting with corporate audiology provider networks (e.g., National Ear Care Plan, HeaRx, Newport Audiology Centers, and Sonus) to provide audiologic services, including hearing aids and costs of repair, to their enrollees (Danhauer, 1998). Thus, audiologists can determine if their patients' HMOs provide hearing plans to their enrollees. If so, audiologists can arrange for these patients to have an appointment with the nearest audiologist affiliated with the provider network, if they are not affiliated themselves. Other plans permit enrollees to acquire services from private-practice audiologists. One should be clear about what benefits each patient's plan covers before initiating provision of services to avoid potential conflicts and billing problems. In addition, audiologists should check to see if any of their patients are veterans who can qualify to receive audiologic services and hearing aids through the nearest Veterans Administration Hospital. These and other sources of funding should be investigated.

As stated earlier, patients who are not covered for audiologic services and hearing aids through their health-care plans must either pay "out-of-pocket" or find some charitable organization to cover the cost of hearing aids. Appendix IV-A lists some service clubs that support programs for persons with disabilities (e.g., Business and Professional Women's Clubs National Federation, Civitan International, Lions Clubs International, Quota International, Sertoma International, Kiwanis International, Pilot International, and Rotary International) (Johnson et al., 1997). Such groups should be contacted as sources for potential hearing aid funding. Lions Club, Quota, Sertoma, and Kiwanis are organizations in which the primary focus is speech and hearing. In addition, the main focus for Pilot Club is neurological disorders, and they may elect to purchase hearing aids for a rehabilitation-hospital patient who has had a cerebral vascular accident. These organizations are listed in the telephone book or they can be reached through the Chamber of Commerce, which will provide the phone numbers of local chapters (Johnson et al., 1997). Service organizations often seek speakers for their meetings that can open the door for audiologists who wish to expand their practices. A sample letter of introduction volunteering to serve as a speaker is provided in Appendix IV-B. These organizations are often willing to fund the charitable causes of professionals who have spoken at their meetings.

Some areas have organizations that provide hearing aids for adults who cannot afford to purchase the devices for themselves. These organizations can have a local, state, or national focus. HEAR NOW, a Denver-based national organization, has a network of almost 2,400 audiologists, hearing instrument specialists, and medical clinics all over the country who have helped more than 7,000 patients with hearing impairment obtain donated hearing instruments, assistive devices, and rehabilitation services (Chartrand, 1998). In addition, more than 100 children and adults have received multichannel cochlear implants with assistance from HEAR NOW, whose address is listed in Appendix IV-A. An example of a statewide organization is the Central Oklahoma Association for the Deaf and Hearing-Impaired (COAD-HI) that provides hearing aids for adults below a certain income level. Hearing aids belonging to individuals who no longer need them are donated to the organization. They are then sent to the John W. Keys Speech and Hearing Center at the University of Oklahoma Health Sciences Center for electroacoustic analysis and classification for appropriateness according to degree of hearing loss. The board of directors reviews potential participants' applications that include proof of income. The organization funds the hearing evaluation as well as the hearing aid evaluation, delivery, and orientation. The staff matches patients to hearing aids; in-the-ear and in-the-canal hearing aids are sent for recasing and reconditioning with a one-year warranty.

Chapter 1 discussed the effects of managed care on aural rehabilitation. Other than the purchase and fitting of hearing aids, aural rehabilitation is generally not reimbursable through hearing plans currently offered through employers and HMOs. Audiologists affiliated with hearing networks must take a proactive approach to managed care by making changes from within the system to expand the scope of services provided to include aural rehabilitation. Unfortunately, those services are considered capitated by most hearing plans. Casey (1997) suggested that in the future, affiliated audiologists may be able to work with their hearing networks to convince rehabilitation hospitals and long-term residential care facilities for the elderly to provide the cost of the hearing plan as part of their patients' fees for individuals who need hearing aids. Clearly, our profession has a long way to go in convincing third-party payers to reimburse for aural rehabilitation services. Audiologists, patients, and their families must begin lobbying insurance companies to provide audiology benefits to their members.

Human Resources

As stated earlier, *the cost of human resources for support programs for patients with hearing impairment lie in the audiologists' time, involvement of support personnel, and the completion of necessary paperwork*. Fortunately, regardless of service-delivery site, efficient support programs should not require a great deal of the audiologists' time because their aural rehabilitation role is mostly one of trainer and manager, rather than direct service-delivery provider. Audiologists providing services to a rehabilitation hospital should spend the majority of their time conducting hearing evaluations, hearing aid evaluations, and hearing aid fittings for patients while relying on audiologic support personnel to keep up with such tasks as hearing aid monitoring, troubleshooting, and documentation. Audiologists may need assistance in providing inservices, visiting patients with malfunctioning hearing aids, and so on. In such cases, they may seek help from local colleges and universities that have graduate-training programs. Most programs would be delighted to have an off-campus practicum site for their students, especially those providing hours in adult aural rehabilitation. Audiologists can make such arrangements with rehabilitation hospitals and long-term residential care facilities for the elderly profitable, provided they are paid for their services, have at least some patients who can afford to pay for hearing aids, and are given latitude in program development by the administration.

Costs for audiologic support personnel are, in most cases, absorbed by the facility. Recall that the selection of a multiskilling model (i.e., who will serve) depends on the unique characteristics of the service-delivery site; this will be covered more in the subsequent chapters. Although dollar amounts may be difficult to estimate on the cost of staff serving as audiologic support personnel because they are usually already employed by the facility, administrators will still want to know how much time will be required for training and subsequent support-program participation.

Audiologists should take confidence in the fact that multiskilling is part of managed care and is well understood by most cost-conscious health administrators. Nevertheless, efficiency is the key! Audiologists must quickly, clearly, and effectively train support personnel to perform assigned tasks competently. Audiologists must design program logistics to minimize the allocation of human resources without sacrificing patient care. The completion of paperwork can drain staff time. Using clear, simple-to-use forms to document visual and listening checks of rehabilitation-hospital patients' hearing aids decreases the hassle of nurses who are frequently expected to "double up" on duties that occur with staff downsizing. Administrators, departmental supervisors, and audiologic support personnel will appreciate anything the audiologist can do to simplify program participation.

Materials

Costs for materials needed to establish, develop, and sustain support programs are less than patient-related and human-resource costs. Chapters 6, 7, and 8 discuss the establishment of support programs in educational settings, rehabilitation hospitals, and long-term residential care facilities for the elderly and the required materials for each service-delivery site. As mentioned earlier, audiologists who are employees of the service-delivery site can have a more direct impact on the annual budget than contract-for-service audiologists. The latter may have to find first-year supplies for support programs from other sources on a probationary status. The service clubs and organizations listed in Appendix IV-A may be willing to provide the required supplies for the first year of a support program in a local nursing home, especially if they are given due recognition for their participation. Appendix IV-C contains a sample letter of request for funding. Again, service clubs and other organizations will be more likely to fund the efforts of audiologists who they know or who have taken the time to speak to their groups. Thus, it pays to establish these relationships ahead of time. Other funding sources include fraternities and sororities at local colleges and universities. After all, if these organizations are willing to adopt stretches of highway to maintain, why not adopt a school, rehabilitation hospital, or nursing home for a year? Audiologists should appeal to the community service portions of such groups.

The most expensive material cost of support programs in rehabilitation hospitals and nursing homes is in supplying the necessary assistive listening devices (ALDs) to these facilities. In reality, the facilities should supply this technology to patients with hearing impairment in order to provide communication accessibility as mandated by the ADA. Because facilities may lean toward purchasing cheap and ineffective ALDs for this purpose, it is important for audiologists to guide them in this area. As part of a viable support program, audiologists should try to establish an ALD center that has quality devices for checkout by patients for their use.

Funding the establishment of ALD centers can be accomplished using several methods. First, audiologists should see if their state has a legislative coalition that can act as a special-interest group to obtain funding for assistive technology (Scott, 1998). For example, the Utah Assistive Technology (AT) Project in Logan, Utah, serves as part of a legislative coalition of AT users, their families, and interested allied-health professionals. The AT Project works with state departments of health and education in lobbying for funding in schools, rehabilitation facilities, and Independent Living Centers (e.g., group homes and nursing homes), and so on (Scott, 1998). Unfortunately, some states may have restrictions in the use of AT under these types of programs. In Utah, AT for rehabilitation must only be used for employment or training purposes. Assistive technology for Independent Living Centers carries no such restrictions. Second, the service organizations listed in Appendix IV-A may be more than willing to purchase one or more ALDs. Third, families of loved ones who were patients at the facility may choose to purchase one or more ALDs in their memory. Charitable donations can be acknowledged with an inscription on a plaque displayed for all to see. Fourth, audiologists can request consignment instruments from ALD manufacturers. Appendix IV-D contains a list of ALD manufacturers' addresses and phone numbers. Appendix IV-E contains a sample letter stating that a nursing home is establishing an ALD center and seeks consignment instruments for patient use. Some manufacturers may comply with such requests. We have successfully used this method in obtaining several devices for our ALD center at the Auburn University Speech and Hearing Clinic. In addition to ALDs, these centers need some space of their own. An ALD center may occupy an entire room or just a simple cart that can be moved from room to room.

Remember that telephone use by individuals with hearing impairment in these service-delivery sites can be quite restrictive. It may be helpful to request assistance from local telephone companies. They may be able to donate telephone amplifiers or telecommunication devices for these facilities, especially if given due recognition for their assistance. Recall that a portion of every telephone bill goes toward telecommunication services and devices for individuals with hearing impairment, so why not solicit their help? The public-relations promotion can be quite attractive to telephone companies. After all, communication is their business.

SUMMARY

This chapter has discussed the funding of support programs for patients with hearing impairment. The practice of "strategic philanthropy" can be used to fund these programs while enhancing audiologists' private practices. Audiologists must know the variables affecting the funding of support programs prior to developing a "game plan." Every support program is unique with regard to funding needs and solutions. Several ideas have been provided for audiologists in establishing, developing, and maintaining support programs. The suggestions for funding sources presented here are not intended to be exhaustive or complete; they are provided as examples that have worked in the past. Audiologists beginning such a program will have to be creative in determining what funding sources may be available in their community, their state, or at the national level.

LEARNING ACTIVITIES

- Interview local audiologists and find as many examples of "strategic philanthropy" in your community as possible.
- Make a resource list of possible support-program sponsors in your community and state.
- Establish an assistive listening device center in your university speech and hearing clinic, hospital, or private practice.
- Volunteer to make a presentation at a local philanthropy group.

REFERENCES

Americans with Disabilities Act of 1990, Public Law 101-336, 42, U.S.C. 12101 *et seq.*: *U.S. Statutes at Large, 104,* 327–378 (1991).

Casey, P. (1997). Personal communication. *National Ear Care Plan.*

Chartrand, M. S. (1998). Growing your practice/business with strategic philanthropy. *The Hearing Review, 5*(7), 35–36.

Danhauer, J. L. (1998). Who are those major multi-office groups moving in on us, and—Is this town big enough for both of us? *Audiology Today, 10*(2), 47–51.

Hosford-Dunn, H., Dunn, D. R., & Harford, E. R. (1995). *Audiology business and practice management.* San Diego, CA: Singular Publishing Group.

Individuals with Disabilities Education Act of 1990 (IDEA), Public Law 101-476, 20, U.S.C. 1400 *et seq.*: *U.S. Statutes at Large, 104,* 1103–1151 (1990).

Johnson, C. D., Benson, P. V., & Seaton, J. B. (1997). *Educational audiology handbook.* San Diego, CA: Singular Publishing Group.

Kochkin, S. (1996). Customer satisfaction and subjective benefit with high performance hearing aids. *The Hearing Review, 31*(2), 16–26.

Mueller, H. G., & Hall, J. W. (1998). *Audiologists' desk reference: Volume II: Audiologic management, rehabilitation, and terminology.* San Diego, CA: Singular Publishing Group.

Reisberg, M., & Frattali, C. (1990). Toward total quality management. *Quality Assurance Digest,* 1–5.

Scott, A. (1998). State legislative coalitions can act as special interest groups to obtain funding for AT. *Advance for Speech-Language Pathologists and Audiologists, 8*(23), 7–8.

Shultz, D., & Mowry, R. B. (1995). Older adults in long-term care facilities. In P. B. Kricos & S. A. Lesner (Eds.), *Hearing care for the older adult: Audiologic rehabilitation* (pp. 167–184). Boston: Butterworth-Heinemann.

Walton, M. (1986). *The Deming management method.* New York: Pedigree/Putnam.

APPENDIX IV-A

Service Clubs and Organizations[1]

(*Organizations that focus philanthropic activities on speech and hearing)

Business and Professional Women's Clubs, National Federation
2012 Massachusetts Avenue NW
Washington, DC 20036
(202) 293-1100

Civitan International
1 Civitan Place
Birmingham, AL 35213-1983
(205) 591-8910
(800) CIVITAN

HEAR NOW*
9745 E. Hampden Avenue, Suite 300
Denver, CO 80231
(303) 695-7797(V/TDD)

Lions Clubs International*
300 22nd Street
Oak Brook, IL 60523-8842
(630) 571-5466

Quota International*
1420 21st Street NW
Washington DC, 20036
(202) 331-9694

Sertoma International*
1912 East Myer Boulevard
Kansas City, MO 64132
(816) 333-8300

Kiwanis International*
3636 Woodview Trace
Indianapolis, IN 46268-3196
(317) 875-8755 Fax
(800) 549-2647

Pilot International
244 College Street
P.O. Box 4844
Macon, GA 31213-0599
(912) 743-7403

Rotary International
1600 Ridge Avenue
Evanston, IL 60201

---

[1]Adapted from "Growing Your Practice/Business With Strategic Philanthropy," by H. S. Chartrand, 1998. *The Hearing Review, 5,* 35–37 and *Educational Audiology Handbook,* by C. D. Johnson, P. V. Benson, & J. B. Seaton, 1997. San Diego, CA: Singular Publishing Group.

APPENDIX IV-B

Letter of Introduction to Local Service Clubs and Organizations

ALL-PRO HEARING SERVICES
"So all can hear…"

June 31, 1999

Pilot International
1100 Deep Pockets Way
Quality of Life City, CA 94545

Dear Pilot Club,

I would like to introduce myself. My name is Starr Audiologist. I am a certified audiologist and the CEO of All-Pro Hearing Services, a member of the Quality of Life City Chamber of Commerce since 1980. All-Pro Hearing Services responds to the hearing-health care needs of the metropolitan area.

Hearing loss is one of our nation's major health problems. Approximately 10% of the American population has some form of hearing loss. I would like to volunteer as a potential speaker for the local chapter of the Pilot Club. I can speak on your choice of several topics, such as hearing, hearing loss, hearing disorders, hearing-loss prevention, effects of hearing loss on communication, hearing aids, and so on. I also could advise your club of current hearing health-care needs in the community that might provide potential philanthropic projects for your members.

I am impressed with the dedication of the Pilot Club in supporting the needs of our community. Please feel free to call me at 555-1122 about the possibility of a future speaking engagement or for information about possible philanthropic projects.

Sincerely,

Starr Audiologist, Ph.D.
Certificate of Clinical Competence in Audiology (CCC-A)
Fellow of the American Academy of Audiology (FAAA)

APPENDIX IV-C

Letter to Request Funding from Local Service Clubs and Organizations

ALL-PRO HEARING SERVICES
"So all can hear..."

June 31, 1999

Pilot International
1100 Deep Pockets Way
Quality of Life City, CA 94545

Dear Pilot Club,

My name is Starr Audiologist, CEO of All-Pro Hearing Services. I spoke to your organization about hearing loss last year. I am writing now to request that your fine service organization consider funding the first year of a support program for the patients at Shady Pines Nursing Home. Shady Pines is a facility in which the residents are primarily low income. Approximately 75% of nursing-home residents have some hearing loss. A hearing support program for individuals at Shady Pines would assist in meeting their hearing health-care needs. It would also improve their quality of life by allowing them to hear and communicate with their doctors and families more effectively.

My practice currently is under contract with Shady Pines to provide audiologic evaluations and fit patients with hearing aids. Most of the residents are transported to my practice for these services. I visit Shady Pines twice a month to assist patients in managing their hearing aids. Unfortunately, sometimes residents must wait for two weeks before I can troubleshoot simple problems.

Support programs involve training nursing-home personnel to communicate with residents with hearing loss and to check and troubleshoot hearing aids. In addition, support programs involve equipping residents' rooms and communal living areas with assistive listening devices. Aural rehabilitation group meetings are also offered for residents and their families.

Shady Pines does not have the funds to establish a support program. However, management has said that if funding for the first year of the program can be found, and if the program is successful, they may consent to funding subsequent years of the program. Costs include staff training, hearing aid check kits, assistive listening devices, and so on. Costs for individual items range from $50 per hearing aid check kit up to $300 for assistive listening devices. The total start-up cost of the support program would be $3000. We are requesting your help in funding the entire amount or any portion of it to establish this much-needed program. Shady Pines would greatly appreciate any help that your organization could provide. If you are interested in this project, please feel free to call me at 555-1122 to schedule a time when we may discuss this joint venture.

Sincerely,

Starr Audiologist, Ph.D.
Certificate of Clinical Competence in Audiology (CCC-A)
Fellow of the American Academy of Audiology (FAAA)

APPENDIX IV-D

Assistive Listening Device Manufacturers

Audex
710 Standard Street
Longview, TX 75604
(800) 237-0716
IR, hardwired devices

Comtek
3572 700 South
Salt Lake City, UT 84115
(801) 466-3463
FM

Oval Window Audio
33 Wild Flower Court
Nederland, CO 80466
(303) 447-3607
Audioloops

Phonic Ear, Inc.
3880 Cypress Drive
Petaluma, CA 94954
(800) 227-0735
FM

Plantronics/Walker Equipment
345 Encinal Street
Santa Cruz, CA 95060
(831) 426-5858
Telephone amplifiers, headsets, etc.

Radio Shack
300 One Tandy Center
Fort Worth, TX 76102
Do-it-yourself ALDs, alerting devices, phone amps; call your local store

Silent Call Corporation
2220 Scott Lake Road
Waterford, MI 48329
Phone: (800) 572-5227 (V/TTY)
FAX: (248) 673-5442
Alerting devices, custom work

Telex Communications, Inc.
9600 Aldrich Ave, South
Minneapolis, MN 55420
(800) 328-8212
FM

Ultratec, Inc.
450 Science Drive
Madison, WI 53711
(800) 482-2424
TTYs, alerting devices

Wheelock, Inc.
273 Branchport Avenue
Long Branch, NJ 07740
auditory and visual fire alarms

Williams Sound Corporation
10399 W. 70th Street
Eden Prairie, MN 55344
(800) 328-6190
FM, hardwired

APPENDIX IV-E

Letter of Request for Consignment Assistive Listening Devices

ALL-PRO HEARING SERVICES
"So all can hear..."

June 31, 1999

HITEC Group International, Inc.
8160 Madison Ave.
Burr Ridge, IL 60521

Dear Hitec Group International,

My name is Starr Audiologist, Ph.D., CCC-A, FAAA, managing audiologist for the Shady Pines Nursing Home in Quality of Life City, CA. Shady Pines has approximately 150 residents. Of those 150 residents, approximately 120 have hearing loss. Shady Pines is currently establishing an Assistive Listening Device Center for residents. We have heard great things about your Sound Wizard Universal Listening System and would like to request two units for consignment so we can make these units available for residents' purchase. We would appreciate any consideration you could provide. Please feel free to call me at 555-1122 if you have any questions.

Sincerely,

Starr Audiologist, Ph.D.
Certificate of Clinical Competence of Audiology (CCC-A)
Fellow of the American Academy of Audiology (FAAA)

Penny Pincher, MHA
Director, Shady Pines Nursing Home

CHAPTER 5

Creating Effective Inservice Programs

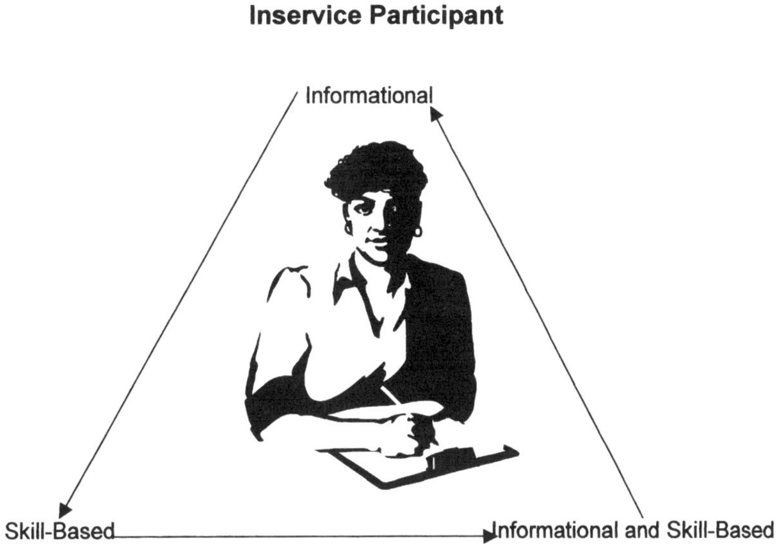

Figure 5-1. Support personnel training includes informational, skill-based, and combination informational and skill-based formats.

INTRODUCTION

Successful support programs require employees in various service-delivery sites to be prepared to facilitate the communication needs of patients with hearing impairment. Recall that *multiskilling* is the training of professionals to perform tasks that typically are carried out by those in other disciplines (Foto, 1996). Multiskilling requires development of inservice programming. Three types of inservice training formats are: (1) informational, (2) skill-based, and (3) a combination of informational and skill-based. Informational inservices are for all individuals who come into contact with patients with hearing impairment and include general information on hearing loss, how to communicate with persons who have a hearing impairment, the Americans with Disabilities Act (1990), and so on. Skill-based and a combination of informational and skill-based inservices teach audiologic support personnel how to perform assigned tasks (e.g., how to perform a visual and listening check on patients' hearing aids, assistive listening devices, and so on). The type and content of the inservice programs will depend on the service-delivery site.

Regardless of service-delivery site, appropriately trained audiologic support personnel are critical to the success of support programs for patients with hearing impairment. Allied-health professionals typically do not have the experience, knowledge, or skills to participate as audiologic support personnel without some amount of inservice training (Johnson, Clark-Lewis, & Griffin, 1998; Johnson, Stein, & Lass, 1992; Johnson, Stein, Lyons, & Lass, 1995).

The "Position Statement and Guidelines of the Consensus Panel on Support Personnel in Audiology" (American Academy of Audiology, 1997) has specific guidelines regarding the criteria for the training and supervision of support personnel. As part of the development of an inservice program, audiologists must decide who will participate as audiologic support personnel, what tasks will be delegated, and the knowledge and skills required to participate competently in the program. Audiologists must be able to create meaningful adult learning experiences that will motivate audiologic support personnel to execute assigned tasks enthusiastically. The purpose of this chapter is to provide the necessary background information, suggestions, and materials for audiologists to create effective inservices for audiologic support personnel.

LEARNING OBJECTIVES

This chapter will enable readers to:

- Familiarize themselves with research findings regarding preparedness of various allied-health professionals to serve as audiologic support personnel
- Select the appropriate models of multiskilling
- Apply the "Position Statement and Guidelines of the Consensus Panel on Support Personnel in Audiology" (AAA, 1997)
- Describe the components of a complete inservice program
- Understand the three different types of inservices
- Create meaningful adult learning experiences
- Use inservice materials provided in the appendices

PREPAREDNESS OF RELATED PROFESSIONALS TO SERVE AS AUDIOLOGIC SUPPORT PERSONNEL

Audiologic support personnel have been used across several service-delivery sites including public schools, hospitals, and hearing-conservation programs to perform tasks such as hearing screenings and hearing aid monitoring. Although individuals both with and without medical training have served as audiologic support personnel in a variety of settings, it is reasonable to expect that nonmedical professionals are not prepared to serve in this capacity without some training. Most regular classroom teachers, for example, have had little or no experience with students who have hearing impairment (Hull & Dilka, 1984). Similarly, Lass, Carlin, Woodford, Campanelli-Humphreys, Joanna, Hushion-Stemple, and Boggs (1986) found that the majority of teachers has never had an academic course that included the topic of hearing or hearing disorders. Unfortunately, research has also shown that potential audiologic support personnel with medical training do not have the necessary skills to participate in a hearing aid monitoring program.

Johnson et al. (1992) surveyed public-school nurses' preparedness to serve as audiologic support personnel in a hearing aid monitoring program. Thirty nurses completed a 19-item questionnaire surveying their prior experience with, attitudes toward, and knowledge of hearing aids, as well as their basic skill level with these devices, hearing aid batteries, and earmolds. The large majority of the nurses (76.7%) had no prior experience with hearing aids, and more than half of these respondents (56.7%) felt uncomfortable handling the devices. In addition, the large majority of the respondents (73.4%) agreed with the statement that, "Children with hearing impairment may not like to wear hearing aids at school because the other children may tease them."

Almost all of the respondents (90.0%) could not identify the parts of a hearing aid. Slightly more than half of the respondents (53.3%) had an understanding of how a hearing aid worked, yet less than half of them (46.7%) felt they could insert or remove a hearing aid from a child's ear. The large majority of the respondents (73.3%) knew that hearing aids could not be washed. Furthermore, although more than half of the respondents (60%) knew what feedback was, only about one-third (33.3%) knew its cause. Finally, most of the respondents (80%) did not know where to send a parent to get a hearing aid repaired.

With regard to batteries, the large majority of respondents (80%) knew that hearing aid batteries came in different sizes, but more than half of the respondents (53.3%) did not know where to purchase them. Furthermore, the large majority of respondents (83.3%) did not know how long hearing aid batteries last, and less than half (46.7%) knew that they were potentially poisonous if swallowed. Similarly, more than one-third of the respondents (36.7%) did not know what an earmold was and more than half (56.6%) felt that they could not attach one to a hearing aid. In conclusion, the results of this survey indicate that nurses employed in public schools may not be prepared to participate as audiologic support personnel in a hearing aid monitoring program. It was not known if similar results would be found for nurses employed in a variety of other work settings.

Johnson et al. (1995) surveyed 100 nurses from a variety of work settings on various aspects of hearing aids including their attitudes toward and academic experience with hearing aids and hearing aid wearers. Of the 91 respondents, 12 worked in the public schools, 61 were employed in hospitals, and 18 worked in telephone-informational settings. The large majority of the nurses (72.5%) had never taken a course that included the topic of hearing aids, and nearly one-third (30.8%) did not know any hearing aid wearers. The large majority of respondents knew some basic information about hearing aids, however. Most respondents agreed that not all persons with a hearing loss can benefit from hearing aids (97.8%), that hearing aids are powered by batteries (90.1%), and that hearing aids can be used by children under five years of age (89.0%). Nonetheless, more than half of the respondents (60.4%) could not identify an audiologist as the nonmedical professional who tests people's hearing and makes recommendations regarding the use of hearing aids. In addition, just over half of the respondents (56.1%) gave a correct answer to the question about where hearing aids could be purchased.

Johnson et al. (1995) also found that the nurses had mixed attitudes toward hearing aids and hearing aid wearers. On a positive note, nearly all of the respondents (98.9%) agreed with the statement, "Hearing aids are a worthwhile expense." Similarly, nearly all of the respondents (96.7%) agreed with the statement, "I would wear a hearing aid if one were recommended to me." In addition, nearly all of the respondents agreed with the statement, "People who wear hearing aids are equally intelligent as those who do not wear hearing aids." The large majority of respondents (83.5%) disagreed with the statement, "People look older when wearing hearing aids." Only about half of the respondents (46.2%) agreed with the statement, "I feel uncomfortable when I talk to people who wear hearing aids." Furthermore, two-thirds of the respondents (67%) agreed with the statement, "People who wear hearing aids tend to be embarrassed about their hearing aids." In summary, this study found that nurses across work settings had limited experience with hearing aids and some deficiencies in their knowledge and attitudes toward these devices. Clearly, nurses across a wide variety of work settings were not prepared to serve as audiologic support personnel. It was not known if similar results would be found for other allied-health professionals.

Johnson et al. (1998) surveyed 155 rehabilitation-hospital staff members from departments of nursing (N = 55), occupational therapy (OT) (N = 48), and physical therapy (PT) (N = 52) on their experience with, attitudes toward, and knowledge of hearing aids and patients with hearing impairment. Most of the respondents estimated that about 25% of their patients wore hearing aids. This estimate does not include patients with undetected or unmanaged hearing loss who are usually identified in the rehabilitation-hospital hearing screening program. Thus, a significant proportion of patients wears hearing aids.

Regarding prior experience with and knowledge of hearing aids and hearing aid batteries, slightly less than half of the nurses (43.6%) and very few of the OT (12.5%) and PT (7.1%) staff reported any previous training on the topic of hearing aids. Few of the respondents (nursing = 25.4%; OT = 8.3%; PT = 9.6%) felt competent performing a simple visual and listening check of a hearing aid. Although more than half of the nurses (65.4%) felt competent changing a hearing aid battery, less than half of the OT (27.1%) and PT staff (25.0%) felt the same way. Similarly, although the large majority of nurses (81.8%) felt competent inserting and removing hearing aids from patients' ears, less than half of the OT (39.6%) and PT (34.6%) staff felt the same way.

Regarding rehabilitation-hospital staff members' attitudes toward patients wearing hearing aids, about half of the respondents (nursing = 58.2%; OT = 47.7%; PT = 59.6%) agreed with the statement, "In general, patients with hearing impairment are more difficult to work with than those with normal hearing." Fortunately, nearly all of the nursing (92.7%), OT (95.8%), and PT (96.2%) staff felt that it was important for patients' hearing aids to be functioning during their hospital stay. Furthermore, about two-thirds of the nursing (69.1%) and OT (66.7%) staff and more than half of the PT (57.7%) staff would be willing to be responsible for maintaining patients' hearing aids or assisting them in caring for these devices. Thus, rehabilitation-hospital staff members recognized how hearing loss can potentially interfere with the rehabilitation process, felt that it is important that patients' hearing aids are functioning during their hospital stay, and were willing to serve as audiologic support personnel.

Johnson et al. (1998) found that rehabilitation staff members had some basic knowledge about hearing aids and hearing aid batteries. The large majority of the nursing (85.5%), OT (85.4%), and PT (80.7%) staff knew that batteries had a positive and negative side and were harmful if swallowed (nursing = 87.3%; OT = 85.4%; PT = 90.4%). Furthermore, nearly all of the respondents could identify appropriate situations for patients to wear hearing aids. Surprisingly, however, approximately half of the nursing (45.5%), OT (50.0%), and PT (55.8%) staff thought that hearing aid batteries lasted for several months. Apparently, the respondents thought that hearing aid batteries were similar to watch batteries. Clearly, rehabilitation-hospital staff members of different allied-health professions had limited experience with hearing aids and some deficiencies regarding their knowledge of these devices and their batteries.

In conclusion, the results of the studies discussed here suggest that allied-health professionals in a variety of work settings have had little or no preservice training on the topic of hearing aids in their academic coursework. Although most of the respondents had some general knowledge about hearing aids and hearing aid batteries, they lacked both skills and critical information to serve competently as audiologic support personnel. Although most respondents knew that hearing aids ran on batteries, for example, they did not know how long the batteries lasted. Furthermore, most respondents were not competent to perform even basic visual and listening checks on hearing aids. Thus, regardless of which professionals are selected to serve as audiologic support personnel, they will need extensive inservice training to be successful in carrying out assigned tasks in a support program.

SELECTION OF THE APPROPRIATE MODEL OF MULTISKILLING

Before initiating inservice training programs, audiologists must select an appropriate model of multiskilling to use for support programs. Chapter 2 defined the three models of multiskilling that use different types of employees. Recall that subordinate multiskilling involves audiology paraprofessionals, collateral multiskilling includes professionals from other disciplines, and collateral-subordinate multiskilling requires support personnel of other professions. Subordinate multiskilling is not generally used in support programs because audiologists rarely enjoy the luxury of having audiology paraprofessionals at their discretion. Thus, collateral and collateral-subordinate multiskilling are used more commonly and involve working with colleagues in other professions and their subordinates. Care must be taken to treat these individuals with respect and to show appreciation for their participation in the support program. Furthermore, when working with the subordinates of other professionals, audiologists must always institute directives through the subordinates' immediate supervisors. Audiologists issuing instructions to nurse's assistants should send them through the head nurse's office, for example.

The model of multiskilling used depends on the setting (e.g., type of educational institution, rehabilitation hospital, or long-term residential care facility for the elderly), population (e.g., age, prevalent etiologies, and disorders), and geographic location (e.g., remote, rural, suburban, urban, or metropolitan) (ASHA, 1996). Selection of the multiskilling model must be the result of a systematic analysis of the service-delivery site in consultation with administrators and consideration of several logistical factors. Several important questions should be answered in this analysis. Which personnel have the most contact with patients with hearing impairment? What is their caseload? Would participation as audiologic support personnel result in a work overload? What are their attitudes toward participation in the support program? Do they meet the criteria for support personnel set forth in the "Position Statement and Guidelines of the Consensus Panel on Support Personnel in Audiology" (AAA, 1997)? Can they be trained and supervised according to the guidelines set forth in the same document?

COMPONENTS OF COMPLETE INSERVICE PROGRAMS

Once audiologists have selected the model of multiskilling, they may begin developing a complete inservice program. Complete inservice programs, regardless of service-delivery site, include components listed in Table 5–1.

First, only certified and/or licensed audiologists can direct inservice training. Second, support personnel trained in those inservices should satisfy the following specific criteria (AAA, 1997):

- have earned a high school degree or equivalent
- possess the communication and interpersonal skills necessary for the tasks assigned
- possess a basic understanding of the needs of the population being served
- meet the training requirements and possess the competency-based skills necessary to perform the assigned tasks
- possess any additional qualifications established by the supervising audiologist to meet the specific needs of the audiology program and the population being served

Guidelines for use of support personnel in specific areas of audiologic practice should be developed as needed. The American Academy of Audiology's Committee on Infant Hearing, for example, has proposed guidelines for the use of support personnel for newborn hearing screening (AAA Committee on Infant Hearing, 1998).

Third, the training for support personnel should be well defined and specific to assigned tasks that do not: (1) require professional judgment, (2) entail the interpretation of results (with the exception of hearing screening), or (3) encompass the generation or change of treatment plans (AAA, 1997). Fourth, the supervising audiologist must verify that the scope and intensity of training encompass all of the activities assigned to support personnel. Fifth, training should be competency

Table 5–1. Components of complete inservice programs.

COMPLETE INSERVICE PROGRAMS ARE

- Directed by licensed and/or certified audiologists
- Specific with regard to support personnel selection criteria
- Well defined and specific to limited tasks
- Appropriate as to the scope and intensity of training
- Competency based
- Developed from support personnel roles and responsibilities
- Well equipped
- Both formal and informal in format
- Ongoing and current
- Well documented
- Evaluated by participants
- Rigorous in evaluating participants' knowledge and skills

Source: Adapted from "Position Statement and Guidelines of the Consensus Panel on Support Personnel in Audiology," 1997, by the American Academy of Audiology, *Audiology Today*, 9(3), 27–28; "Experiences, Attitudes, and Competencies of Audiologic Support Personnel in a Rehabilitation Hospital," 1998, by C. E. Johnson, S. Clark-Lewis, & D. Griffith. *American Journal of Audiology*, 7(2), 26–31; and "Dimensions of Multiskilling: Considerations for Educational Audiology," 1999, by C. E. Johnson, *Language, Speech, and Hearing Services in Schools*, 30, 4–10.

based, which means that support personnel learn skills that are directly related to their roles and responsibilities in the program. Audiologists should list those roles and responsibilities for support personnel. Johnson et al. (1998) determined that OT, PT, and nursing staff in a rehabilitation hospital should be given the following roles and responsibilities as audiologic support personnel:

- performing daily visual and listening checks of patients' hearing aids
- troubleshooting patients' hearing aids when necessary
- assisting or possibly retraining stroke patients in the insertion and removal of their hearing aids
- contacting the managing audiologist when necessary
- helping patients use assistive listening devices (ALDs)
- structuring interactions with patients who have hearing impairments for optimal communication (e.g., face-to-face communication, minimizing speaker-to-listener distance, eliminating background noise, using "clear speech" [Schum, 1997], and so on)

Sixth, those roles and responsibilities should serve as a basis for formulating topics and the behavioral objectives for the inservices. Johnson et al. (1998) found the following topics appropriate for inservices in the rehabilitation hospital: roles and functions of support personnel, types of hearing aids, hearing aid parts and their function, insertion and removal of hearing aids, Universal Precautions, visual and listening checks of hearing aids, troubleshooting hearing aids, program documentation and logistics, ALDs, and characteristics of optimal communication situations. Similarly, Johnson et al. (1998) formulated behavioral objectives for the inservice that are presented in Table 5–2. Seventh, inservices should be well equipped. Table 5–3 lists the required equipment to achieve the behavioral objectives listed in Table 5–2. In addition, inservices should have appropriate overheads, audio-visual equipment, and handouts for each participant. Eighth, training should be provided in formal and informal formats. Formal training is defined as scheduled, mandatory inservices and supervised practicum. Informal training includes support personnel peer assistance, e-mail communications with the supervising audiologist, and so on. Ninth, inservices should be ongoing and current to ensure that an ever-changing pool of support personnel has the most up-to-date information and skills. Completely-in-the-canal (CIC) hearing aids, for example, are relatively new technology, and even experienced audiologic support personnel need training in their insertion, removal, and maintenance.

Tenth, inservices should be documented. Documentation of inservices may include announcements in staff newsletters, letters to the administration, listing in quarterly support program reports, and so on. A sample letter to administrators documenting inservice activities appears in Appendix V-A. The letter should include the topic of inservice (e.g., hearing aid checks and troubleshooting), the specific audience (e.g., OT and PT staff), the number of participants, and the direct impact on patient care. Documentation also includes information in participants' personnel folders regarding their inservice attendance and performance on evaluation measures. A Staff Inservice Participation Documentation Form is provided in Appendix V-B.

Eleventh, participants should have an opportunity to evaluate inservices as part of Continuous Quality Improvement (CQI) (Hosford-Dunn, Dunn, & Harford, 1995; Reisberg & Fratalli, 1990; Walton, 1986). An Inservice Participant Evaluation Form is provided in Appendix V-C. Twelfth, participants should be tested after each inservice. Participant evaluation ensures that participants pay attention, obtain necessary knowledge, and can perform requisite skills. Thus, there should be a hands-on practicum component to the evaluation to ensure that each participant can perform all tasks before completing the inservice training. Evaluation tools vary based on the different types of inservice formats and accompany each inservice topic in the appendices.

TYPES OF INSERVICE FORMATS

Recall that there are at least three types of inservice formats: (1) informational, (2) skill-based, or (3) a combination of informational and skill-based. Informational and a combination of informational and skill-based formats are the most commonly used. Skill-based only formats are usually for training new skills with new technology (e.g., CIC hearing aids) to otherwise knowledgeable and experienced audiologic support personnel. Table 5–4 shows relevant topics for support program inservices subdivided by format type.

Informational inservices are usually presented in didactic lectures, cover a specific topic,

Table 5–2. Behavioral objectives for an inservice for rehabilitation-hospital staff.

Participants will be able to:

Objective Area 1: Overall Hearing Aid Monitoring Program

- With regard to the hearing aid monitoring program:
  ⇒ Describe its importance.
  ⇒ Describe the role and function of support personnel
  ⇒ Describe the logistics of the program.
  ⇒ Describe how to complete necessary documentation.

Objective Area 2: Hearing Aids and their Parts

- With regard to different types of hearing aids:
  ⇒ Identify different types of hearing aids.
  ⇒ Identify their parts.
  ⇒ Describe the function of the parts.
  ⇒ Distinguish between right and left earmolds and hearing aids.

Objective Area 3: Hearing Aid Batteries

- With regard to batteries:
  ⇒ Distinguish between different sizes of hearing aid batteries based on style of hearing aid.
  ⇒ Describe battery use (e.g., how long they last and so on).
  ⇒ Insert and remove batteries from hearing aids.
  ⇒ Check the voltage with a battery checker.
  ⇒ Replace dead batteries with fresh ones.

Objective Area 4: Insertion and Removal of Hearing Aids

- With regard to insertion and removal of hearing aids:
  ⇒ Insert and remove from patients' ears with proper manipulation of the volume-control wheels.
  ⇒ Have an awareness of Universal Precautions.
  ⇒ Reteach stroke patients how to manipulate their hearing aids.

Objective Area 5: Troubleshooting Hearing Aids

- With regard to troubleshooting hearing aids:
  ⇒ Perform visual and listening checks on hearing aids.
  ⇒ Troubleshoot minor problems on hearing aids (e.g., cleaning earmold bores, and so on).
  ⇒ Know when to contact an audiologist for repairs.

Objective Area 6: Manipulating and Troubleshooting ALDs

- With regard to assistive listening devices:
  ⇒ Describe major provisions of the Americans with Disabilities Act (ADA) (1990).
  ⇒ Identify ALD parts and state their function.
  ⇒ Manipulate ALDs available for use at the rehabilitation hospital.
  ⇒ Troubleshoot ALDs when necessary.
  ⇒ Teach patients how to use ALDs.

Source: From "Experiences, Attitudes, and Competences of Audiological Support Personnel in a Rehabilitation Hospital," by C. E. Johnson, S. Clark-Lewis, and D. Griffin, 1998, p. 30, *American Journal of Audiology, 7*(2). Reprinted with permission.

and are attended by both audiologic support personnel and all individuals that interact with patients with hearing impairment. Pertinent informational inservices include: (1) the Americans with Disabilities Act (1990) (Appendix V-D), (2) "Hearing Loss and its Effect on Communication" (Appendix V-E), and (3) "How Do You Communicate with Someone with a Hearing Loss?" (Appendix V-F). Readers should consider supplementing these inservices with materials used in specific service-delivery sites. The inservice on communicating with an individual who has a hearing loss presented to nursing-home personnel can be supplemented with specific suggestions for dealing with Alzheimer patients (see Chapter 8), for example.

The instructor-to-participant ratio can be large using the informational format providing

Table 5-3. Equipment needed to accomplish the behavioral objectives.

Objective Area	Equipment Needed
1. Overall Hearing Aid Monitoring Program	■ Overhead projector ■ Charts depicting program logistics ■ Appropriate forms
2. Hearing Aids and their Parts	■ Models of behind-the-ear hearing aids ■ Models of body hearing aids ■ Models of in-the-canal hearing aids ■ Models of in-the-ear hearing aids ■ Models of completely-in-the-canal hearing aids ■ Appropriate earmolds (behind-the-ear and body hearing aids)
3. Hearing Aids and their Batteries	■ Battery checkers ■ Different sizes of hearing aid batteries ■ Different sizes of hearing aids demonstrating the correct insertion of batteries
4. Insertion and Removal of Hearing Aids	■ Hearing aids ■ Earmolds ■ Plastic ears on stands ■ Volunteer models ■ Alcohol wipes ■ Plastic surgical gloves
5. Troubleshooting Hearing Aids	■ "Booby-trapped" hearing aids ■ Hearing aid check kits ■ Hearing aid check sheets
6. Maintaining and troubleshooting ALDs	■ ALDs used in the rehabilitation hospital ■ Appropriate batteries

Source: From "Experiences, Attitudes, and Competencies of Audiologic Support Personnel in a Rehabilitation Hospital," by C.E. Johnson, S. Clark-Lewis, & D, Griffin, 1998, p. 31. *American Journal of Audiology, 7*(2). Reprinted with permission.

Table 5-4. Example topics for informational and informational and skill-based formats.

Informational Format

- Americans with Disabilities Act (ADA) (1990)
- Hearing Loss and its Effect on Communication
- How Do You Communicate with Someone with a Hearing Loss?

Informational and Skill-Based Format

- Understanding Hearing Aids, Their Care and Their Use
- Understanding Cochlear Implants, Their Care and Their Use
- Understanding Personal FM Systems, Their Care and Their Use
- Understanding Sound-Field FM Amplification Systems, Their Care and Their Use

---

that all attendees can see and hear the presentation. Important points made in the lecture can be emphasized using demonstrations, videotapes, or audience-participation techniques. Rosenberg and Blake-Rahter (1995) suggested demonstrating sound-field FM amplification to teachers during the inservice to show how an increase in the signal-to-noise ratio (S/N) can improve understanding. Similarly, the American Speech-Language-Hearing Association provides a short yet informative videotape on the Americans with Disabilities Act (ADA) (1990) that can provide interest to an inservice on the same topic. Furthermore, requiring audience members to participate in role-play situations can reinforce communication tips to be used with persons who have hearing impairment. Participants are given a short, multiple-choice quiz at the end of the inservice to assess their retention of information. Suggestions, lists of required materials, ready-to-copy overheads, appropriate handouts, and post-inservice quizzes can be found in the appendices as indicated above.

The combination informational and skill-based format involves both didactic lecture and supervised practicum. Important content information is presented first, followed by a "hands-on" practicum that allows participants to practice new skills while being supervised by knowledgeable instructors. Only audiologic support personnel attend these types of inservices. Pertinent combination informational and skill-based inservices included in this chapter are: (1) Understanding Hearing Aids, Their Care and Their Use (Appendix V-G) and (2) Understanding Cochlear Implants, Their Care and Their Use (Appendix V-H). Similar inservices on personal FM systems, sound-field FM amplification systems, and assistive listening devices should be developed. Readers can use the principles presented in this chapter with established inservice protocols on selected topics. Blake-Rahter and Rosenberg (1994) provided suggestions for developing an inservice for sound-field amplification systems, for example.

As with the informational format, the informational portion of the inservice can have a large instructor-to-participant ratio. *The supervised practicum must have an instructor-to-participant ratio of no more than 1:4, however.* In addition, the instructional space is arranged differently for the supervised practicum than for the didactic lecture. Johnson et al. (1998) found that setting up a series of four to five learning stations is an effective method of providing ample practice for participants to learn several skills. To accomplish the behavioral objectives listed in Table 5–2, Johnson et al. (1998) set up the following five learning stations focusing on: (1) different styles of hearing aids and their parts; (2) hearing aid batteries (e.g., checking voltage and proper insertion); (3) insertion and removal of patients' hearing aids; (4) troubleshooting hearing aids; and (5) using, checking, and troubleshooting ALDs. At each of the learning stations were one or two learning guides to supervise participants in practicing new skills. Figure 5–2 shows use of a learning station during an inservice. Participants rotated from station to station every 15 to 20 minutes, having ample time to practice all skills within an hour and a half. In addition, instructors assess participants on the knowledge and skills learned in both portions of the inservice. Johnson et al. (1998) required that participants pass a short quiz on material from the informational portion of the inservice and a

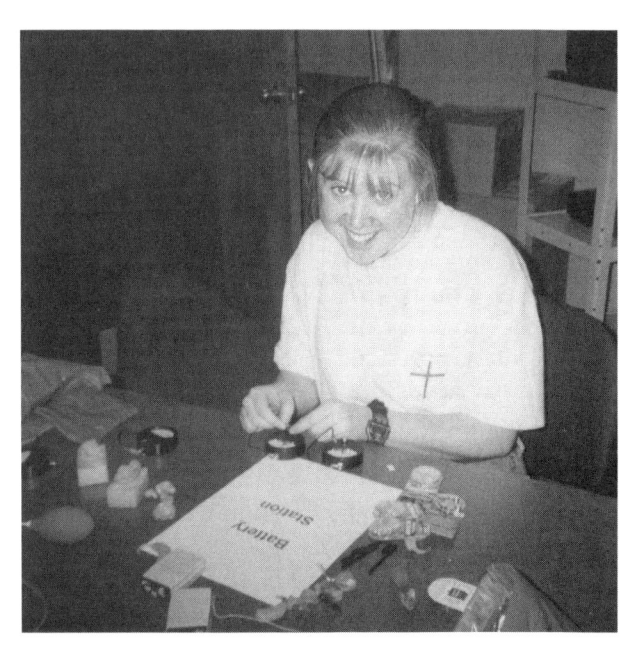

Figure 5–2. Inservice utilizing stations to teach specific skills.

practical examination from the informational and skill-based portion. Participants must achieve scores of 80% or higher on both portions of the examination in order to pass. Suggestions, lists of required materials, appropriate handouts, and post-inservice quizzes can be found in the appendices as indicated above.

CREATING MEANINGFUL ADULT LEARNING EXPERIENCES

Audiologists must consider the following questions in order to create meaningful adult learning experiences through their inservices: Who? What? Where? When? Why? How? and How long? First, audiologists must address *who* they are professionally and within the institution or system in which they are establishing a support program. For example, audiologists must have a strong professional image in order to motivate the audience to learn the information and skills necessary to participate competently as audiologic support personnel.

In addition, audiologists' relationships to the health-care facility, institution, or school system can affect their ability to provide effective inservices. These relationships often depend on the service-delivery model. For example, there are two basic service-delivery models in educational audiology: (1) school-based and (2) contracted services (Johnson, Benson, & Seaton, 1997). In the school-based service-delivery model, the audiologist is an employee of the school system and more than likely considered an "insider" by other educational personnel who may be enthusiastic in learning from their colleague. In the contracted-services model, however, audiologists are hired from year-to-year to provide services to a specific population. These audiologists may face hostile educational personnel who resent being told what to do and how to do it by an "outsider." Thus, audiologists must consider who their audience is and be prepared for any response. Furthermore, the educational level of the audience must be considered so that the content can be geared up or down as needed. Often, audience educational levels will be mixed so audiologists must be skilled in making a connection with a variety of people on some level. It also may be necessary to have an interpreter present for the inservice. We have given numerous inservices to staff at nursing homes in Alabama and California where more than half of the participants spoke very little English. These participants usually sat through an inservice and smiled or nodded approvingly, but when it came to the practicum, we found that they failed to grasp the concepts. In such cases, presenting inservices without an interpreter would be fruitless. This is another reason why audiologists must know characteristics about the audience before an inservice.

Another question for audiologists to consider is *what* they will be teaching in their inservices. *Inservice content varies from situation to situation even across similar service-delivery sites.* Audiologists who give inservices to several different long-term residential facilities for the elderly may find that each needs information on different topics. One nursing home may already be in compliance with the ADA, while another facility may need extensive training on the topic. Audiologists should modify suggested inservice protocols provided at the end of this chapter to meet their needs. Audiologists may find that the handout on the ADA provided by the American Speech-Language-Hearing Association that appears in Appendix V-D is too long and detailed to be covered in a 45-minute presentation, for example. In this case, audiologists may select key points from the handout and make their own abbreviated handout for the inservice.

Other important considerations are *where* and *when* the inservices are to take place. Selection of the instructional facility and scheduling of the inservice are key to the success of the learning experience. Johnson (1999) stated that the instructional facility should be comfortable (e.g., temperature, lighting, and acoustics) and have adequate seating so that all participants can see and hear the presentation. If part of the inservice has a skill-based format, the room should be large enough and equipped with moveable tables and chairs so that audiologists can arrange the room as needed for setting up learning stations and so on. Similarly, inservice sessions should never be scheduled during staff's break, lunch, or at the end of a long day of other inservices. Participants cannot learn how to troubleshoot hearing aids with a cafeteria tray in front of them. Similarly, otherwise cooperative rehabilitation staff may appear hostile to audiologists who try to convey information during their coffee breaks. If inservices are only allowed to be scheduled during staff "free time," then audiologists should question administrators' and area supervisors' commitment to the support program. Audiologic support personnel need to be alert, motivated, and interested for facilitated learning.

To remain engaged, participants need to know why they are learning the content of the inservice. Attendance may be mandatory, but long-term success depends on audiologists' ability to obtain participants' cooperation. Participants need to make the connection between improving patients' ability to communicate and the facilitation of patient care. Johnson et al. (1998) found that PT, OT, and nursing staff in a rehabilitation hospital were eager to learn how to assist patients in managing their hearing aids. Rehabilitation-hospital staff members felt that patients who can hear are easier to deal with and progress more rapidly in therapy. Nonetheless, audiologists may find it difficult to convince already overworked employees that participation as audiologic support personnel is important to positive patient outcomes. Participants need to hear this several times during a presentation: in the introduction, during instruction, and at the end of the presentation.

How the instructor presents information is almost as important as the content (Johnson, 1999). Johnson et al. (1997) suggested that presenters personalize the information, be flexible, and alert to physical and mental limits, and use "ice-breakers" with the audience, such as humor. Prior to an inservice, skillful audiologists will investigate particular problems that a nursing-home staff experiences in meeting the communication needs of their patients with hearing impairment. Not only does prior investigation assist audiologists in selecting appropriate topics for the inservice, but the information will provide insight as to specific examples to be used that will captivate the interest of the audience. Audiologists also must be flexible if participants would rather focus on specific problems within their service-delivery site. Skillful instructors should be able to teach content information and skills even when there is a change of format. Furthermore, the use of handouts and overheads in inservices is another important consideration. Johnson et al. (1997) suggested the following for handouts:

- Describe to participants how the handouts will be useful.
- Make handouts easy to read and use.
- Consider color-coding handouts for future reference.
- Provide a handout that restates critical information presented in the inservice, with the name, e-mail address, office address, and phone number of the audiologist.

Allen (1998) suggested the following for overheads:

- Use a large enough font so that the words can be read easily from across the room.
- Avoid using all capital letters.
- Use easy-to-read fonts.
- Use only one or two fonts for an entire presentation.
- Match the font with the presentation.
- Avoid always using your favorite font.
- Avoid overusing a bold style that can be fatiguing for large amounts of text.
- Use bullets to help separate items.
- Consider your audience.
- Strive to use a 12th-grade reading level.

Regardless of service-delivery site and the type of audience involved, audiologists must always remember to make arrangements to have the information delivered in the language of and at the appropriate level for each participant. The need to reduce the complexity of information down to a lay-person's level goes without saying. Instructors must remember that English may not be the most appropriate language for communicating the critical points of an inservice. In our 20-year experience providing audiologic services to more than 100 long-term residential care facilities in Alabama, central Oklahoma, and Southern California, we have learned that the caregivers who most often interact with patients are nurse's assistants. They are the ones who are actually aware of each patient's daily needs (including hearing and communication) and can be helpful serving as audiologic support personnel. Unfortunately, many do not possess a good working use of the English language; Spanish and various Asian languages are common, but several others are also prevalent. Therefore, it is necessary to have appropriate interpreters present for an inservice when necessary.

Another important consideration is *how long* inservices should last. Audiologists must ensure that the inservice is long enough to accomplish the behavioral objectives, but not too long so that participants get fatigued. At one extreme, audiologists must be wary of administrators not allowing sufficient time for inservices. To administrators, employee time is money. Sometimes requesting more time than is required for the inservice is a good strategy because administrators will allocate less time than requested. Suggested time allocations are provided for each inservice appearing in the appendices. At the other extreme, audiologists should be sensitive to audience attentional limitations. Johnson et al. (1998) found that participants find it difficult to attend to presentations lasting longer than one hour unless they have a break. Beyond one hour, audiences tend to get fatigued and hostile.

SUMMARY

This chapter discussed how to develop effective inservice programs. Innovative inservice programs are the cornerstones for developing support programs for patients with hearing impairment. Readers should possess the background to select an appropriate model of multskilling, understand the components of a complete inservice program, differentiate the three types of inservice formats, and create meaningful adult learning experiences regardless of service-delivery site. Useful inservice topics using different formats are provided in the appendices. Each topic contains suggestions (i.e., time allotment, materials, equipment, and so on), handouts, participant quizzes, and other useful information that audiologists can quickly and efficiently use to present an inservice.

LEARNING ACTIVITIES

- Volunteer to give an inservice at a local school, rehabilitation hospital, or nursing home using the materials provided in the appendices.
- Critique previous inservices in which you have taken part using the criteria in this chapter.

REFERENCES

Allen, L. (1998). Presentation and publication tips. *Educational Audiology Review, 15*(2), 10.

American Academy of Audiology. (1997). Position statement and guidelines of the consensus panel on support personnel in audiology. *Audiology Today, 9*(3), 27–28.

American Speech-Language-Hearing Association. (1996, Spring). Technical report of the ad hoc committee on multiskilling. *Asha, 38*(Suppl. 16), 53–61.

Americans with Disabilities Act of 1990, Public Law 101-336, 42, U.S.C. 12101 et seq.: *U.S. Statutes at Large, 104,* 327–378 (1991).

Anderson, K. (1996). Thirteen facts on the impact of hearing loss on education. *The Hearing Review, 3*(9), 19.

Cochlear Corporation. (1995). *Teacher guide.* Inverness, CO: Author.

Cochlear Corporation. (1996). *Issues and answers.* Inverness, CO: Author.

Edwards, C. (1995). Listening strategies for teachers and students. In C.C. Crandell, J.J. Smaldino, & C. Flexer (Eds.), *Sound-field FM amplification: Theory and practical applications* (pp. 191–200). San Diego, CA: Singular Publishing Group.

Foto, M. (1996). Multiskilling: Who, how, when, and why? *The American Journal of Occupational Therapy, 50,* 1.

Hosford-Dunn, H., Dunn, D. R., & Harford, E. R. (1995). *Audiology business and practice management.* San Diego, CA: Singular Publishing Group.

Hull, R. H., & Dilka, K. L. (1984). *The hearing-impaired child.* Orlando, FL: Grune & Stratton.

Johnson, C. D., Benson, P. V., & Seaton, J. B. (1997). *Educational audiology handbook.* San Diego, CA: Singular Publishing Group.

Johnson, C. E. (1999). Dimensions of multiskilling: Considerations for educational audiology. *Language, Speech, and Hearing Services in the Schools, 30,* 4–10.

Johnson, C. E., Clark-Lewis, S., & Griffin, D. (1998). Experience, attitudes, and competencies of audiologic support personnel in a rehabilitation hospital. *American Journal of Audiology: A Journal of Clinical Practice, 7*(2) 26–31.

Johnson, C. E., Stein, R. L., & Lass, N. J. (1992). Public school nurses' preparedness for a hearing aid monitoring program. *Language, Speech, and Hearing Services in the Schools, 23,* 141–144.

Johnson, C. E., Stein, R. L., Lyons, R., & Lass, N. J. (1995). Nurses' views on hearing aids and hearing aid wearers: A survey. *The Hearing Journal, 48*(2), 29–31.

Lass, N., Carlin, M., Woodford, C., Campanelli-Humphreys, A., Joanna, J., Hushion-Stemple, E. & Boggs, J. (1986). A survey of professionals' knowledge of and exposure to hearing loss. *The Volta Review, 88*(7), 333–338.

Reisberg, M., & Frattali, C. (1990). Toward total quality management. *Quality Assurance Digest,* 1–5.

Rosenberg, G., & Blake-Rahter, P. (1995). Inservice training for the classroom teacher. In C. C. Crandell, J. J. Smaldino, & C. Flexer (Eds.) *Sound-field FM amplification: Theory and practical applications* (pp. 149–190). San Diego, CA: Singular Publishing Group.

Schum, D. J. (1997). Beyond hearing aids: Clear speech training as an intervention strategy. *The Hearing Journal, 50*(10), 36–38, 40.

Walton, M. (1986). *The Deming management method.* New York: Pedigree/Putnam.

Wayner, D., & Abrahamson, J. (1996). How to gain a larger slice of the "communication pie." *The Hearing Review, 3*(9), 32–34.

APPENDIX V-A

Letter to Administrators Documenting Inservice Activity

ALL-PRO HEARING SERVICES
"So all can hear..."

June 31, 1999

Dr. R.E. Habilitate
XYZ Rehabilitation Hospital
1144 Recovery Way
Quality of Life City, CA 94545

RE: Report of Inservice Activity

Dear Dr. Habilitate,

This letter is to inform you that an inservice was provided by All-Pro Hearing Services on Thursday, June 25, 1999 from 9:00 am to 12:00 pm on the topic of assisting patients with their hearing aids. A skillful staff is the foundation of an effective support program for patients with hearing impairment.

The inservice consisted of a one-hour lecture about hearing aids and a two-hour supervised practicum to teach troubleshooting skills. The participants were 12 members of the occupational-therapy staff, 10 members of the physical-therapy staff, and 14 members of the nursing staff. The names of the participants are on the attached sheet along with the scores on their inservice performance evaluation. You will note that 30 out of 36 participants achieved the recommended passing score of 80%. In addition, participants evaluated the inservice experience. The results of that evaluation will be sent to you shortly.

I appreciate your commitment to our efforts to maintain an exemplary support program for patients with hearing impairment. If you have any questions, please feel free to schedule an appointment or call me at 555-1122.

Sincerely,

Starr Audiologist, Ph.D.

Certificate of Clinical Competence in Audiology (CCC-A)
Fellow of the American Academy of Audiology (FAAA)

Participants in Hearing Aid Monitoring Inservice

Occupational-Therapy Staff	Score
XXXXXX XXXXXX	XX%
XXXXXX XXXXXX	XX%
XXXXXX XXXXXX	XX%
XXXXXX XXXXXX	XX%
XXXXXX XXXXXX	XX%
XXXXXX XXXXXX	XX%
XXXXXX XXXXXX	XX%
XXXXXX XXXXXX	XX%
XXXXXX XXXXXX	XX%
XXXXXX XXXXXX	XX%

Physical-Therapy Staff	Score
XXXXXX XXXXXX	XX%
XXXXXX XXXXXX	XX%
XXXXXX XXXXXX	XX%
XXXXXX XXXXXX	XX%
XXXXXX XXXXXX	XX%
XXXXXX XXXXXX	XX%
XXXXXX XXXXXX	XX%
XXXXXX XXXXXX	XX%

Nursing Staff	Score
XXXXXX XXXXXX	XX%
XXXXXX XXXXXX	XX%
XXXXXX XXXXXX	XX%
XXXXXX XXXXXX	XX%
XXXXXX XXXXXX	XX%
XXXXXX XXXXXX	XX%
XXXXXX XXXXXX	XX%
XXXXXX XXXXXX	XX%
XXXXXX XXXXXX	XX%
XXXXXX XXXXXX	XX%
XXXXXX XXXXXX	XX%
XXXXXX XXXXXX	XX%

APPENDIX V-B

Staff Inservice Participation Documentation Form

Name: _____   Department: _____

DATE	TOPIC	SCORE ON EXAM	PASS OR FAIL

NOTES:

APPENDIX V-C

Inservice Participant Evaluation Form

Topic of Inservice: _____

Date: _____

Instructor(s): _____

Your department: _____

Instructions: Please circle your degree of agreement for each statement below:

1. Inservice objectives were clear.

    Agree   1   2   3   5   6   7   8   9   10   Disagree

2. Instructors were knowledgeable about the topic presented.

    Agree   1   2   3   5   6   7   8   9   10   Disagree

3. Instructors were actively helpful.

    Agree   1   2   3   5   6   7   8   9   10   Disagree

4. Instructors spoke clearly and audibly.

    Agree   1   2   3   5   6   7   8   9   10   Disagree

5. Information was clearly presented.

    Agree   1   2   3   5   6   7   8   9   10   Disagree

6. Visual and teaching aids used were effective.

    Agree   1   2   3   5   6   7   8   9   10   Disagree

7. Information was useful and relevant to working with individuals who have hearing impairment.

    Agree   1   2   3   5   6   7   8   9   10   Disagree

8. Time was used efficiently.

    Agree   1   2   3   5   6   7   8   9   10   Disagree

Please list three things you learned during the inservice.

How could this inservice be improved?

APPENDIX V-D

Inservice for the Americans with Disabilities Act (1990)

Behavioral Objectives

Through participation in this inservice, attendees will be able to:
- Define the Americans with Disabilities Act (ADA) (1990)
- Identify the five sections (titles) of the law
- Know the pertinent aspects of the law with regard to speech-language and hearing disabilities
- Distinguish among the different types of assistive listening devices (ALDs)

Suggested Time Allotment

About 2 hours, 30 minutes
- Introduction (10 minutes)
- ASHA Video and Questions (20 minutes)
- Communication and the ADA (50 minutes)
- Break: ALD Show and Tell (20 minutes)
- Group Activity (40 minutes)
- Quiz (10 minutes)

Format

Informational

Suggested Materials

- Overhead projector
- VCR and monitor
- ADA Kit available from: ASHA Products
  c/o The American Speech-Language-Hearing Association
  10801 Rockville Pike
  Rockville, MD 20852
- Appropriate handouts
- Appropriate overheads
- Examples of ALDs from each of the following categories:
  ⇒ devices for telephone communication
  ⇒ devices for environmental sounds
  ⇒ devices for face-to-face communication or television listening

Suggested Participant Activities

- Form discussion groups:
  ⇒ to perform a facility communication accessibility audit. Create a fictional patient with a hearing impairment and have the groups determine necessary steps to ensure that the patient's communication accessibility is provided.
  ⇒ to discuss statements about the ADA and determine whether they are true or false.
- Use role-play scenarios to have participants display their knowledge of the ADA. For example, a participant can portray a patient with hearing impairment who must explain the ADA to a skeptical rehabilitation-hospital administrator who is reluctant to provide any type of ALD for the patient's room.
- Ask for volunteers to demonstrate the use of the ALDs on hand.

HANDOUTS

WHAT IS THE AMERICANS WITH DISABILITIES ACT?

The Americans with Disabilities Act (ADA) is a federal law (Public Law 101-336) that was passed in 1990 to provide protection from discrimination based on an individual's disability. This law is patterned after an earlier law, the Rehabilitation Act of 1973 (Public Law 93-380), which was considered the civil rights act for the handicapped. It prohibits those receiving federal funds from discriminating against otherwise qualified persons with a handicap.

The ADA is different from the Rehabilitation Act of 1973 in at least two ways:

- The word "handicap" is replaced by the term "disability."
- The law pertains to all employers, not just those receiving federal funds.

WHAT ARE THE MAJOR SECTIONS OF THE ADA?

The law has five major sections or titles. They are:

- Employment
- Public Services and Transportation
- Public Accommodations and Commercial Facilities
- Telecommunications
- Miscellaneous Provisions

WHAT DOES THE ADA HAVE TO DO WITH SPEECH-LANGUAGE AND HEARING DISABILITIES?

The American Speech-Language-Hearing Association has determined some important aspects of the ADA as it relates to communication. The attached handout summarizes those aspects. We will now discuss them.

COMMUNICATION AND THE ADA
(Effective Communication and Accessibility)

What is EFFECTIVE COMMUNICATION under ADA?

- **Taking steps to ensure** that people with communication disabilities
  - Have **access to goods, services, and facilities**
  - Are **not excluded, denied services, segregated or otherwise treated differently** than other people
- **Making information accessible to and useable** by people with communication disabilities

What is required to achieve EFFECTIVE COMMUNICATION under ADA?

- **Providing any necessary auxiliary communication aids and services**
  - Unless an undue burden or a fundamental change in the nature of the goods, services, facilities, etc. would result
  - Without a surcharge to the individual
- **Making aurally (via hearing) delivered information available** to persons with hearing and speech impairments (including alarms, nonverbal speech, and computer-generated speech)
- Personally prescribed devices such as hearing aids are **not** required.

How do you determine NECESSARY AUXILIARY COMMUNICATION AIDS AND SERVICES?

- Consideration of:
  - **Expressed preference of the individual with disability**
  - **Level and type of the communication exchange** (complexity, length, and importance of material). For example, interpreter services might not be necessary for a simple business transaction such as buying groceries, but they might be appropriate in lengthy or major transactions such as purchasing a car or provision of legal or medical services.
- **Selection of appropriate aids and services** from available technologies and services (low-tech as well as high-tech) based on facility resources and communication needs (individual's and type of material)

What are STRATEGIES for achieving EFFECTIVE COMMUNICATION?

- **Establishing appropriate attitudes and behaviors:**
  - Assuming that persons with communication disabilities can express themselves if afforded the opportunity, respect, and the necessary assistance to do so
  - Consulting the person with the disability how best to communicate with him or her, and asking about the need for aids and services
  - Training staff to communicate more effectively
- **Modifying the communication setting**, for example, reducing noise levels. Improving the communication setting can also reduce the need for assistive devices in some cases.
- **Providing auxiliary aids and services**
- **Responding to auxiliary aids and services requests**
- **Providing materials in accessible formats** (e.g., written transcripts)
- **Keeping written materials simple and direct**
- **Providing visual as well as auditory information**
- **Providing a means for written exchange of information**
- **Informing public of available accommodations**
- **Maintaining devices in good working condition**
- **Consulting a professional** (audiologist, speech-language pathologist)

What are examples of COMMUNICATION (SPEECH AND HEARING) AIDS AND SERVICES?

- **In assembly areas, meetings, conversations:**
  - Assistive listening devices and systems (ALDs), communication boards (word, symbol), qualified interpreters (oral, cued speech, sign language), real-time captioning, written communication exchange and transcripts, computer-assisted note taking, lighting on speaker's face, preferential seating for good listening and viewing position, electrical outlet near accessible seating, videotext displays
- **In telecommunications:**
  - Hearing aid compatible telephones, volume control telephone handsets, amplified telephone mouthpieces (for person with weak voice) (to amplify speech for a hard-of-hearing listener), telecommunication device for the deaf (TDD) or text telephone, facsimile machines (that use visual symbols), computer/modem, interactive computer software with videotext
  - TDD/telephone relay systems
- **In buildings:**
  - Alerting, signaling, warning, and announcement systems using amplified auditory signals, visual signals (flashing, strobe), vibrotactile (touch) devices, videotext displays
- **In prepared (non-live) materials:**
  - Written materials in alternate formats (e.g., symbols, pictures)
  - Aurally-delivered materials in alternate formats (e.g., captioned videotapes, written transcript, sign interpreter)
  - Notification of accessibility options (e.g., alternative formats)

What are COMMUNICATION BARRIERS?

- Factors that hinder or prevent information coming to and/or from a person
- **Visually-related barriers**
  - Inadequate or poor lighting/poor background that interferes with ability to speechread or see signing
  - Unreadable signage (too small, not in line of vision of people in wheelchairs or of short stature)
  - Lack of visual information (For example, not showing speaker's face)
  - Lack of signage and accessibility symbols
- **Acoustically-related barriers**
  - High noise levels
  - High reverberation levels
  - Lack of aurally-delivered information to supplement visual information (For example, not using amplified auditory as well as visual signals in emergency alarms, partitions that block sound between speaker and listener)
- **Attitudinal and prejudicial barriers**
- **Information complexity** (such as difficult reading level)

What is required for COMMUNICATION ACCESSIBILITY under ADA?

- **Providing TDD and accessible telephone or alternative service**
  - When telephone service is regularly provided to customers/patients on more than just an incidental basis (e.g., hospitals, hotels)
  - When building entry requires aural or voice information exchange (e.g., closed circuit security telephone)

COMMUNICATION ACCESSIBILITY under ADA *continued*

- **Providing means for two-way communication in emergency situations** (e.g., elevator emergency notification system) that does not require hearing or speech for communication exchange
- **Providing closed caption decoders**, upon request, in hospitals that provide televisions, and in places of lodging with televisions in five or more guest rooms
- **Removing structural communication barriers** in existing buildings when readily achievable (inexpensively and easily removed)
- **Providing alternative service** when barriers are not easily removed (For example, preferential seating area)
- **Following accessibility standards** for new construction/alterations (ADA Accessibility Guidelines, Uniform Federal Accessibility Standard)

What are some READILY ACHIEVABLE STRUCTURAL BARRIER REMOVAL STRATEGIES?

- **Installing sound buffers** to reduce noise and reverberation
- **Installing flashing alarm lights** in restrooms, any general usage areas, hallways, lobbies, and any other common usage areas
- **Integrating visual alarms** into facility alarm systems
- **Removing physical partitions** that block sound or visual information between employees and customers
- **Providing directional signage** with symbols to indicate available services

What is needed for SIGNAGE AND SYMBOLS OF COMMUNICATION ACCESSIBILITY?

- **Symbols** for:
  - **Telephone** accessibility:
    - blue grommet between cord and handset—"hearing aid compatible"
    - telephone handset with radiating soundwaves—"volume control"
  - **TDDs** or text telephones—the international TDD symbol
- **Signage:**
  - **Directional signage** indicating nearest TDD or accessible telephone
  - **Messages for availability of Assistive Listening Devices** (ALDs) in announcements, in key building areas
  - **Messages for communication aids and services** (e.g., interpreters)

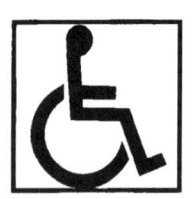

International Symbol of Accessibility

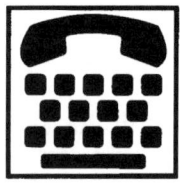

International TDD Symbol

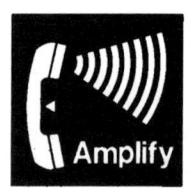

Telephone Handset Amplification Symbol

What types of POLICIES AND PRACTICES NEED TO BE MODIFIED?

- Discriminatory policies such as prohibiting hearing assistance dogs
- Discriminatory eligibility criteria such as restricting access to goods and services unless necessary for the provision of goods and services

What is the best way to ensure COST-EFFECTIVE ADA COMPLIANCE?

- **Perform a facility accessibility audit** that includes identification of communication barriers
- **Determine auxiliary aids and services needs**
- **Develop a plan to remove barriers and acquire assistive devices**
- **Perform ongoing audit and maintenance of accessibility features**
- **Modify discriminatory policies, practices, and procedures**
- **Obtain technical assistance and consult** with rehabilitation professionals, disability organizations, consumers, federal agencies as appropriate

The BOTTOM LINE

- **Ask people about their needs, show respect and sensitivity, use what works (not necessarily what is most expensive), use your resources creatively and effectively.**

This document is available in the following formats: large print, audiotape, computer disk, braille, electronic bulletin board (202-514-6193).

This document provides general information to promote voluntary compliance with the Americans with Disabilities Act (ADA). It was prepared under a grant from the U.S. Department of Justice. While the Office on the Americans with Disabilities Act has reviewed its contents, any opinions or interpretations in the document are those of the American Speech-Language-Hearing Association and do not necessarily reflect the views of the Department of Justice. The ADA itself and the Department's ADA regulations should be consulted for further, more specific guidance.

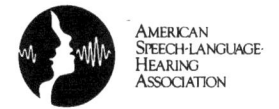

AMERICAN SPEECH-LANGUAGE-HEARING ASSOCIATION

Produced by American Speech-Language-Hearing Association,
10801 Rockville Pike, Rockville, MD 20852,
1-800-638-8255 (V/TDD), 301-897-5700(V); 301-897-0157 (TDD).

INSTRUCTOR OVERHEADS

THE AMERICANS WITH DISABILITIES ACT (ADA) (1990)

I. Introduction

   A. What is it?

   B. In what ways does it differ from previous laws?

   C. What are the major sections (titles) of the law?

      1. Employment
      2. Public Services and Transportation
      3. Public Accommodations and Commercial Facilities
      4. Telecommunications
      5. Miscellaneous Provisions

What is EFFECTIVE COMMUNICATION under ADA?

- **Taking steps to ensure:**
  ⇒ **Access to goods, services, and facilities.**
  ⇒ **No segregation, exclusion, or differential treatment.**

- **Making information accessible and useable.**

What is required to achieve EFFECTIVE COMMUNICATION under ADA?

- **Providing any necessary auxiliary communication aids and services**

- **Making aurally (via hearing) delivered information available**

Personally prescribed devices such as HEARING AIDS are NOT required.

How do you determine NECESSARY AUXILIARY COMMUNICATION AIDS AND SERVICES?

Consider:

- **Expressed preference of the individual with disability**

- **Level and type of communication exchange**

- **Selection of appropriate aids and services**

What are STRATEGIES for achieving EFFECTIVE COMMUNICATION?

- **Establishing appropriate attitudes and behaviors**
- **Modifying the communication setting**
- **Providing auxiliary aids and services**
- **Responding to auxiliary aids and services requests**
- **Providing materials in accessible formats**
- **Keeping written materials simple and direct**
- **Providing visual as well as auditory information**
- **Providing a means for written exchange of information**
- **Informing the public of available accommodations**
- **Maintaining devices in good working condition**
- **Consulting a professional**

What are examples of COMMUNICATION (SPEECH AND HEARING) AIDS AND SERVICES?

- **In assembly areas, meetings, and conversations**

- **In telecommunications**

- **In buildings**

- **In prepared (non-live) materials**

What are COMMUNICATION BARRIERS?

- **Visually related barriers**

- **Acoustically related barriers**

- **Attitudinal and prejudicial barriers**

- **Information complexity**

What is required for COMMUNICATION ACCESSIBILITY under the ADA?

- **Providing TDD and accessible telephone or alternative service**
- **Providing means for two-way communication in emergency situations**
- **Providing closed-caption decoders**
- **Removing structural communication barriers**
- **Providing alternative service**
- **Following accessibility standards**

What are some READILY ACHIEVABLE STRATEGIES FOR REMOVAL OF STRUCTURAL BARRIERS?

- **Installing sound buffers**

- **Installing flashing alarm lights**

- **Integrating visual alarms**

- **Removing physical partitions**

- **Providing directional signage**

What is needed for SIGNAGE AND SYMBOLS OF COMMUNICATION ACCESSIBILITY?

- **Symbols for:**
  ⇒ **Telephone accessibility**
  ⇒ **TDDs**

- **Signage:**
  ⇒ **Directional signage**
  ⇒ **Messages for availability of Assistive Listening Devices**
  ⇒ **Messages for communication aids and services**

What is the best way to ensure COST-EFFECTIVE ADA COMPLIANCE?

- **Perform a facility accessibility audit**
- **Determine aids and services needs**
- **Develop a plan to remove barriers and acquire assistive devices**
- **Perform ongoing audit and maintenance of accessibility features**
- **Modify discriminatory policies, practices, and procedures**
- **Obtain technical assistance and consultation**

What is the BOTTOM LINE?

- **Ask people about their needs**

- **Show respect and sensitivity**

- **Use what works**

INSERVICE QUIZ ON THE ADA

Score: _____   Name: _____

Pass   Fail   (Circle one)   Dept: _____

                                 Date: _____

Multiple Choice: Please circle the most appropriate answer for each item.

1. What year was the ADA passed?

    A. 1970
    B. 1980
    C. 1990
    D. none of the above

2. The ADA protects persons with disabilities in

    A. places of employment that receive federal funds.
    B. all places of employment.
    C. federal job situations only.
    D. none of the above

3. What is not required to achieve effective communication under the ADA?

    A. providing necessary auxiliary communication aids and services
    B. making aurally (via hearing) delivered information available
    C. making personally prescribed devices such as hearing aids available
    D. none of the above

4. Communication barriers can be

    A. visually related barriers.
    B. acoustically related barriers.
    C. attitudinal and prejudicial barriers.
    D. A and B
    E. all of the above

5. Which is/are acoustically related barriers?

    A. high noise levels
    B. lack of visual information
    C. high reverberation levels
    D. A and C
    E. all of the above

6. Closed-caption decoders are found on

    A. telephones.
    B. televisions.
    C. fire alarms.
    D. none of the above

7. Which of the following is the International Symbol of Accessibility?

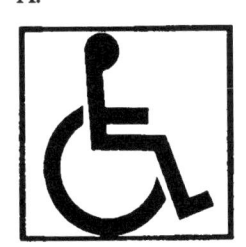

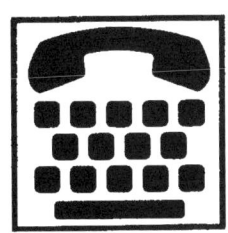

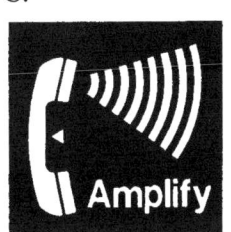

   A.   B.   C.

8. A TDD is used

    A. for television viewing.
    B. as an alerting device.
    C. for telephone communication.
    D. none of the above

9. Hearing assistance dogs

    A. are sometimes discriminated against.
    B. should be allowed the same accessibility as visual assistance dogs.
    C. are less important than visual assistance dogs.
    D. both A and B
    E. none of the above

10. The bottom line with the ADA involves

    A. asking people about their needs.
    B. showing respect and sensitivity.
    C. using what works.
    D. all of the above

APPENDIX V-E

Inservice on Hearing Loss and Its Effect on Communication

Behavioral Objectives

Through participation in this inservice, attendees will be able to:
- Identify the three parts of the ear and describe their function
- Describe at least two pathological conditions in each part of the ear
- Understand the audiogram with regard to:
  ⇒ Frequency
  ⇒ Intensity
  ⇒ Decibel (dB)
  ⇒ Air-conduction testing
  ⇒ Bone-conduction testing
  ⇒ Normal hearing
  ⇒ Conductive hearing loss
  ⇒ Sensorineural hearing loss
  ⇒ Mixed hearing loss
  ⇒ Speech banana
  ⇒ Normal conversational level
- Conceptualize the "Audiogram of Familiar Sounds"
- Explain the lifestyle effects of hearing loss

Suggested Time Allotment

About 1 hour, 30 minutes
- Introduction (10 minutes)
- Anatomy of the ear (15 minutes)
- Audiogram (20 minutes)
- Break (10 minutes)
- Lifestyle effects of hearing loss (15 minutes)
- Group activity (10 minutes)
- Quiz (10 minutes)

Format

Informational

Suggested Materials

- Audiogram from your facility depicting a moderate hearing loss. (Make handout and overhead of the audiogram to include with inservice materials in this appendix.)
- Overhead projector
- VCR and monitor
- Slide projector
- CD player or tape recorder
- Slides illustrating auditory pathologies
- Appropriate handouts
- Appropriate overheads
- Earplugs
- Audiometer earphones
- Bone conduction oscillator
- Screening audiometers

Selected Participant Activities

- Ask for a few volunteers at the beginning of the inservice to wear earplugs for five minutes during the introduction and to discuss their experiences and feelings with the audience.
- Videotape a favorite sitcom and play the sample to the audience without any sound and ask them what is going on in the episode.
- Play commercially available audio materials (e.g., CD or audiotape) that simulate hearing loss.
- Pass out earplugs and ask participants to wear them for 10 minutes while talking to each other. Edwards (1995) suggested demonstrating some of the following concepts during the simulation by having participants:

  ⇒ vary speaker-to-listener distance,
  ⇒ restrict visual cues,
  ⇒ converse in a background of noise,
  ⇒ change the topic of conversation with every other communication turn, and
  ⇒ compare the understandability of vowels to consonants.

HANDOUTS

WHAT IS HEARING LOSS AND HOW DOES IT AFFECT COMMUNICATION?

- **How does the ear work?**

    ⇒ First, a picture:

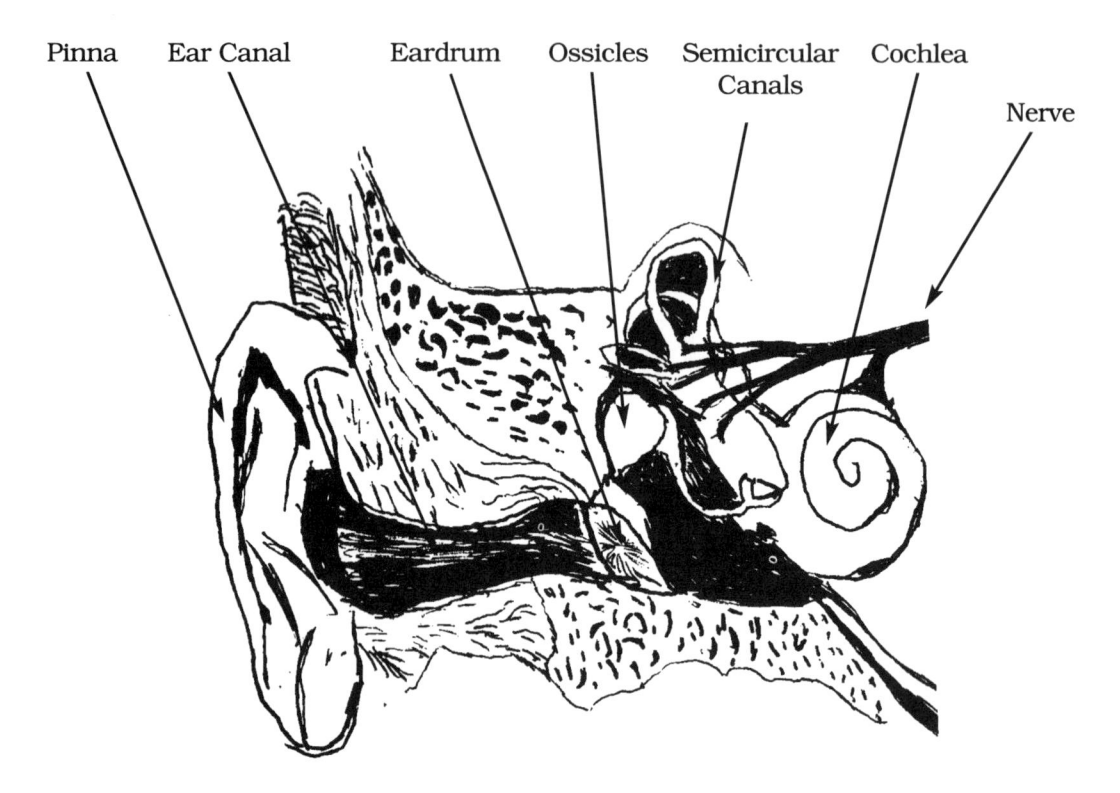

    Pinna   Ear Canal   Eardrum   Ossicles   Semicircular Canals   Cochlea   Nerve

    (Note: Drawing is not to scale)

    ⇒ The ear has three parts:
    - ➢ The outer ear consists of the pinna and the ear canal. The pinna collects sound, and the ear canal funnels it toward the eardrum.
    - ➢ The middle ear consists of the eardrum, ossicles (ear bones), middle ear space, muscles, tendons, and ligaments. The eardrum changes the sound energy into mechanical-vibrational energy that travels across the ossicles. The first bone is the malleus (hammer), the second is the incus (anvil), and the last is the stapes (stirrup). The stapes vibrates in and out of a window that leads to the fluid-filled inner ear.
    - ➢ The inner ear consists of three main parts: the vestibule, the semicircular canals, and the cochlea. The movement of the stapes sets up waves in the inner ear fluid. Hair cells sense the waves and cause electrical impulses to be sent up the VIIIth nerve (or hearing and balance nerve) to the brain for meaning.

- **What are some auditory problems and what types of hearing loss can they cause?**

  ⇒ Conductive hearing loss occurs when there is a problem in the outer ear, the middle ear, or the parts of the ears responsible for sending sound to the inner ear. Outer ear problems include impacted earwax (cerumen), or an infection that causes blockage in the external ear canal. Middle-ear problems include fluid in the middle ear caused by an ear infection or perforations in the eardrum. Many conductive hearing losses can be corrected through medical intervention.

  ⇒ Sensorineural hearing loss occurs when there is a problem in the inner ear. Most often, sensorineural hearing losses are the result of the hair cells dying from such things as noise exposure, certain types of drugs, or the aging process. In most cases, sensorineural hearing losses cannot be corrected through medical intervention, and patients require use of hearing aids and aural rehabilitation.

  ⇒ Mixed hearing loss occurs when there is a problem in both the conductive and the sensorineural mechanism. Again, in most cases, the problem in the conductive mechanism can be corrected, but the problem involving the sensorineural mechanism cannot.

- **How is hearing sensitivity measured?**

Hearing is measured with an instrument called an audiometer. The audiometer can present tones of varying frequencies and intensities to the patient via earphones (air conduction) or through a bone oscillator that is placed on the mastoid bone behind the ear. Air conduction tests all three parts of the ear. Bone conduction directly tests the inner ear by vibrating the bones of the skull and bypassing the conductive mechanism.

Patients press a button or raise their hands when they hear a tone. Patients' thresholds are obtained for both ears via air conduction and bone conduction. Threshold is the softest tone in decibels (dB) that a patient hears 50% of the time. Decibels are used to measure the intensity of a sound.

Thresholds are obtained for different frequencies, measured in Hertz (Hz), that indicate different pitches. The frequencies of 250 through 8000 Hz are assessed for air conduction and 250 through 4000 Hz for bone conduction.

Patients' thresholds are recorded on an audiogram, which is a graph with two axes. The horizontal axis represents frequency, and the vertical axis represents intensity. Patients' thresholds are plotted using special symbols. For example, for a patient who hears a 1000 Hz tone, at 10 dB 50% of the time via air conduction in the right ear, a red circle will be placed at the intersection point of 1000 Hz and 10 dB. The air-conduction symbol for the left ear is a blue "X." As can be seen from the legend, there is a variety of symbols that can be used, most of which we will not cover today. Although a complete audiogram includes both air and bone conduction, hearing sensitivity is classified on the basis of air-conduction thresholds. Straight lines connect the air-conduction symbols for the right ear and for the left ear as in the example. It is important to note that the relationship between patients' air and bone conduction assists the audiologist in differentially diagnosing the type of hearing loss, which will not be covered here. However, patients with a conductive or mixed hearing loss must be referred for medical management.

■ What is considered normal hearing?

Normal hearing sensitivity is defined as thresholds that range from −10 dB to +10 dB. Thresholds falling out of this range are considered abnormal or consistent with a hearing loss. Hearing loss has degrees of severity based on the dB range where thresholds are found. Stach (1998) listed the following degrees of hearing impairment based on specific dB ranges:

Degree of Loss	Range in dB
Normal	−10 to 10
Minimal	11 to 24
Mild	25 to 39
Moderate	40 to 54
Moderately severe	55 to 69
Severe	70 to 89
Profound	90 plus

Usually, a patient's overall classification of hearing sensitivity for each ear is based on the average thresholds taken at 500, 1000, and 2000 Hz, which is known as the pure-tone average. Consider an example from the attached audiogram. The pure-tone average for both ears is 45 dB, so the patient has a moderate degree of hearing loss.

■ What are the functional effects of hearing loss?

So far, we have considered the audiometric effects of hearing loss. Stach (1998) has determined the communication effects of different degrees of hearing loss as follows:

Degree of Loss	Communication Problem
Minimal	Difficulty hearing faint speech in a noisy environment
Mild	Difficulty hearing faint or distant speech, even in a quiet
Moderate	Hears conversational speech only at a close distance
Moderately severe	Hears loud conversational speech
Severe	Cannot hear conversational speech
Profound	May hear loud sounds; hearing is not the primary communication channel

The patient in our example can hear conversational speech only at a close distance.

A more specific way to determine the effect of hearing loss on communication is to use the "Audiogram of Familiar Sounds." The Audiogram of Familiar Sounds places sounds we encounter everyday onto the audiogram taking into consideration their frequency and intensity characteristics. For example, loud sounds, such as a chain saw, are toward the bottom of the audiogram, whereas very soft sounds, such as leaves rustling, are at the top. When the audiometric symbols of our patient are placed on this audiogram, the familiar sounds that the patient can hear fall below the audiometric symbols (toward the bottom of the page) and the inaudible sounds are above the audiometric symbols (toward the top of the page).

THE IMPACT OF HEARING LOSS ON EDUCATION: THIRTEEN FACTS[1]

- Hearing screening procedures identify less than 50% of children with significant hearing loss.
- Medically, a child is not considered to have a hearing loss until hearing is worse than 25 dB. A 25 dB hearing loss is similar to going through life with your fingers plugging your ears.
- Middle ear infections also cause a "plugged ear effect." Consider these statistics:
  ⇒ 66% of preschoolers have at least one episode of ear problems.
  ⇒ 16% of preschoolers have six or more episodes.
  ⇒ 50% of all episodes of ear problems go undetected by parents and teachers.
  ⇒ Preschoolers can still continue to have ear problems even with excellent medical intervention.
- Children in the fourth grade who have 25 dB hearing losses are two grade levels behind in reading when compared to their peers with normal hearing.
- Children with hearing loss also experience delayed language development when compared to their peers with normal hearing. As can be seen from the following, the greater the hearing loss, the greater the delay:

Degree of Loss	*Language Delay in Years*
15–26 dB	1.2
27–40 dB	2.0
41–55 dB	2.9
56–70 dB	3.5 +

- Twenty-five percent of children with learning disabilities have histories of or ongoing ear problems, and 38% have been found to have abnormal audiometric thresholds.
- Eighty-nine percent of children with hyperactivity have had three or more episodes of ear problems, and 74% of these children have had 10 or more episodes.
- Hearing loss may be more common in children with other developmental delays. For example, the incidence of hearing loss in the Down Syndrome population ranges from 23 to 90%, and 40 to 50% have hearing loss greater than 25 dB in both ears.
- Chronic hearing loss can limit the achievement of gifted children.
- Children who have a hearing loss of at least 30 dB in one ear have 10 times the risk for failing a grade in school. In addition, 50% of these children have failed one or more grades or are receiving special services.
- Noise-induced hearing loss is a serious concern in the school-age population. The incidence of this type of hearing loss is 22% in the high school population.
- The efficacy of hearing aids for children with hearing loss is severely restricted in classrooms that have high noise levels and hard surfaces that increase reverberation time.

---

[1]Adapted from "Thirteen Facts on the Impact of Hearing Loss on Education," 1996, by K. Anderson, *The Hearing Review*, *3*(9), 28.

INSTRUCTOR OVERHEADS

What does the ear LOOK LIKE?

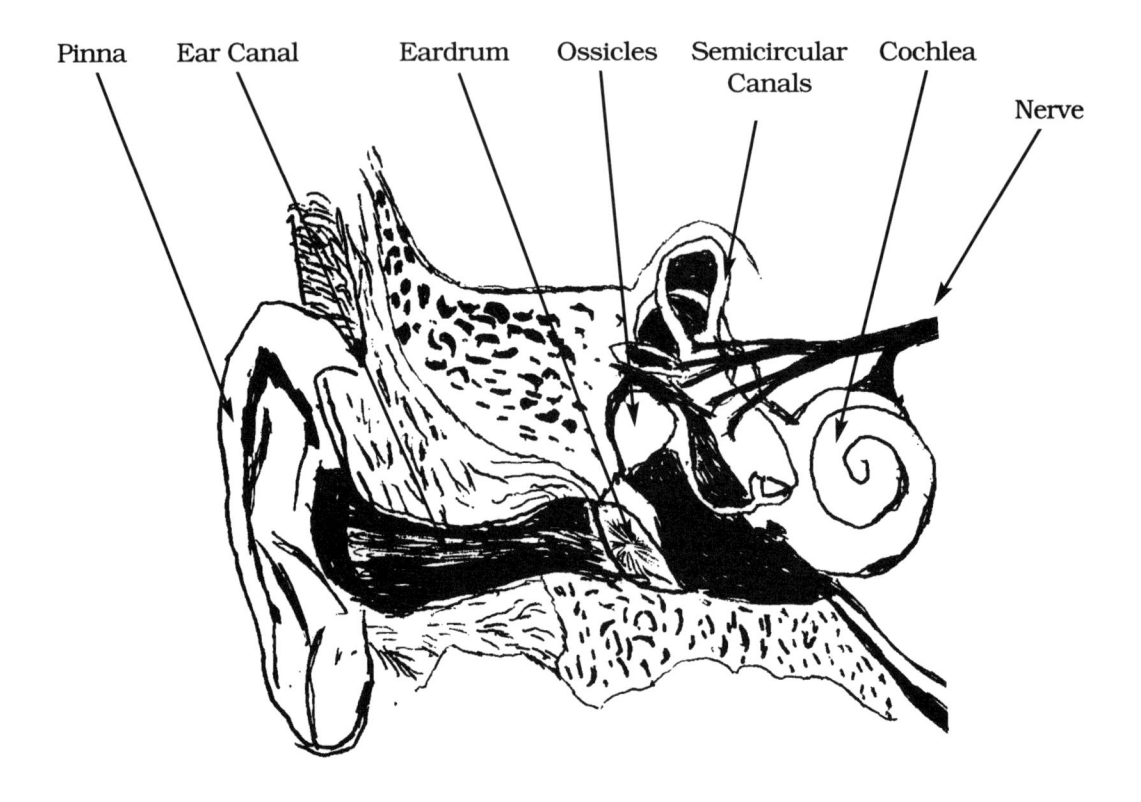

Pinna · Ear Canal · Eardrum · Ossicles · Semicircular Canals · Cochlea · Nerve

(Note: Drawing is not to scale)

How does the ear WORK?
The ear has three parts, each with a job:

- **Outer ear**
    - ⇒ **Pinna—collects sound**
    - ⇒ **Ear canal—channels sound**

- **Middle ear**
    - ⇒ **Eardrum—changes sound to vibrations**
    - ⇒ **Ossicles—carry vibrations to fluid of inner ear**

- **Inner ear**
    - ⇒ **Cochlea—hearing**
        - ✓ **Hair cells—change wave energy to electrical impulses**
    - ⇒ **Semicircular canals—balance**
    - ⇒ **Vestibule—balance**

What are some AUDITORY PROBLEMS and the types of HEARING LOSS that they cause?

- **Conductive hearing loss**
    - ⇒ **Outer ear: impacted earwax, severe infection**
    - ⇒ **Middle ear: eardrum perforations, middle ear fluid**

- **Sensorineural hearing loss: hair cell death due to noise exposure, aging**

- **Mixed hearing loss: combination of conductive and sensorineural hearing loss**

How is hearing sensitivity MEASURED?

- **Audiometer—an instrument that emits tones of varying frequencies and intensities via:**
  ⇒ **Earphones, which use air conduction to assess outer, middle, and inner ear**
  ⇒ **Bone oscillator, which uses bone conduction to assess inner ear directly**

- **Audiogram—thresholds are plotted using special symbols on this graph that has two axes:**
  ⇒ **The horizontal axis plots frequency (pitch) in Hertz (Hz) from 250 to 8000 Hz.**
  ⇒ **The vertical axis plots intensity (loudness) in decibels (dB) from –10 to 120 dB.**

- **Differential diagnosis—requires an analysis of the relationship between air-conduction and bone-conduction thresholds.**

What is NORMAL HEARING?

Degree of Loss	Range in dB
Normal	–10 to 10
Minimal	11 to 24
Mild	25 to 39
Moderate	40 to 54
Moderately severe	55 to 69
Severe	70 to 89
Profound	90 plus

What are the COMMUNICATION EFFECTS of hearing loss?

Degree of Loss	*Problem*
Minimal	Difficulty hearing faint speech in a noisy environment
Mild	Difficulty hearing faint or distant speech, even in a quiet environment
Moderate	Hears speech at a conversational level only at a close distance
Moderately severe	Hears loud conversational speech
Severe	Cannot hear conversational speech
Profound	May hear loud sounds; hearing is not the primary communication channel

Audiogram of Familiar Sounds

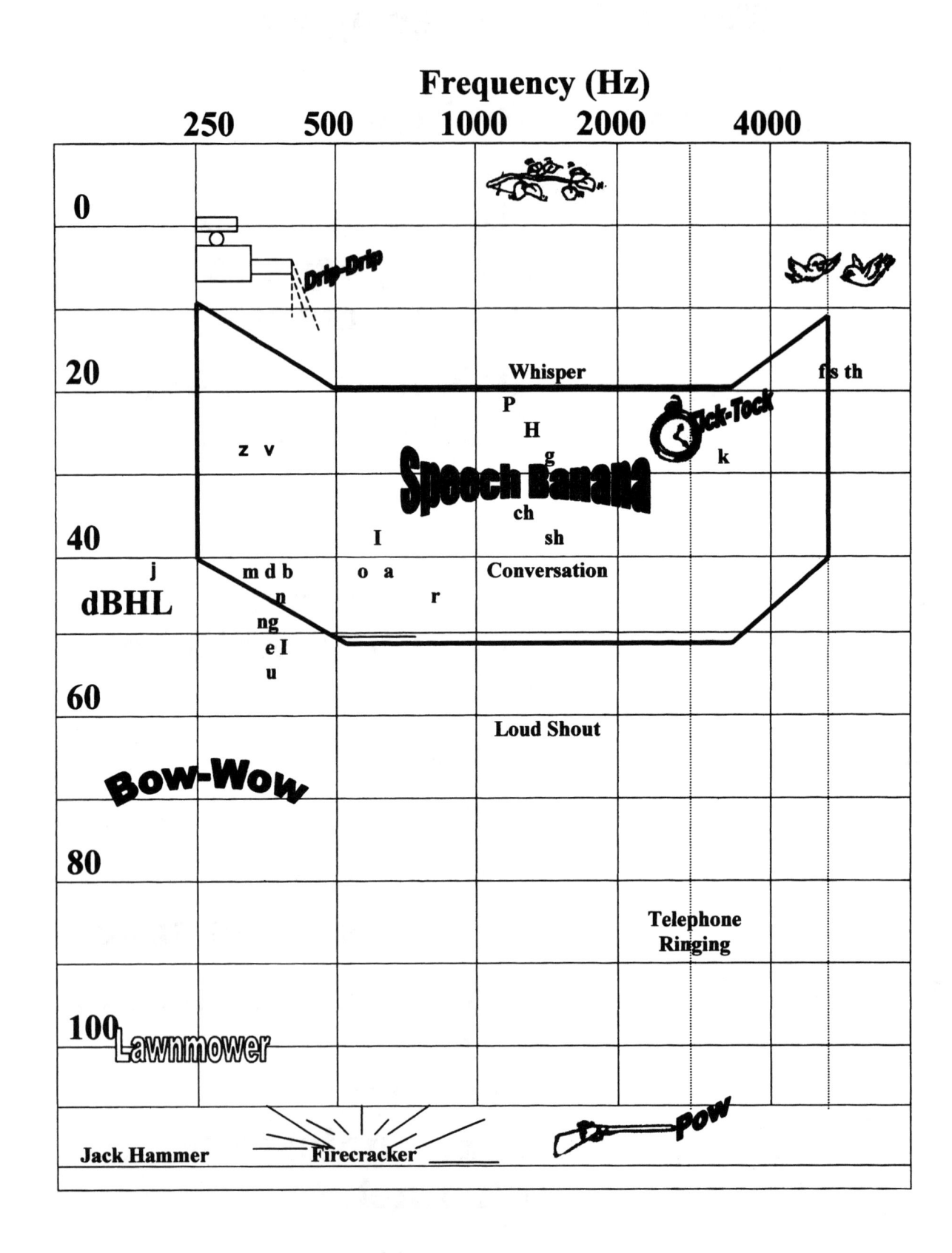

Frequency (Hz)

	250	500	1000	2000	4000

0

Drip-Drip

20 — Whisper — f s th

P
H g
z v — Speech Banana — Tick-Tock k
ch
40 — I — sh
j — m d b — o a — Conversation
n — r
dBHL — ng
e I
u

60

Bow-Wow — Loud Shout

80

Telephone Ringing

100 Lawnmower

Jack Hammer — Firecracker — Pow

INSERVICE QUIZ ON HEARING LOSS AND ITS EFFECT ON COMMUNICATION

Score:_____   Name: _____
Pass   Fail   (Circle one)   Dept: _____
                                 Date: _____

Multiple Choice: Please circle the most appropriate answer for each item.

1. The ossicles are found in the

    A. outer ear.
    B. middle ear.
    C. inner ear.
    D. none of the above

2. The function of the eardrum is to

    A. collect sound.
    B. change sound to mechanical-vibrational energy.
    C. funnel sound.
    D. none of the above

3. The sensorineural mechanism consists of the

    A. outer ear.
    B. middle ear.
    C. inner ear.
    D. both A and B
    E. none of the above

4. Testing by air conduction

    A. requires earphones.
    B. assesses outer, middle, and inner ears.
    C. assesses inner ear only.
    D. A and B
    E. none of the above

5. A perforated eardrum may result in a

    A. conductive hearing loss.
    B. sensorineural hearing loss.
    C. either
    D. none of the above

6. Which statement(s) is/are false about the audiogram?

    A. Frequency is represented on the horizontal axis.
    B. Intensity is represented on the horizontal axis.
    C. Straight lines connect air conduction symbols in each ear.
    D. B and C
    E. none of the above

7. For which of the following is hearing usually not the primary channel for communication?

    A. moderate
    B. moderately severe
    C. severe
    D. none of the above

8. Which of the following will a patient with a severe hearing loss not be able to hear?

    A. whispering
    B. a dog barking at very close range
    C. leaves rustling
    D. A and C
    E. none of the above

9. Pure-tone average

    A. is an average of the air-conduction thresholds taken at 500, 1000, and 2000 Hz.
    B. is used to determine degree of hearing loss.
    C. is the average of all the air-conduction thresholds.
    D. A and B
    E. none of the above

10. The speech banana

    A. is also called the speech boat.
    B. is the area where most of the speech sounds can be found.
    C. is the area in which conversational speech has most of its energy.
    D. all of the above

APPENDIX V-F

Inservice on, "How Do You Communicate With Someone With a Hearing Loss?"

Behavioral Objectives

Through participation in this inservice, attendees will be able to:
- Use appropriate communication strategies with persons who have hearing impairment
- Understand the effects of noise and reverberation on speech recognition
- Implement strategies to decrease communication barriers in the environment

Suggested Time Allotment

About 1 hour, 20 minutes
- Introduction (5 minutes)
- Communication Tips (15 minutes)
- Acoustic Barriers to Communication (15 minutes)
- Strategies for Removing Communication Barriers (15 minutes)
- Questions and Answers (5-10 minutes)
- Group Activity (20 minutes)

Format

Informational

Suggested Materials

- Overhead projectors
- Appropriate handouts
- Portable tape recorder and multitalker tape

Suggested Participant Activities

- Form discussion groups to analyze the appropriateness of acoustic environments within the facility
- Practice "clear speech"
- Problem solve difficult communication situations

HANDOUTS

HOW DO YOU COMMUNICATE WITH SOMEONE WITH A HEARING LOSS?[1]

Communication Barriers

- *Visually related barriers*

  ⇒ Lack of visual aspects of speech

  ⇒ Lack of appropriate signage directing individuals with hearing impairment to devices for communication accessibility

- *Acoustically related barriers*

  ⇒ **Reverberation** is the continuation of sound in a room due to reflections off of room surfaces that distorts speech energy.

  ⇒ **Noise** is any unwanted sound and is of three types:

  ✔ **External noise:** comes from outside the building (e.g., traffic noise)

  ✔ **Internal noise:** comes from inside the building, but not from inside the room (e.g., people walking in the hallway)

  ✔ **Room noise:** comes from inside the room

- *Attitudinal and prejudicial barriers*

  ⇒ Negative attitudes toward persons with disabilities

  ⇒ Failure to modify communication style for persons with hearing impairment

- *Information complexity*

  ⇒ Presence of unimportant details

  ⇒ Overly complicated syntax

  ⇒ Unfamiliar vocabulary

The Communication Process

Communication is a two-way process. Both the listener and speaker must cooperate to optimize communication.

---

[1]Adapted from *Communication and the ADA (Effective Communication and Accessibility)*, 1995, by the American Speech-Language-Hearing Association, pp. 1–4. Rockville, MD: Author; and "How to gain a larger slice of the "communication pie," 1996, by D. Wayner and J. Abrahamson, *The Hearing Review*, 3(9), 32–34.

The listener with hearing loss can:

- **Provide feedback.** If listeners can tell their communication partner what they have heard, both parties will know if the message was understood.

- **Pay attention.** Listener concentration is very important.

- **Develop good listening skills.** The listener must concentrate on what is being said.

- **Observe the talker.** The listener needs both the visual and auditory information to understand the message.

- **Plan ahead.** The listener should anticipate potential communication challenges and obstacles.

- **Take breaks if needed.** If fatigued, the listener may need to take some time out from communication to improve concentration.

- **Make specific suggestions.** The listener should ask the speaker to make a modification in the manner of communication to improve speech understanding.

- **Double check details:** Listeners should repeat what the speaker has said, especially dates and times, to confirm understanding.

- **Set realistic expectations:** Listeners must realize that communication may be impossible in some situations with excessive background noise.

- **Should not bluff:** Listeners should not pretend to understand when they do not.

The speaker can:

- **Get the listener's attention.** If you wait until the listener is ready to begin talking, you may not have to repeat yourself.

- **Not shout.** Talking louder does not help.

- **Slow down a bit:** Talking just a little slower can help, but talking too slow can make matters worse.

- **Get close.** Moving closer to your listener before speaking reduces the urge to shout and makes you easier to understand.

- **Speak clearly.** Don't over exaggerate pronunciation, but do finish all of the sounds of one word before beginning the next.

- **Rephrase.** If your listener doesn't understand you the first time, use different words to express the same idea.

- ***State the topic.*** Inform your listener of the topic of conversation and whenever the topic changes.

- ***Use gestures.*** This can help your listener understand better.

- ***Notice background noise.*** Turn televisions and radios down or move to a quiet area. Be extra vigilant of your communication style in a noisy place.

- ***Confirm details.*** Politely double check to make sure your listener has understood the details of the message (i.e., meeting times and places).

- ***Be visible.*** Make sure your listener can see your face when you speak.

- ***Simplify the message.*** Eliminate useless details; use simple syntax and familiar vocabulary.

INSTRUCTOR OVERHEADS

COMMUNICATION BARRIERS

- **VISUALLY related barriers**

- **ACOUSTICALLY related barriers**
    - ⇒ **Reverberation**
    - ⇒ **Noise**
        - ✓ **External**
        - ✓ **Internal**
        - ✓ **Room**

- **ATTITUDINAL and PREJUDICIAL barriers**

- **INFORMATION complexity**

COMMUNICATION IS A TWO-WAY PROCESS

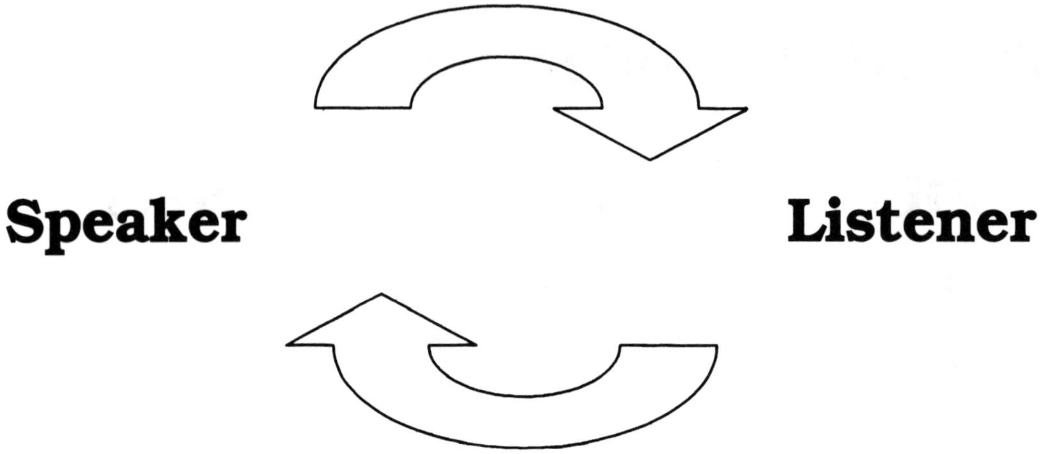

Speaker ⟷ **Listener**

LISTENERS can:

- **Provide feedback.**

- **Pay attention.**

- **Develop good listening skills.**

- **Observe the talker.**

- **Plan ahead.**

- **Take breaks if needed.**

- **Make specific suggestions to the speaker on how to communicate.**

- **Double check details.**

- **Set realistic expectations.**

- **Not bluff.**

SPEAKERS can:

- **Get the listener's attention.**
- **Not shout.**
- **Slow down a bit.**
- **Get close.**
- **Speak clearly.**
- **Rephrase.**
- **State the topic.**
- **Use gestures.**
- **Notice background noise.**
- **Confirm details.**
- **Be visible.**
- **Simplify the message.**

INSERVICE QUIZ ON COMMUNICATION TIPS

Score:_____   Name: _____

Pass   Fail   (Circle one)   Dept: _____

                                 Date: _____

True and False: Put "T" for true and "F" for false.

_____ 1. Communication is a two-way process involving both the speaker and the listener.

_____ 2. Visually related barriers refer to inaccessibility of the visual aspects of speech only.

_____ 3. Internal noise originates from inside the room.

_____ 4. Reverberation is the continuation of sound in a room due to reflections off of room surfaces that distorts speech energy.

_____ 5. Noise is any unwanted sound.

_____ 6. Overarticulating greatly improves listener's speech understanding.

_____ 7. People walking in the hallway is an example of external noise.

_____ 8. Using simple syntax and familiar vocabulary words reduces the complexity of information.

_____ 9. Listeners should pretend they understand the speaker even when they don't.

_____ 10. Attitudinal and prejudicial barriers include people's negative attitudes toward the disabled.

APPENDIX V-G

Inservice on Understanding Hearing Aids, Their Care, and Their Use

Behavioral Objectives

Covered in chapter

Suggested Time Allotment

Covered in chapter

Format

Combination informational and skill-based

Suggested Materials

- Overhead projectors
- Other materials covered in chapter

Suggested Participant Activities

- Set up five learning stations with learning guides
- Participants rotate throughout all stations learning skills

HANDOUTS AND OVERHEADS

STATION 1: DIFFERENT TYPES OF HEARING AIDS AND THEIR PARTS

All hearing aids work on the same principle. They also have the same three basic parts.

- Microphone: changes acoustic energy to electric energy
- Amplifier: amplifies sound
- Receiver: changes electric energy into acoustic energy

The illustration below shows a generic hearing aid:

BLOCK DIAGRAM OF A GENERIC HEARING AID

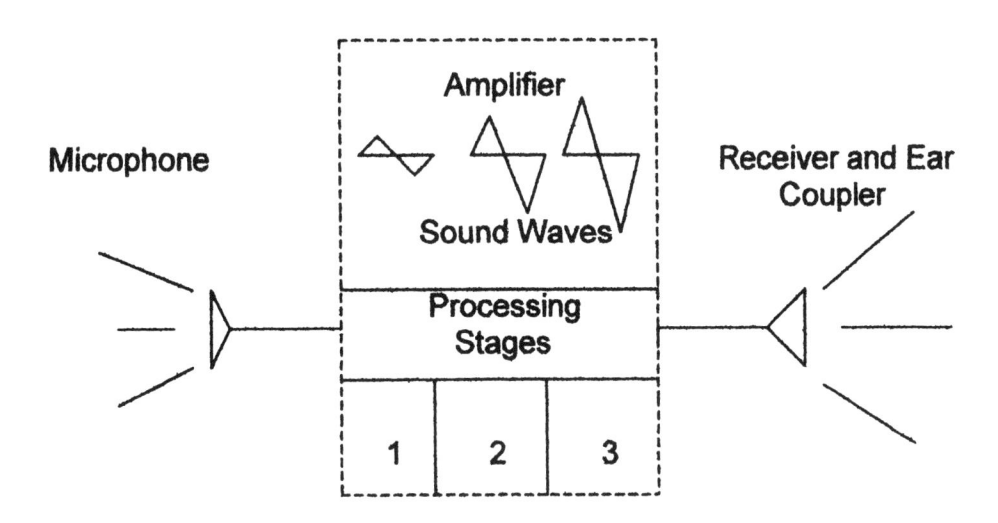

There are several styles of hearing aids. We will review the three most common types and their parts:

- Behind-the-ear hearing aid: has an earmold to attach the hearing aid to ear. The hearing aid is situated behind the pinna.
- Classic In-the-ear hearing aid: has its components built into an ear piece. The hearing aid is situated in the concha.
- In-the-canal hearing aid: has its components built into an ear piece. The hearing aid is situated in the ear canal.

Behind-the-ear Hearing Aid[1]

Internal Parts — External Parts

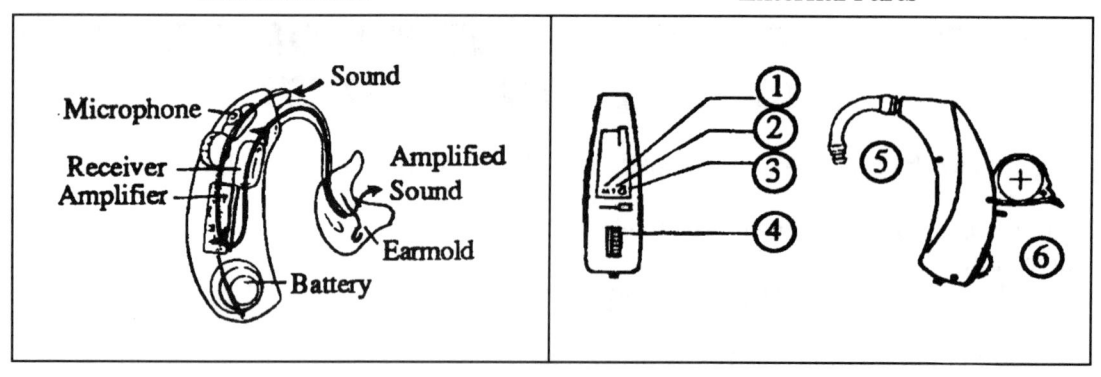

Legend
3 Position Telecoil Switch
1. Microphone
2. Telephone
3. Off
4. Volume Control
5. Earhook
6. Battery Compartment

In-the-Ear Styles of Hearing Aids

Classic In-the-Ear Style — In-the-Canal Style
Outside — Inside

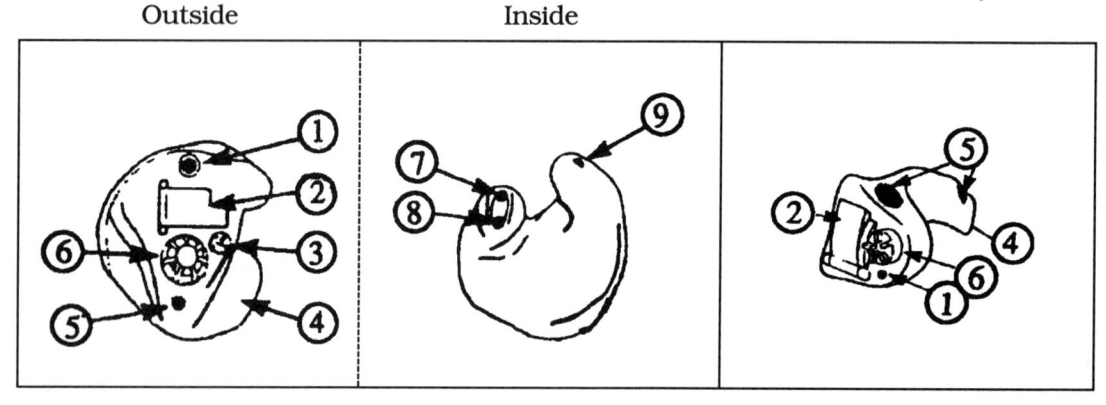

Legend
1. Microphone
2. Battery Compartment
3. Control (optional)
4. Canal portion
5. Vent
6. Volume control
7. Sound bore
8. Vent
9. Identification

---

[1]Pictures on this page are from *Hearing Aids: A User's Guide* by W. J. Staab, 1991, pp. 60–61. Phoenix, AZ: Author. Reprinted with permission.

STATION 2: HEARING AID BATTERIES

All hearing aids run on batteries. Each hearing aid runs on a particular size of battery that is designated by a number. Each battery has a positive and a negative side. The positive side is smooth and marked with a "+," whereas the unmarked negative side has a ridge. The life of a hearing aid battery depends on several factors, such as the strength of the hearing aid, the volume-wheel setting used by the patient, and the number of hours per day the hearing aid is in use. Generally, hearing aid batteries last between 10 to 14 days. Battery checkers should be available in the hearing aid check kits; one is pictured below. Batteries should have at least 1.4 volts. Batteries are poisonous and should be kept away from children and pets. Furthermore, hearing aids should be shut off with the battery drawer open at night. Your learning guide will show you how to check the battery and how to insert and remove it from a hearing aid. Zinc air batteries are commonly used in hearing aids. Remember to remove the paper-tape tab from the battery before inserting it into the battery compartment.

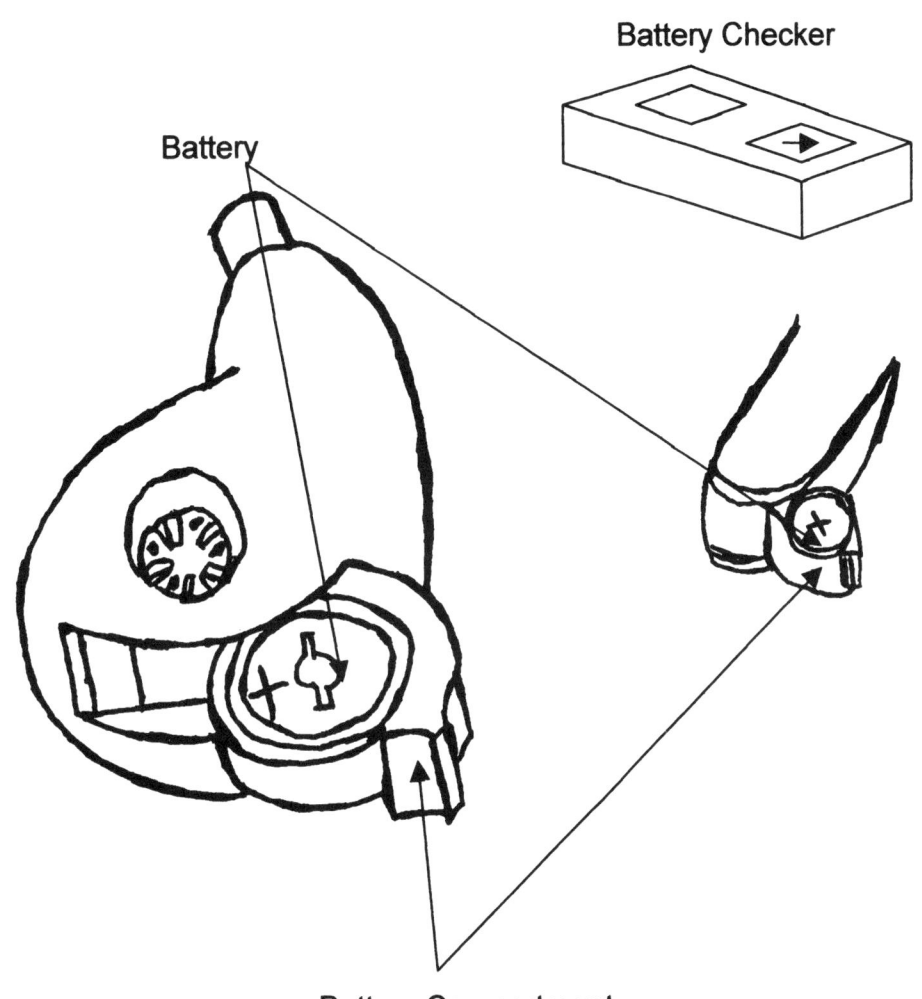

STATION 3: INSERTION AND REMOVAL OF A HEARING AID FROM AN EAR

Insertion and removal of a hearing aid from a person's ear is not as difficult as it looks. First, you must realize that hearing aids are made specifically for the left or for the right ear. Second, the in-the-ear and the in-the-canal hearing aids for the right ear are usually marked with a red dot, and those for left ear are marked with a blue dot. Third, although earmolds for behind-the-ear hearing aids are not marked in this way, they too are specifically made for either the right ear or the left ear. Your learning guide will show you how to tell a right from a left earmold.

Now that you can distinguish between right and left, you're ready to practice insertion and removal of the hearing aid from an ear. If persons are incapacitated, you will have to do this for them. The first thing to remember is that neither the hearing aid nor the patient's ear are extremely fragile. It is OK to pull on the pinna to straighten out the ear canal for hearing aid insertion. Here is a list of steps to follow:

- Wear gloves for Universal Precautions, when necessary.

- Make sure that the volume-control wheel is rolled all the way down when inserting or removing the hearing aid from an ear. Otherwise, the hearing aid will whistle loudly into the patient's ear, which could be painful.

- Try to orient the hearing aid. Hold it in one hand as it would be positioned in the patient's ear. Your other hand should be free to manipulate the pinna.

- The hearing aid should slip right into the ear. If not, pull backward and upward on the pinna to straighten out the ear canal so the hearing aid can slide into place.

- Once the hearing aid is in the ear, try rolling the volume-control wheel up very slowing. Gently experiment with the volume-control wheel by talking to the patient and asking which setting sounds best.

- Now try on a pretend ear. Let your learning guide assist you.

- Insertion of behind-the-ear hearing aids is similar to in-the-ear hearing aids except you are placing an earmold in the ear. When the earmold is securely in place, simply slip the behind-the-ear hearing aid behind the pinna. Try it! Your learning guide will assist you.

STATION 4: TROUBLESHOOTING HEARING AIDS

You may be asked to try to determine why a patient's hearing aid is not working. There are several causes of hearing aid malfunction that you can check for and correct.

- Check the battery:
  ⇒ Open the battery drawer and make sure the battery is inserted properly. If not, the hearing aid will be inoperable. In most cases, the battery drawer will not close if the battery has been placed incorrectly into the drawer.
  ⇒ Remove the battery from the drawer and check it with the battery tester. If the battery is weak (< 1.4 volts) or dead, replace it.
- Listen to a hearing aid with a stethoscope:
  ⇒ Connect the end of the hearing aid stethoscope to the part of the hearing aid that goes into the patient's ear.
  ⇒ Turn the hearing aid on.
  ⇒ Gently talk into the hearing aid.
  ⇒ Slowly turn the volume wheel up.
    ✓ Does the aid sound loud enough?
    ✓ Does it have any strange sounds coming out?
    ✓ Do you hear any humming or buzzing?
  ⇒ If everything sounds OK, you have succeeded. If not, continue on.
- Check the part of the hearing aid that goes into the patient's ear. If it is blocked with earwax, gently remove it with a small brush or wax loop.
- Look at the earmold or hearing aid to determine if it is properly inserted into the ear. If not, try reinserting it.
- Make sure that the hearing aid is "ON." Behind-the-ear hearing aids have an "MTO" switch. Make sure the switch is on "M" for microphone. The "T" is for telephone listening only and "O" is off.
- If none of the above strategies work, contact the audiologist

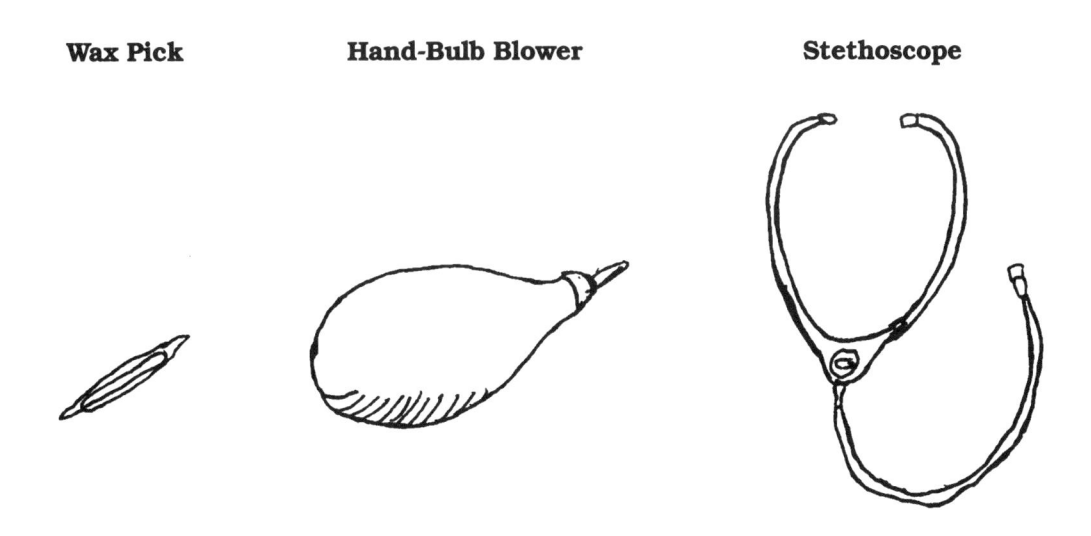

Wax Pick   **Hand-Bulb Blower**   **Stethoscope**

STATION 5: ASSISTIVE LISTENING DEVICES

The Americans with Disabilities Act (ADA), which requires that assistive devices be made available for persons with disabilities, was passed in 1990. One category of assistive devices is assistive listening devices for persons with hearing impairment. Assistive listening devices can be especially critical for patients in an acute-care hospital, rehabilitation hospital, or long-term residential care facility who need to communicate with others (e.g., family members, occupational therapists, physical therapists, physicians, speech-language pathologists, etc.) but don't have hearing aids. Assistive listening devices can also assist patients when they are talking on the telephone or watching television. Your learning guide will show you the assistive listening devices available at your facility.

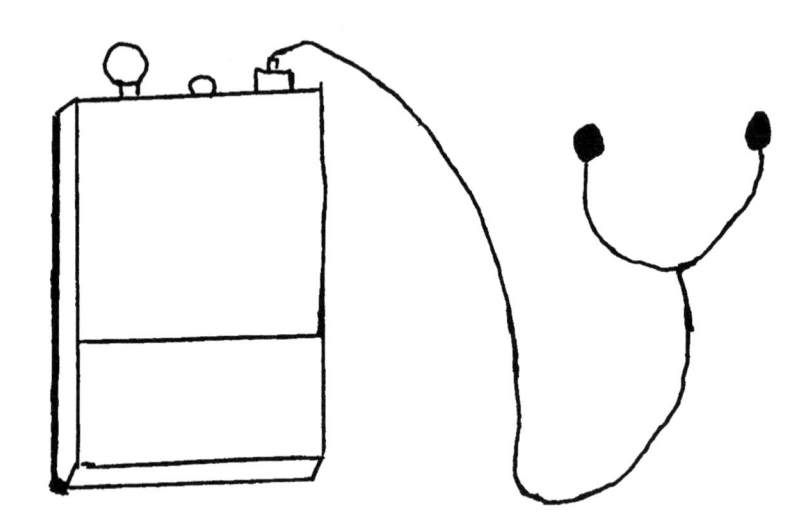

Assistive Listening Device

INSERVICE QUIZ ON UNDERSTANDING HEARING AIDS, THEIR CARE, AND THEIR USE

Score:_____   Name: _____
Pass   Fail   (Circle one)   Dept: _____
                               Date: _____

Multiple Choice: Please select the most appropriate answer for each item.

1. Which of the following is not a standard part for a generic hearing aid?

    A. microphone
    B. receiver
    C. AC adapter
    D. none of the above

2. The microphone changes

    A. acoustic energy to electric energy.
    B. electric energy to acoustic energy.
    C. acoustic energy to mechanical energy.
    D. none of the above

3. Batteries should last

    A. 1 to 4 days.
    B. 10 to 14 days.
    C. 4 to 5 weeks.
    D. none of the above

4. Which statement is true?

    A. Behind-the-ear hearing aids require use of an earmold.
    B. Batteries should have 1.0 volts.
    C. Hearing aids for the right ear are usually designated by a blue dot.
    D. none of the above

True and False: Put "T" for true and "F" for false.

____ 5. Batteries have only a positive side.

____ 6. Batteries are poisonous if swallowed.

____ 7. It may be necessary to pull backward and upward on the pinna to insert a hearing aid into the ear.

____ 8. The hearing aid should be left on when not in use.

____ 9. The receiver is the part of the hearing aid where the sound comes out.

____10. The volume wheel should be rolled down when inserting or removing a hearing aid from a patient's ear.

APPENDIX V-H

Inservice on Understanding Cochlear Implants, Their Care, and Their Use

Behavioral Objectives

Through participation in this inservice, attendees will be able to:
- Define and describe a cochlear implant
- List and explain patient-selection criteria for adults and children
- Identify internal and external parts of the cochlear implant and their function
- Describe how a cochlear implant works
- Describe potential benefits of a cochlear implant
- Describe and demonstrate how to check a cochlear implant
- Describe and demonstrate how to troubleshoot a cochlear implant
- Describe factors to check when a child is wearing a cochlear implant
- Describe important things to remember for cochlear implant use in the classroom

Suggested Time Allotment

Approximately 2 hours
- Introduction (5 minutes)
- Lecture (40 minutes)
- Questions (5 minutes)
- Break (10 minutes)
- Practicum (50 minutes)
- Quiz (10 minutes)

Format

Combination informational and skill-based

Suggested Materials

- Overhead projectors
- Appropriate handouts
- Instructor overheads
- Cochlear implants, checking equipment, and accessories (e.g., batteries, cords, extra microphones, etc.)

Additional Suggestions

Ask children with cochlear implants to volunteer to attend the inservice.

Suggested Participant Activities

- Set up four learning stations with learning guides
  ⇒ Station 1: Cochlear Implants and Their Parts
  ⇒ Station 2: Checking Cochlear Implants
  ⇒ Station 3: Troubleshooting Cochlear Implants
  ⇒ Station 4: FM Systems and Cochlear Implants

- Participants rotate throughout all stations learning skills

HANDOUTS

UNDERSTANDING COCHLEAR IMPLANTS, THEIR USE AND THEIR CARE
(Cochlear Corporation, 1995, 1996)

What is a cochlear implant?

A cochlear implant is an electronic device designed to provide sound information to children and adults with profound sensorineural hearing loss in both ears that receive little or no benefit from traditional hearing aids. More than 21,000 people worldwide have received cochlear implants, with more than 7,000 of those being children.

Who can benefit from a cochlear implant?

There are several patient-selection criteria for adults and children that determine candidacy for cochlear implants.

For adults:
- Profound or severe-to-profound sensorineural hearing loss in both ears
- Hearing loss acquired after learning oral speech and language
- Limited benefit from appropriate hearing aids
- No medical contraindications
- A desire to be part of the hearing world

For children:
- Profound sensorineural hearing loss in both ears
- 18 months through 17 years of age
- Little or no benefit from hearing aids
- No medical contraindications
- High motivation and appropriate expectations (both child and family)
- Placement in an educational program that emphasizes development of auditory skills after the implant has been fitted

What are the parts of a cochlear implant?

Cochlear implants have internal and external components.

- ***Internal components*** are surgically implanted completely under the skin and include:

    ⇒ ***A receiver/stimulator,*** which is positioned under the skin in a shallow "bed" made in the bone behind the ear.

    ⇒ ***A flexible biocompatible electrode array,*** which consists of 22 tiny electrode bands and is inserted approximately 1 inch into the cochlea.

- **External components** are worn by the individual and include:

    ⇒ **A speech processor,** which looks like a pocket calculator.

    ⇒ **A headset,** which includes:

        ✓ **A directional front-facing microphone,** which looks like a small behind-the-ear hearing aid.

        ✓ **A transmitting coil,** which is about 1 inch in diameter and is held in place behind the ear over the implanted receiver/stimulator by small magnets in both the transmitting coil and receiver/stimulator.

        ✓ **Two cables (cords),** which connect the microphone, speech processor, and transmitting coil.

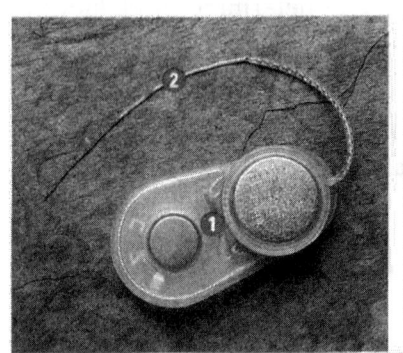

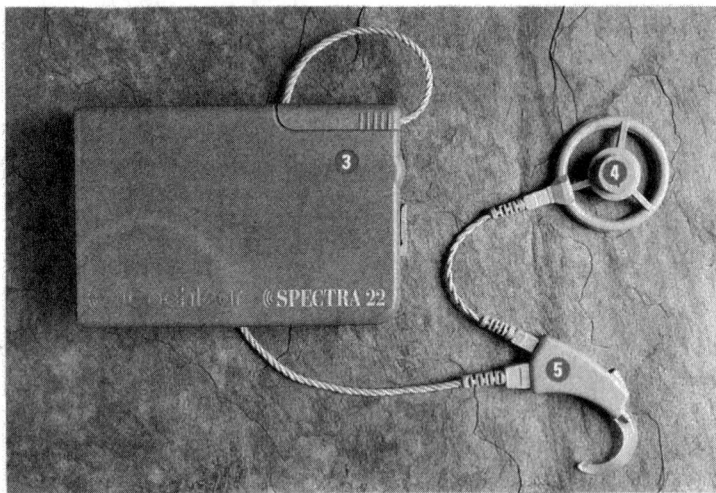

Legend:

1. Receiver/stimulator
2. Electrode array
3. Speech processor
4. Transmitting coil
5. Microphone

How does the cochlear implant work?

1. Sounds in the environment are picked up by the microphone.

2. A thin cable (cord) sends the sound from the microphone to the speech processor, a powerful miniaturized computer.

CREATING EFFECTIVE INSERVICE PROGRAMS **137**

3. The speech processor filters, analyzes, and digitizes sound into coded signals.

4. These coded signals are sent from the speech processor to the transmitting coil via the cables.

5. The transmitting coil sends the signals across the skin to the implanted receiver/stimulator via an FM radio signal.

6. The receiver/stimulator delivers the correct amount of electrical stimulation to the appropriate electrodes on the array.

7. The electrodes along the array stimulate the remaining auditory nerve fibers in the cochlea.

8. The resulting electrical signal (sound) information is sent through the auditory system to the brain for interpretation.

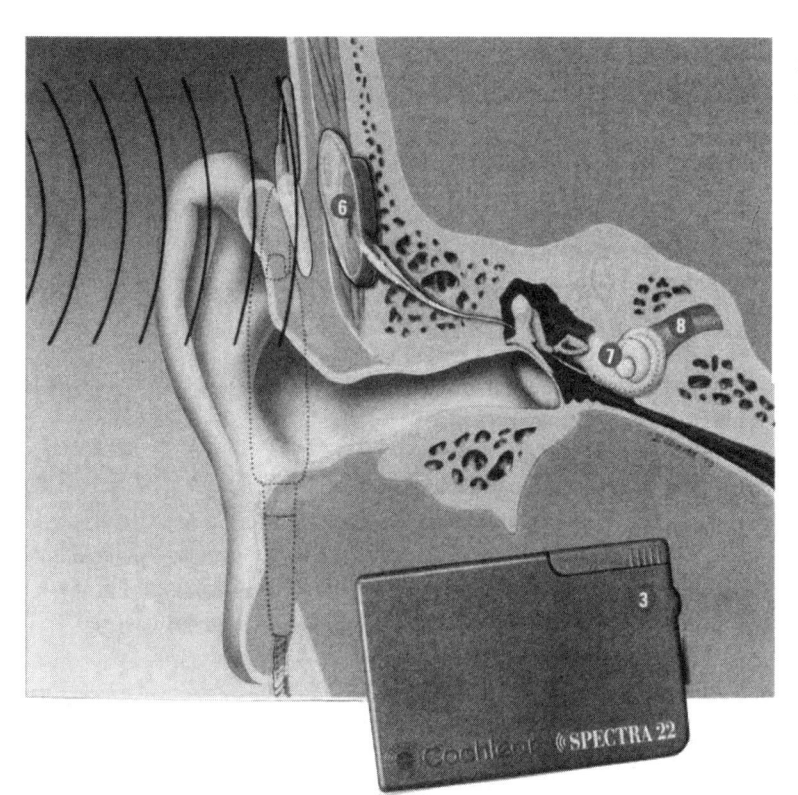

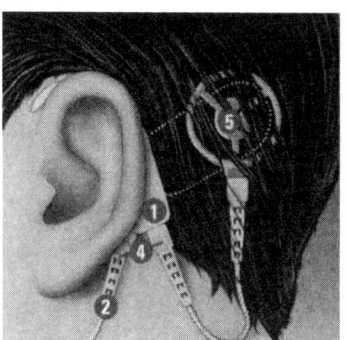

What are potential benefits from a cochlear implant?

- Children are able to detect conversational-level environmental sounds, including speech, at comfortable loudness levels.

- Some children can identify everyday sounds, such as car horns, doorbells, and birds singing, from a set of alternatives.

- Many children can distinguish among different speech patterns.

- Many children can identify words from a set of alternatives without lipreading.

- Some children exhibit improved lipreading.

- After training and experience with the device, many children demonstrate improvements in speech.

How do I check a cochlear implant?

Cochlear implants should be checked daily by performing the following steps:

- ***Turn the function knob to "T" (test).***

    ⇒ The "M" (microphone) light should glow if the battery has enough power.
    ⇒ If the "M" light does not glow, or if it flashes slowly, check or change the battery.

- ***Hold the signal check next to the transmitting coil. The signal check light should glow if the speech processor and coil are working.***

- ***Switch the function knob to "N" (normal) and turn the sensitivity control knob to the child's usual setting, generally 3 to 5.***

    ⇒ The "M" light should flash while you speak.
    ⇒ The signal check light should remain on.

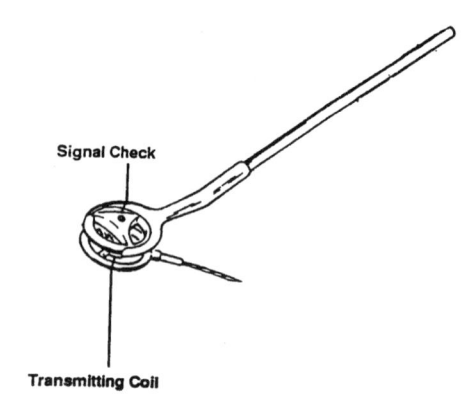

■ *How to change the battery:*

⇒ Remove the belt clip if the child uses it.
⇒ Slide the speech processor's battery cover off by pressing your thumb down on the thumb slot and sliding the cover back.
⇒ Remove the old battery, using the cloth strip to lift out the battery.
⇒ Insert a new AA battery (fully charged NiCad or disposable alkaline battery), making sure to match the plus and minus ends of the battery and battery compartment.
⇒ Replace the battery cover.

■ *How to change the cables:*

⇒ There are two cables: the long Tricord cable (speech processor to microphone) and the short transmitting cable (microphone to transmitting coil).
⇒ When replacing cables, be sure to grasp the end of the plug, not the cable.
⇒ Replace each cable separately.

■ *How to clean the battery contacts inside the speech processor:*

⇒ Slide off the battery cover and remove the battery.
⇒ Very slightly moisten a foam (or cotton) swab with alcohol and gently rub the ends of the rechargeable batteries and the battery contacts. If they are excessively dirty, use a clean pencil eraser.
⇒ Do not touch the row of six pins in the battery compartment with your finger or a swab.

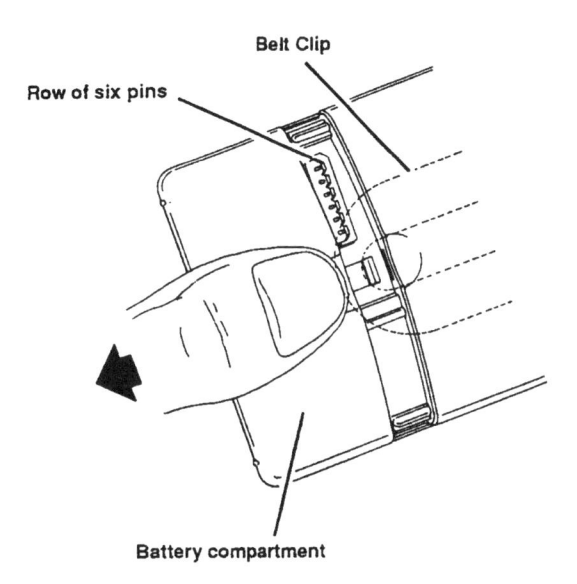

How do I troubleshoot the cochlear implant?

You will need to keep spare long and short cords, a microphone, and transmitting coil to sufficiently troubleshoot the speech processor. Perform the following steps in sequence to determine which part of the system may be malfunctioning:

- **STEP 1:** Set the function knob to the "T" (test) position. The "M" (microphone) light will illuminate continuously if the battery is sufficiently charged. If the "M" light blinks once per second, the battery may not be charged. Replace it with either a fully charged NiCad battery, or a new AA alkaline battery. If the "M" light still does not illuminate steadily, then consider:

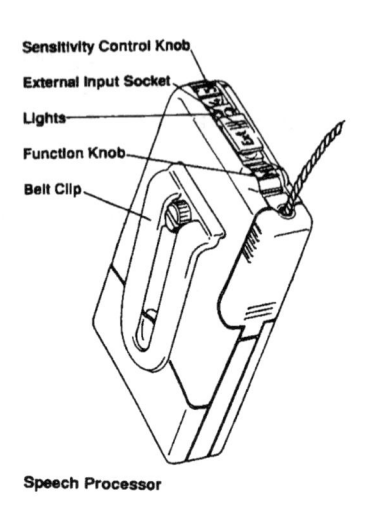

    ⇒ Is the battery inserted properly?
    ⇒ Are the battery contacts clean?

- **STEP 2:** Set the function knob to "N" (normal) and the sensitivity knob to 4 or 5. Then place the transmitting coil against the front center of the speech processor. Both the "M" and "C" (coil) lights will flash when an audio signal is present if the entire system is working.

- **STEP 3:** If the "M" light stays on steadily when the function knob is in the "T" position, but does not flicker when in the "N" position, replace the long Tricord cable that connects the speech processor to the microphone. Make sure the dots line up on the microphone and the straight end plug. Repeat Step 2. If the "M" light still does not flicker with an audio signal present, go to Step 4.

- **STEP 4:** Replace the short coil connecting cable that connects the microphone to the transmitting coil. Repeat Step 2. If the "M" light still does not flicker with an audio signal present, go to step 5.

- **STEP 5:** Replace the microphone and repeat Step 2. If you do not have a spare microphone, the child's accessory kit has a lapel microphone. Plug it into the speech processor's external input socket and repeat Step 2. If Step 2 now works, the headset microphone may not be functional, although the problem could be a faulty speech processor. The child should be able to use the lapel microphone until the speech processor can be evaluated at the child's implant center. If neither the replacement microphone (if available) nor the lapel microphone solves the problem, go to Step 6.

- **STEP 6:** Replace the transmitting coil and repeat Step 2. If this step still does not solve the problem, notify the child's parents. The speech processor should be taken to the implant center for evaluation.

What are some things to check when a child is wearing a cochlear implant?

- Make sure the speech processor is worn securely.

- Tuck the cords under child's clothing.

- Make sure the child wears a hooded raincoat or other waterproof clothing when going out in the rain.

- Discuss guidelines for sports and energetic play with parents and the child.

- Protect the child from activities that might result in a head injury.

- Keep spare batteries and spare cords on hand.

- Wrap the speech processor in a small plastic bag to protect it from food or drink if the processor is worn in front of the child.

What are some important things to remember for cochlear implant use in the classroom?

- *Reduce background noise:*
  ⇒ Try to teach in a quiet listening environment.
  ⇒ Seat the child as close as possible to the speaker.
  ⇒ Seat the child as far away as possible from noise sources.
  ⇒ Set the speech processor to "S" to activate the noise suppression switch.

- *Maximize opportunities for lipreading:*
  ⇒ Maintain a 3-to-5 foot distance from the child.
  ⇒ Make sure the child can see your face.

- *Remember the directional microphone:*
  ⇒ Sound source should be in front of the child.
  ⇒ Sound source should be not on the non-implanted side of the child.

- **Use FM systems, if needed.**
  ⇒ Due to the variability of among FM systems, the child should be fitted and tested with an FM system by an implant center audiologist.
  ⇒ To attach the child's speech processor to the FM receiver:
      ✓ Turn the speech processor and FM receiver OFF.
      ✓ Attach the connecting cable from the FM receiver to the external input socket of the speech processor.
      ✓ Set the tone control and volume control of the FM receiver to the level stipulated by the implant center audiologist.
      ✓ Turn the sensitivity control of the speech processor to the child's usual setting.
      ✓ Turn the speech processor and FM receiver ON.

NOTE: When an FM receiver is connected to the child's speech processor, the headset microphone will automatically be disconnected. The sounds coming through the teacher's microphone will be the only ones heard by the child. If the child needs to hear his own voice or the voices of other children around him/her, the environmental microphone on the FM receiver must be used.

How do I troubleshoot the FM system?

If the child reports that the FM system is producing **static or a buzzing sound**, try these steps:

- Have the child move to another place in the room.
- Turn the FM receiver to a different position.
- Move the FM receiver away from the speech processor.
- Change the FM channel.
- Try different lengths of implant transmitting cables, which connect the implant microphone to the speech processor.

If the child reports that the **sound quality is poor** through the FM system, refer the child to the implant center.

INSTRUCTOR OVERHEADS

COCHLEAR IMPLANTS

- What is a COCHLEAR IMPLANT?

- Who can BENEFIT from a cochlear implant?

- What are the PARTS of the cochlear implant?

    ⇒ Internal parts
    ⇒ External parts

- How does the cochlear implant WORK?

- What are the POTENTIAL BENEFITS of a cochlear implant?

- How do I CHECK a cochlear implant?

- How do I TROUBLESHOOT a cochlear implant?

- What are some things to CHECK when a CHILD WEARS a cochlear implant?

- What are some important things to REMEMBER for cochlear implant use in the CLASSROOM?

INSERVICE QUIZ ON UNDERSTANDING COCHLEAR IMPLANTS, THEIR CARE, AND THEIR USE

Score:_____   Name:_____

Pass   Fail   (Circle one)   Dept:_____

                                  Date:_____

Multiple choice: Please select the most appropriate answer for each item.

1. Generally, cochlear implants are most appropriate for persons with a

   A. moderate sensorineural hearing loss.
   B. severe sensorineural hearing loss.
   C. profound sensorineural hearing loss.
   D. none of the above

2. Which of the following skills is generally not possible with a cochlear implant?

   A. awareness of environmental sounds at about conversational level
   B. understanding conversational speech without visual cues
   C. distinguishing among the sound of a horn, bells, and bird songs
   D. None of the above

3. Which of the following are internal parts of the cochlear implant?

   A. speech processor
   B. electrode array
   C. receiver/stimulator
   D. microphone
   E. B and C

4. Cochlear implants should be checked

   A. daily.
   B. weekly.
   C. monthly.
   D. none of the above

5. Cochlear implants use a(n)

   A. AA battery.
   B. AAA battery.
   C. C battery.
   D. none of the above

6. Directional microphones

    A. pick up sound best from the front and the side of the child.
    B. pick up sound from the implanted side of the child.
    C. pick up sound equally from all directions.
    D. A and B.
    E. all of the above

True and False: Put "T" for true and "F" for false.

____ 7. FM systems can be used with cochlear implants.

____ 8. The "S" switch is for suppression of background noise.

____ 9. A child can go swimming wearing the internal and external parts of a cochlear implant.

____ 10. Any audiologist can fit FM systems to children with cochlear implants.

CHAPTER 6

Establishing Support Programs in Educational Settings

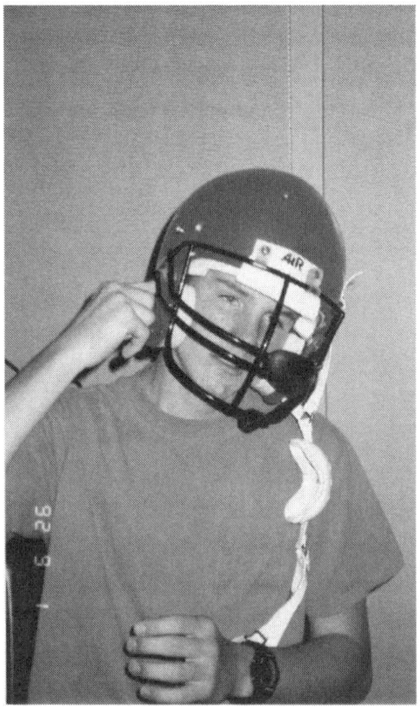

Figure 6-1. Chris, a boy who beat the odds. Despite having a severe hearing loss, Chris was an excellent student and athlete. He was quarterback for his high school football team and is shown here adjusting his hearing aids that had to be fit into his helmet.

"Silence" by Chris Mauldin

Silence was my world
Until I was three
The sounds of life
Were all deprived from me

The whispers of my mother
The laughter and joy
The sounds of early life
Never reached this little boy

All that I had
Was what I could see
What I felt, what I smelt
Were the things that brought glee

Despite the destruction
Inside of my ears
Through dark and frustration
Some sounds I could hear

These sounds that I heard
The amount was so few
Rang through this lost sense
Whose purpose I never knew

The sound of pots clanging
Often made me upset
Or the rumble of my dad's truck
A sound I knew best

The drone of a bass
Or the lonely drum beat
Was the only music
To reach and comfort me

But the words of my parents
Were just lip motions to me
So I taught myself to read lips
At the early age of three

This is the reason
I remained isolated until three
I read lips and talked
Giving my parents no worry

But still they wondered
Why I acted so strange
Why I had fits of rage
Like short bursts of rain

They wondered why when faced
Their order I'd repeat
But when my back turned
To their call I didn't speak

Why with my cousins
I was a calm, dead sea
But then all of a sudden
I'd attack violently

So there came a day
When I went for a test
To my parent's surprise
I was over 80% deaf

Then we set an appointment
To get my first set
Of hearing aids that is
For the time, I got the best

And when they arrived
The doc gave them to me
After putting them in
My face shown with glee

My mouth dropped in wonder
As sound raced through my brain
Like the opening of a closed door
Or the sun shining through rain

Indeed it was an opened door
For it gave a new way to see
My brain was a cold, dark lock
And my hearing aids the key

That day lead to school
And my life went a whirl
And this curious deaf boy
Went out and faced the world

INTRODUCTION

The poem "Silence" was written by Chris Mauldin (pictured in Figure 6–1), a boy with hearing loss who beat the odds to excel in school and sports. Chris' success depended not only on the efforts of his audiologist and amplification, but on the support systems made available to him by his family and schools.

Currently, there is a nationwide shortage of educational audiologists (Johnson, Benson, & Seaton, 1997) and caseloads far exceed the recommended practitioner-to-child ratio of 1:12,000 (ASHA, 1993). For example, the nationwide, full-time equivalent ratio of educational audiologists to children ages 3 to 21 years was 1:68,804 in 1994 (Johnson et al., 1997; U.S. Department of Education, 1994). Many school districts do not employ an audiologist on a full-time basis. Rather, these districts choose to contract for all or part of necessary audiologic services to specific populations. In addition, there is a mandate for cost-efficiency in our nation's school districts. With large caseloads, audiologists cannot meet all children's hearing health-care needs without delegating some responsibilities to audiologic support personnel. It is not cost efficient, for example, for audiologists to perform daily visual and listening checks on all children's hearing aids or FM listening systems. A more cost-efficient use of resources would involve an audiologist managing a system-wide, amplification device support program for children with hearing impairment.

Unlike rehabilitation hospitals and long-term residential care facilities for the elderly discussed in this textbook, description of a single support program for educational settings could not suffice, considering the unique characteristics of audiologic service delivery within each school district. Furthermore, support programs in educational settings can be both informal and formal. Informal support programs are the interrelationships, ties of communications, and overall attitudes of school districts toward providing a seamless system (English, 1998) to manage the hearing health-care needs of and to ensure accommodations for children with hearing impairment in all aspects of their educational careers. Formal support programs involve specific areas of service delivery. Thus, the focus of this chapter is on establishing both informal and formal support programs in key areas of educational settings to offer stellar audiologic service delivery, often in less than optimal situations. The purpose of this chapter is to review the law, discuss current realities in educational audiology, and provide suggestions for establishing support programs both informally and formally in key areas of amplification devices, family counseling, central auditory processing disorders (CAPD) service delivery, and for postsecondary educational institutions.

LEARNING OBJECTIVES

This chapter will enable the reader to:

- Be familiar with current legislation regarding audiologic services in public schools
- Acknowledge the current realities regarding audiologic service delivery in education
- Understand the dynamics of establishing both formal and informal support programs in key areas of educational settings

---

THE LAW

Recently, there has been an active history of legislation aimed at ensuring a free and appropriate public education for all children with disabilities. The presentation of the legislation is beyond the scope of this textbook, and the reader is referred to Johnson et al. (1997) for a complete history of this legislation. The current law, the Individuals with Disabilities Education Act (IDEA) (1990), will be discussed in some detail here.

The IDEA combines all of the amendments to PL 94-142 or the Education for all Handicapped Children's Act and PL 99-457, the Education of Handicapped Act Amendments (EHA) of 1986 (Johnson et al., 1997). Part H of the IDEA, the Early Intervention Program for Infants and Toddlers with Disabilities, contains the amendments made in 1991 and describes services for children with disabilities from birth through 5 years of age (Johnson et al., 1997). Section 34CFR303.12(D) contains this definition of audiology:

(i) Identification of children with impairments, using at-risk criteria and appropriate audiological screening techniques;
(ii) Determination of the range, nature, and degree of hearing loss and communication functions, by use of audiologic evaluation procedures;
(iii) Referral for medical and other services necessary for the habilitation and rehabilitation of children with auditory impairment;
(iv) Provision of auditory training, aural rehabilitation, speech reading and listening device orientation and training, and other services;
(v) Provision of services for the prevention of hearing loss; and
(vi) Determination of the child's need for individual amplification, including selecting, fitting, and dispensing of appropriate listening and vibrotactile devices, and evaluating the effectiveness of those devices.

Similarly, Part B of the IDEA, the Education of Children with Disabilities Program applies to preschool (Part 301) and school-age children (Part 300) (Johnson et al., 1997). Section 34CFR300.13(B) contains this definition of audiology:

(i) Identification of children with hearing loss;
(ii) Determination of the range, nature, and degree of loss, including referral for medical or other professional attention for the habilitation of hearing;
(iii) Provision of habilitation activities, such as language habilitation, auditory training, speech reading, (lipreading), hearing evaluation, and speech conservation;
(iv) Creation and administration of programs for prevention of hearing loss;
(v) Counseling and guidance of pupils, parents, and teachers regarding hearing loss; and
(vi) Determination of the child's need for group and individual amplification, including selecting, fitting, and dispensing of appropriate listening and vibrotactile devices, and evaluating the effectiveness of those devices.

Part B of the IDEA has a section on the "Proper Functioning of Hearing Aids" (34CFR300.303) that states that, "Each public agency shall ensure that the hearing aids worn by children with hearing impairment, including deafness, in school are functioning properly."

Johnson et al. (1997) stated that several additions were added to this law on September 29, 1992, that had important applications to audiology, the most important of which was the definition of the "assistive technology device" and "assistive technology service." These additions to the law were made to Parts B and H of the IDEA in sections called "Assistive Technology" (34CFR300.4-6; 34CFR303.12):

Assistive technology devices and services are necessary if a child with a disability requires the device and services in order to receive a free and appropriate education (FAPE); the public agency must ensure that they are made available.

"Assistive technology device" means any item, piece of equipment, or product system, whether acquired commercially off of the shelf, modified, or customized, that is used to increase, maintain, or improve the functional capabilities of children with disabilities.

"Assistive technology service" means any service that directly assists a child with a disability in the selection, acquisition, or use of an assistive technology device. The term includes:
(a) The evaluation of the needs of a child with a disability, including a functional evaluation of the child in the child's customary environment;
(b) Purchasing, leasing, or otherwise providing for the acquisition of assistive technology devices by children with disabilities;
(c) Selecting, designing, fitting, customizing, adapting, applying, retaining, repairing, or replacing assistive technology devices;
(d) Coordinating and using other therapies, interventions, or services with assistive technology devices, such as those associated with existing education and rehabilitation plans and programs;
(e) Training or technical assistance for a child with a disability or, if appropriate, that child's family; and

(f) Training or technical assistance for professionals (including individuals providing education or rehabilitation services), employers, or other individuals who provide services to, employ, or are otherwise substantially involved in the major life functions of children with disabilities.

Audiologists must realize that federal laws (e.g., the IDEA) are constantly changing and that it is imperative to keep up-to-date with changes in legislation.

Federal laws provide only frameworks for audiologic service provisions in the schools. For example, the laws are often interpreted differently by educational administrators. The director of special education for a school district may interpret Part B of the IDEA, "Proper Functioning of Hearing Aids" (34CFR300.303), to mean that teachers should check children's hearing aids and FM systems once a week by making sure that they squeal. Fortunately, most audiologists are aware of the various practice guidelines and position statements that provide "gold standards" of care for educational audiology. Table 6–1 lists some related guidelines, one of which is the "Guidelines for Fitting and Monitoring FM Systems" (ASHA, 1994). This document recommends that daily checks on children's personal hearing aids and FM systems be completed by the audiologist or other appropriately trained educational personnel.

There is one item in Table 6–1, "Guidelines for Audiology Services in the Schools," that pertains specifically to educational audiology (ASHA, 1993). Those guidelines have a suggested list of roles and responsibilities for educational audiologists that appear in Table 6–2.

CURRENT REALITIES IN EDUCATIONAL SETTINGS

As mentioned in the introduction, *there is a severe shortage of audiologists who are practicing in the schools.* Currently, only about one fifth of the recommended number of audiologists is practicing in educational settings. Furthermore, the severity of the practitioner shortage varies greatly from state to state. Some states, such as Iowa (reported ratio of 1:13,413), almost meet the suggested full-time equivalent ratio of one audiologist employed in the schools to 12,000 children aged 3 to 21 years of age (U.S. Department of Education, 1994). Unfortunately, many other states do not come close to meeting this ratio. Obviously, these statistics do not bode well for the ability of public agencies to meet the hearing health-care needs of their students.

As stated previously, there are two service-delivery models in educational audiology: (1) school-based and (2) contracted audiology services (Johnson et al., 1997). In a *school-based service-delivery model*, the audiologist is an employee of the school district. The school district purchases and maintains all necessary equipment and materials. In a *contract service-delivery model*, the audiologist is a completely autonomous employee who provides services to a specific caseload that is defined by a contract. The contract-for-service audiologist is most likely in private practice or employed by a hospital or other agency and is responsible for supplying all necessary equipment and materials. Although Johnson et al. (1997) stated that the contract service-delivery model is common within small, rural school districts, the statistics re-

Table 6–1. Some practice guidelines from the American Speech-Language-Hearing Association pertaining to educational audiology.

- Acoustics in Educational Settings
- Amplification as a Remediation Technique for Children with Normal Peripheral Hearing
- Amplification for Infants and Children with Hearing Loss
- Audiologic Screening of Newborns Who Are at Risk for Hearing Impairment
- Guidelines for Audiology Services in Schools
- Guidelines for Fitting and Monitoring FM Systems
- Guidelines for Identification Audiometry
- Guidelines for Screening for Hearing Impairment and Middle-Ear Disorders
- Guidelines for the Audiologic Assessment of Children from Birth through 36 Months of Age
- The Use of FM Amplification Instruments for Infants and Preschool Children with Hearing Impairment

Table 6–2. Responsibilities of educational audiologists.

- Provide community leadership to ensure that all infants, toddlers, and youth with impaired hearing are promptly identified, evaluated, and provided with appropriate intervention service.
- Collaborate with community resources to develop a high-risk registry and follow-up.
- Develop and supervise a hearing screening program for preschool and school-aged children.
- Train audiometric technicians or other appropriate personnel to screen for hearing loss.
- Perform follow-up comprehensive audiological evaluations.
- Assess central auditory function.
- Make appropriate referrals for further audiological, communication, educational, psychosocial, or medical assessment.
- Interpret audiological assessment results to other school personnel.
- Serve as a member of the educational team in the evaluation, planning, and placement process, to make recommendations regarding placement, related service needs, communication needs, and modification of classroom environments for students with hearing impairments or other auditory problems.
- Provide in-service training on hearing and hearing impairments and their implication to school personnel, children, and parents.
- Educate parents, children, and school personnel about hearing loss prevention.
- Make recommendations about use of hearing aids, cochlear implants, group and classroom amplification, and assistive listening devices.
- Ensure the proper fit and functioning of hearing aids, cochlear implants, group and classroom amplification, and assistive listening devices.
- Analyze classroom noise and acoustics and make recommendations for improving the listening environment.
- Manage the use and calibration of audiometric equipment.
- Collaborate with school, parents, teachers, special support personnel, and relevant community agencies and professionals to ensure delivery of appropriate services.
- Make recommendations for assistive devices (radio/television, telephone, alerting, convenience) for students with hearing impairment.
- Provide services, including home programming if appropriate, in the areas of speechreading, listening, communication strategies, use and care of amplification, including cochlear implants, and self-management of hearing needs.

Source: From "Guidelines for Audiology Services in Schools," by American Speech-Language-Hearing Association, 1993, p. 29. *Asha, 35*(Suppl. 10), 24–32.

---

garding the shortage of audiologists suggest otherwise. If most states are not employing audiologists in educational settings, how are children's hearing health-care needs being met? Most likely, the contract service-delivery model is being used across different types of school districts. Unfortunately, many contracts fall short of the recommended "gold standards" of audiologic service delivery in educational settings.

Audiologists must be careful before entering into a contract to provide audiologic services in educational settings for several reasons. First, audiologists are contracted to provide very specific services (e.g., hearing screenings, audiologic evaluations, amplification device monitoring, and so on) to specific caseloads. Situations may arise in which audiologists feel compelled to provide assistance for ethical reasons, but cannot due to limitations in contract coverage. Audiologists contracted to manage children's hearing aids and FM systems in self-contained classrooms may not be reimbursed after supplying batteries for the hearing aids of mainstreamed children with hearing impairment, for example.

Second, as stated earlier, audiologists may find that contracts provide for less than optimal hearing health-care for children. Audiologists may find, for example, that administrators have only allowed one hour of inservice time to instruct 50 public-school nurses on appropriate hearing screening techniques.

Third, audiologists may find that they are spending more time and using more resources than are covered in the contract. Audiologists may have only allotted two hours per week to visit the self-contained classrooms for children with hearing impairment, but they may find that four to five hours per week are needed to provide the necessary services.

Fourth, contract-for-service audiologists may have a difficult time achieving acceptance and respect from other educational personnel. Some school employees may resent serving as audiologic support personnel who must answer to an "outsider." Furthermore, contract-for-service audiologists are often viewed as "transient" employees in some school districts. Also, the itinerant nature of a "transient" educational audiologist means that much time can be wasted in the car traveling from school to school. Audiologists must carefully plan to minimize commute time.

The "Guidelines for Audiology Services in the Schools" (ASHA, 1993) suggested that the contract should specify the nature of the services to be provided, the name and credentials of the provider, when and how services will be provided, and the nature of the reporting and consultation activities. Audiologists who are contemplating providing services through a contract in educational settings should take the following precautions:

- Investigate the history of audiologic service provision within the school district. What service-delivery model has been used? If the school district previously employed a school-based audiologist, why did he or she leave? Why is the school district changing to a contract service-delivery model?
- Find out the areas of service provision to be provided for in the contract.
- Estimate the total cost of providing "gold standard" services.
- Fully "cost" the contract to meet the needs of the school district, as well as the fiscal responsibilities of your own practice or employer.
- Refuse to compromise the quality of hearing health-care services just to secure a contract.
- Try to include clauses within the contract that offer flexibility in coverage for unforeseen program needs.
- Check personal liability coverage.
- Develop cost-efficient ways of providing "gold standards" of care.

One way of accomplishing the last objective is to establish support programs for children with hearing impairment in educational settings. Because of the many roles and responsibilities served by educational audiologists, there are several critical areas in which support programs can be beneficial. Recall that support programs are areas in which multiskilling and the use of support personnel can result in a delegation of some tasks so that audiologists' time can be spent in more critical aspects of service delivery. Support programs can be informal or formal, with the latter being designated for key areas.

INFORMAL SUPPORT PROGRAMS

Informal support programs are those professional interrelationships, lines of communication, and overall attitudes of school districts toward providing a seamless system of managing the hearing health-care needs of and providing necessary accommodations for children with hearing impairment. Unfortunately, this is not always possible, as exemplified by Sali, who found that no such program seems to exist at her new school.

Sali—a first grader with a bilateral, moderate-to-severe sensorineural hearing impairment—moved to a new city with her family when her father was transferred. Sali's parents were particularly concerned about her transition to a new school. In their old town, Sali was able to attend the neighborhood elementary school, which contained the program for elementary students with hearing impairment. Unfortunately, Sali now would have to travel across town to attend Carver Elementary. On the first day of school, Sali's mom drove her to her new school. She parked the car, and they walked into the school together. The school secretary walked with them to Mrs. White's classroom. Mrs. White welcomed Sali and showed her to her seat. Sali noticed that all of the other children had FM receivers or hearing aids like she had worn at her other school. Mrs. White introduced Sali to the class and continued on with the morning lesson.

Soon it was time for recess. All the children in Sali's class lined up at the door and walked to the playground. The children with normal hearing often teased the children with hearing impairment. Several of these children on the playground stared at Sali. One child said, "Who is the new kid with gum in her ear?" One boy kept pointing and laughing at her. Sali said, "Stop, stop!" Sali's articulation errors made her sound like a younger child. The bully tormented Sali by pointing and yelling, "Baby talk, baby talk!" Sali ran inside, sat at her desk, and put her head down. She missed her old school because none of the children teased her there. Now she felt awful.

After recess, it was time for music class. All of the children in Mrs. White's class lined up and walked to Mrs. Brubaker's music class. Mrs. Brubaker was always happy to see the children from Mrs. White's classroom. Sali liked Mrs. Brubaker because she seemed so friendly and enthusiastic. Unfortunately, she often spoke with her back to the children, and she didn't wear the FM transmitter like Mrs. White. It was very difficult for Sali to understand. All of Sali's teachers at her old school used the FM transmitter and made sure that students could see their faces when they talked.

Unfortunately, the teachers and students at Sali's new school did not understand or were not sensitive to the needs of children with hearing impairment. Clearly, the educational audiologist needed to enlighten these individuals regarding hearing, hearing loss, its effects, and the roles and responsibilities of everyone in meeting the needs of these children, perhaps through an educational audiology marketing campaign. Marketing educational audiology is critical for school administrators, teachers, ancillary educational personnel (e.g., public-school nurses, school psychologists, social workers, and so on), and students to understand the roles and responsibilities of hearing health-care providers. Chapter 3, "Defining and Marketing Support Programs," provided numerous suggestions that can be used to market audiology in educational settings. Educational audiology marketing campaigns should not only secure necessary support program funding, but they also should ensure that everyone understands the importance of hearing health care and is considerate of the needs of children with hearing impairment.

Communication is the single most important component in informal support programs. Everyone needs to know who the educational audiologist is and what he or she does. Figure 6–2 illustrates a model of communication used in informal support programs.

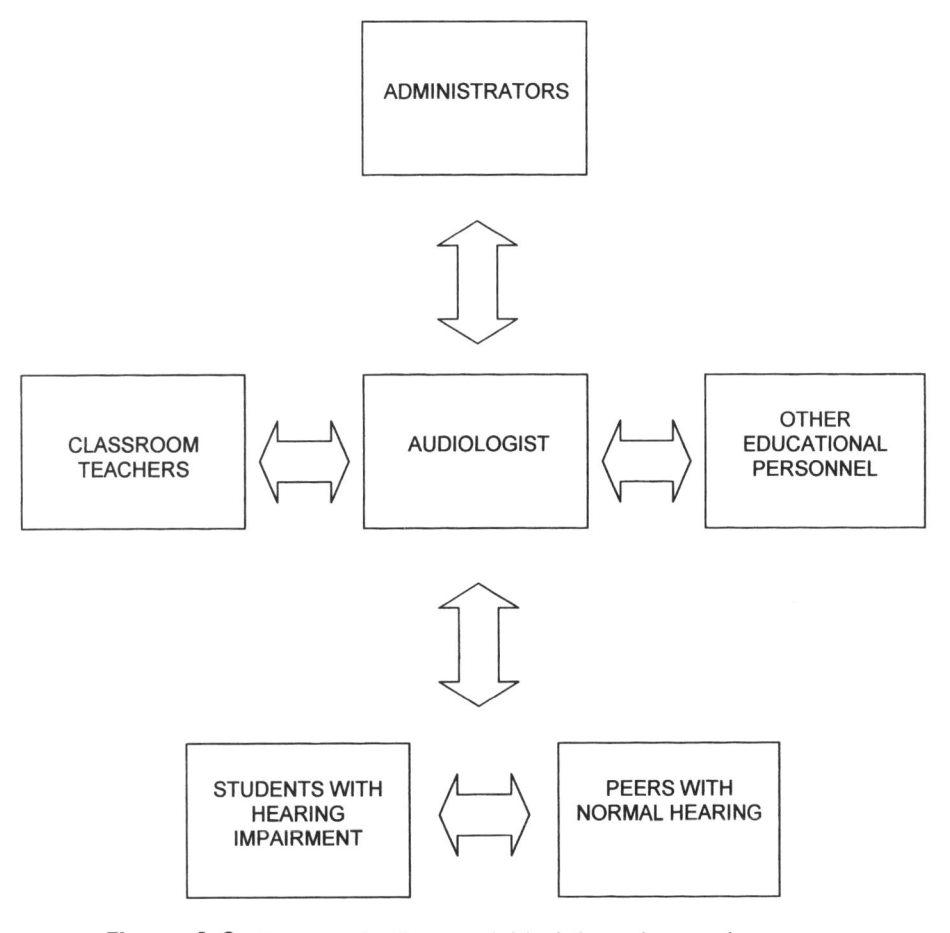

Figure 6–2. Communication model for informal support programs.

Communication should be top-down (e.g., from administrators to educational audiologist to students), bottom-up (i.e., from students to educational audiologist to administrators), and side-to-side (i.e., from one administrator to another, from educational audiologist to other educational personnel, and among students).

Informal support programs can exist within individual schools or can be district wide. For example, informal support programs can be established in elementary schools that serve as a school district's primary educational site for young children with hearing impairment. A successful elementary-school program, for example, required that all teachers and personnel attend informational inservices on the effects of hearing loss on communication and on how to communicate with students who have hearing impairment. With this added knowledge and sensitivity, all school personnel collaborated to enhance the communication potential of these students. Furthermore, teachers provided lessons to all children regarding hearing, hearing loss, hearing aids, communication tips, and sign language. Instead of being ridiculed, children with hearing impairment were now thought of as "cool." Some of their peers with normal hearing even wanted to have their own FM receivers! Clearly, programs such as these are the best of all possible scenarios. Informal support programs augment formal support programs established in areas of amplification devices, CAPD service delivery, and counseling.

AMPLIFICATION DEVICE SUPPORT PROGRAMS

Support programs for amplification devices are needed in school districts, especially those utilizing contract-for-service audiologists. Audiologists must have an organized plan to establish a support program for monitoring and maintaining amplification devices in educational settings. If not, audiologists may find themselves in a predicament like Starr's. Starr, a newly hired audiologist at a local hospital, initially was excited when her boss told her that she would be providing services to the local school district on a contract basis. She looked forward to her first day out of the office and in the public schools. Educational audiology was one of her favorite classes in graduate school. She carefully consulted her class notes and her textbook, the *Educational Audiology Handbook* (Johnson et al., 1997), in preparation for her first day.

Starr started her new adventure as an educational audiologist at about 9:00 a.m. Her boss had given her a map showing the location of the three schools she was to visit that day, first the elementary school, then the high school, then the junior high school. She felt well prepared with her portable hearing aid analyzer (complete with a real-ear probe-tube microphone measurement system), her black bag full of supplies, hearing aid check kits, and documentation forms for audiologic support personnel. Starr assumed that the teachers would be pleased to serve as audiologic support personnel. To impress her boss, Starr had ordered all of the materials for the hearing aid check kits on her own.

After 45 minutes and realizing that she should have checked a map first, Starr finally found the elementary school and reported to the principal's office. Starr was surprised when the secretary said, "There you are! You were suppose to be here two hours ago!" Embarrassed, Starr was escorted to the program for children with hearing impairment. Before Starr could introduce herself, the teacher pointed to a box of FM receivers and a pile of last year's audiograms and said, "Adjust and label those auditory trainers. After that, we have eight children who need earmold impressions." Starr prepared the portable hearing-aid analyzer to perform both electroacoustic analyses and real-ear probe-tube microphone measurements. Starr felt uneasy when she noticed that the teacher was staring at her. She was even more surprised when the teacher said, "We don't have time for you to do that. Last year, the other girl set the auditory trainers with just a screwdriver!" Starr explained that she could not do it that way. Frustrated, the teacher reluctantly brought the students in, one-by-one. The time flew. Starr could only set FM receivers for five children who did not have personal hearing aids. It would take much longer for the others. At noon, Starr said she needed to be off to the high school and would return next week. Before leaving, she gave each teacher a hearing aid check kit to perform daily visual and listening checks on children's hearing aids. The teachers told Starr they didn't know how, nor did they have the time to participate as support personnel, and that it was her job to check the hearing aids. Starr proceeded to perform a visual and listening check on all the children's hearing aids, half of which were not working.

Starr arrived at the high school at 1:30 p.m. Starr had attended Northwest High School, so she knew that the program for students with hearing impairment was in the back of the school on the third floor. To save time, Starr went through the backdoor and up the stairwell. "Hey! Hey you! Where do you think you're going?" Starr realized that the security guard was talking to her. Starr, who looked young for her 24 years, explained that she was the new audiologist and that she was on her way to the program for students with hearing impairment. The security guard said, "Yeah, sure. Where is your visitor's tag? Let's go to the principal's office." Starr knew she had made a bad decision. She was relieved when the principal laughed at the incident and said, "Well, you've learned your lesson." Starr looked at her watch as she left the office and was surprised to find that it was 2:15 p.m. As she entered the classroom, she found that the students were gone and the teacher was at her desk reading a textbook. Starr introduced herself. Without looking up from her book, the teacher said, "The students have left for the day. Next week, knock on the door so that I can give you students' hearing aids to check in the empty classroom down the hall. Also, you're going to have to get here before 2:00 p.m. Now, if you'll excuse me." Starr was bewildered. She also realized that the junior high school let out in 15 minutes. Using her cellular phone, Starr called the junior high school and said she would be there next week. Starr had had a difficult day. She returned to the hospital to find that her boss had received numerous complaints from the schools and bills totalling $300 for hearing aid stethoscopes, battery checkers, forced-air blowers, and so on. Also, Starr had a message on her voicemail from a troubled parent saying that her child has her own audiologist and to not check her hearing aids.

Starr's situation is not uncommon for contract-for-service audiologists in educational settings. Starr's first day could have been less hectic had she had an organized plan for establishing a amplification device support program.

Amplification devices in schools include personal hearing aids, personal FM systems, sound-field FM classroom amplification systems, assistive listening devices, and cochlear implants. Audiologists can establish support programs for amplification devices by: (1) assessing program needs, (2) setting up the program, and (3) acknowledging children's role as audiologic support personnel.

Establishing a Need

Children's hearing aids and personal FM systems are often found to be nonfunctional (e.g., Bess, Sinclair, & Riggs, 1984; Gaeth & Lounsbury, 1966; Kemker, McConnell, Logan, & Green, 1979; Maxon & Brackett, 1981; Smedley & Plaplinger, 1988). Reichman and Healey (1989) found that less than 50% of schools surveyed across the nation had adequate systems for monitoring and maintaining amplification devices. They indicated that successful programs required:

- daily visual and listening inspections of hearing aids and auditory trainers (i.e., personal FM systems);
- periodic electroacoustic analysis of hearing aids and auditory trainers;
- availability of hearing aids and auditory trainers as loaners on the day a malfunction is detected;
- procedures for replacing earmolds and other accessories including equipment provisions and fiscal responsibility; and
- teacher, parent, and student instruction in monitoring and maintenance.

These preferred practices are supported by "Guidelines for Fitting and Monitoring FM Systems" by the American Speech-Language-Hearing Association (ASHA, 1994).

Preferred practices for cochlear implants and sound-field FM classroom amplification systems are similar and include:

- daily visual and listening checks of the devices;
- periodic electroacoustic checks of the devices by manufacturers;
- availability of loaners on the day malfunction is detected;
- procedures for replacing accessories; and
- teacher, parent, and student instruction in monitoring and maintenance.

Most educational audiologists cannot complete daily visual and listening checks on all personal hearing aids, personal FM systems, cochlear implants, or sound-field FM amplification systems within a school district. Obviously, it is more cost efficient and feasible to delegate some of those responsibilities to audiologic support personnel. Implementing an adequate monitoring program requires careful planning, use of audiologic support personnel, and selection of an appropriate model of multiskilling.

Amplification Device Monitoring Program Set Up

Program set up requires a(n):

- inventory of amplification devices (e.g., owner, make, model, serial numbers, warranty status, children's personal audiologists, equipment representative, and so on);
- receipt of informed consent from parents;
- selection of multiskilling model and training support personnel;
- requisition of necessary equipment and materials; and
- consideration of program logistics.

Inventory of Amplification Devices

At the beginning of the school year, audiologists should visit classrooms that (1) are self-contained (i.e., children with hearing impairment), (2) use sound-field FM amplification systems, or (3) mainstream children with hearing impairment. Audiologists should schedule formal appointments with each teacher. These visits provide opportunities to: (1) observe the class, (2) assess immediate needs, (3) meet teachers and students, and (4) inventory amplification devices.

Audiologists should send a letter like the one shown in Appendix VI-A to all teachers. The letter should introduce the audiologist (including phone number and e-mail address), request an appointment to visit the classroom, state the reason for the visit, and request that children bring their hearing aids (whether working or not) to school on the day of the visit. The letter should be followed by a phone call to the teacher to schedule the actual appointment. In addition, audiologists should try to schedule appointments with all teachers in the same school on the same day to increase efficiency and minimize travel time.

Educational audiologists must follow protocol when visiting a school. Never make a surprise visit. Always check in at the front office before venturing to classrooms. School principals can be very territorial—especially when security is a problem at their schools, and is unfortunately becoming more common across the country. Educational audiologists, like Starr, may find themselves escorted to the principal's office by a security guard for slipping in the side entrance of the school.

When visiting a class for the first time, educational audiologists should take mental notes regarding the following:

- Are there any FM systems used in the class? If so, are they being used appropriately? If not, where are the FM units? Why aren't they being used?
- Is the teacher's style of presenting information optimal for students with hearing impairment?
- Are the acoustical conditions poor (i.e., poor signal-to-noise ratio and excessive reverberation)? Are there some easy acoustic modifications that can be made (e.g., artwork on the walls, windows to the playground closed, draperies closed to cover windows, and so on)?

Educational audiologists should explain their roles and responsibilities and how they might be of service to teachers. Likewise, teachers should be asked about any special needs, concerns, or difficulties they might have or that they may have in the future. Audiologists should listen carefully and take note of issues that require follow-up. For example, teachers may inquire about different styles of microphones that can be used with FM transmitters. Audiologists can discuss different microphone options with the manufacturer and then e-mail information to teachers. Teachers appreciate this personal contact with audiologists. In addition, teachers should be asked if they are able to interface FM systems with audio-visual equipment or classroom computers. Audiologists also should ask teachers if any children come from non-English speaking households. In California, many parents in Spanish-speaking households may not be able to read English, for example. All correspondence with these parents must be either written in their native language or interpreted by a social worker or other school personnel.

In addition, audiologists should spend a few minutes with each student. Audiologists should introduce themselves, explain their job, and ask each child his or her name and a general question (e.g., What did you do for your summer vacation?) to establish rapport. At this time, audiologists should take inventory of hearing aids, noting students' names, ear(s) fit, makes, models, serial numbers, battery sizes, and general notation of their condition. Appendix VI-B shows an inventory sheet that catalogues children's hearing aids and other amplification devices used in the classroom.

Obtaining Informed Consent

Audiologists may find it odd to have to obtain parents' informed consent to check their children's personal hearing aids. However, some parents do not want ANYONE touching their children's hearing aids for any reason. Many of these parents have a personal audiologist who manages their children's hearing health-care needs and may not want a "stranger" checking the hearing aids. Thus, audiologists should send a letter home to parents introducing themselves, explaining the amplification device support program, and explaining the purpose of the informed-consent forms. In addition, the letter should include audiologists' office phone numbers and e-mail addresses. Appendix VI-C shows an example of a letter and informed-consent form. On the form, audiologists should inquire whether children have personal audiologists and if their hearing aids are covered under warranty. As suggested in Chapter 4 (i.e., "Funding Support Programs"), audiologists should also inquire about any third-party billing information. Audiologists should not be shy in asking if families qualify to receive Medicaid. If possible, they should request all information necessary for filing claims for hearing aid repairs.

Selection of a Model of Multiskilling and Training Support Personnel

Several models of multiskilling may be appropriate for implementation in an amplification device monitoring program. Chapter 2 discussed the various dimensions of multiskilling. Any one or a combination of the following may be appropriate: (1) collateral multiskilling (e.g., public-school nurses, speech-language pathologists, classroom teachers, and so on), (2) subordinate multiskilling (e.g., audiology assistants), and/or (3) collateral-subordinate multiskilling (e.g., speech-language pathology assistants, teacher's assistants, and so on).

As stated in Chapter 5, selection of a model of multiskilling should be done after a careful systematic analysis of the audiologists' caseload, logistical factors, and administrative concerns. First, what personnel have daily contact with children who wear hearing aids, personal FM systems, and cochlear implants? Second, would participation in the amplification device monitoring program result in a work overload? Third, what are the attitudes of those personnel about participating as audiologic support personnel? Fourth, do these personnel meet the criteria for audiologic support personnel set forth in the "Position Statement and Guidelines of the Consensus Panel on Support Personnel in Audiology" (AAA, 1997)? Fifth, can those personnel be trained and supervised according to the guidelines set forth in that same document?

As previously mentioned, one or all models of multiskilling may be applicable for use in an amplification device monitoring program. The multiskilling model may be different in self-contained classrooms for students with hearing impairment than for regular classrooms with a few mainstreamed students. It may be more efficient for teachers of the deaf (i.e., collateral multiskilling) to perform visual and listening checks of the hearing aids used in their classrooms than for speech-language pathology assistants (i.e., collateral-subordinate multiskilling) who serve mainstreamed children with hearing impairment. Selection of a multiskilling model is followed by development of effective inservice programs to train audiologic support personnel. Chapter 5 presented tips and effective protocols for this purpose, which are not repeated here. Musket (1995) suggested including the following guidelines for training audiologic support personnel for hearing aid monitoring programs in educational settings:

- Keep extra batteries and hearing aids out of reach of children.
- Dispose of batteries properly and away from children.
- Do not incinerate or burn old batteries because they can explode.
- Do not change batteries in front of children.
- Do not put batteries in your mouth for any reason.
- Secure the battery compartment of hearing aids that belong to younger children.

- Check medications because batteries look like tablets.
- If a battery is swallowed:
  ⇒ Find a battery exactly like the one swallowed to obtain the identification number.
  ⇒ Call the school nurse, the child's parents, and a pediatrician.
  ⇒ Call the battery-ingestion hotline on the back of the package.

Successful multiskilling in the practice of educational audiology requires:

- commitment of the educational audiologist;
- commitment of multiskilled personnel;
- cooperation and support of administrators;
- consistent implementation of facility, professional organization, state, and federal guidelines; and
- ongoing review of the effects on children and educational staff (e.g., Runnels, 1994; Werven, 1993).

Commitment of multiskilled personnel and administrators is earned over time. Educational audiologists must work toward mutual respect with other educational personnel. Audiologists should treat others as they wish to be treated. Once administrators, children, parents, and teachers realize the benefits of a quality support program, audiologists should easily gain the respect and support of all involved. Having a solid plan from the beginning is a big help. To secure the cooperation of others, audiologists must try a little harder and be especially careful to use the appropriate channels of communication for accomplishing goals. Audiologists should first consult the head of nursing, for example, prior to requesting that public-school nurses perform the daily visual and listening checks of all personal hearing aids belonging to children with hearing impairment who are mainstreamed into regular classrooms. There are certain "dos" and "don'ts" to consider when using multiskilling and support personnel (Johnson, 1999). Educational audiologists should:

- Know provisions within the "Position Statement and Guidelines of the Consensus Panel on Support Personnel in Audiology" (AAA, 1997).
- Consult federal laws, state licensure requirements, the codes of ethics for professional organizations, and other professional guidelines.
- Communicate with and seek the support of school administrators prior to implementing new programming or changes in existing programming.
- Fully cost-out school contracts to account for adequate inservice training and necessary equipment.
- Define specific roles and functions of audiologic support personnel.
- Design effective and meaningful inservice training experiences.
- Motivate, respect, and appreciate audiologic support personnel.
- Provide ongoing evaluation of all aspects of the program.

On the other hand, educational audiologists should not:

- Act without consulting administrators.
- Take any unnecessary risks that may compromise student care.
- Assume that audiologic support personnel know what to do without appropriate training.
- Assume that audiologic support personnel can operate independently without any supervision.
- Treat audiologic support personnel as subordinates.
- Cut necessary costs to secure contracts.

Obtaining Necessary Equipment and Materials

Recall that contract-for-service audiologists must supply the equipment and the supplies for amplification device support programs. Regardless of the service-delivery model, audiologists should have access to the latest equipment and clinical protocols for fitting high-technology hearing aids discussed in Chapter 7. Aside from a functioning and currently calibrated audiometer, the most important piece of equipment for itinerant audiologists is a portable hearing aid analyzer/real-ear probe-tube microphone measurement system such as the AUDIOSCAN. The AUDIOSCAN is equipped with the Desired Sensation Level (DSL) software (Cornelisse, Seewald, & Jamieson, 1994). DSL is ideal for setting the gain and output of children's hearing aids and FM systems.

Audiologists' materials for amplification device support programs should include a portable hearing aid laboratory that can easily be carried from classroom to classroom in a bag. The bag should contain: a hearing aid stethoscope, battery checker, forced-air bulb, wax picks, pipe-cleaners, hearing aid brushes, earmold/hearing aid cleaner, disinfectant, alcohol pads, surgical gloves, battery contact spray, extra battery doors, tubing of all sizes, batteries of all sizes, ear hooks, earmold impression materials, FM system transducers and cords, mailing boxes with labels, glue, portable drill, scissors, and so on. As most audiologists are aware, cerumen can be a common cause for failure in children's hearing aids and personal FM systems. Thus, depending on state licensure and scope of practice guidelines, most audiologists should also have portable cerumen management equipment available. Audiologists should have an approved cerumen management protocol agreed upon by administrators, school personnel, and, if appropriate, supervising physicians, however. Informed consent is a requirement here and should not be overlooked. In addition, all audiologic support personnel should have hearing aid check kits (e.g., a hearing aid stethoscope and adapter; a battery checker [voltmeter]; a forced-air bulb; a wax pick or pipe cleaners; a soft, small brush; a small, lighted magnifying class; extra batteries; plastic bags; and a drying agent [Musket, 1995]). Material costs for amplification device support programs can be considerable. In some cases, school systems will not be able to afford these expenses. Chapter 4, "Funding Support Programs," lists some suggestions for covering these necessary costs.

Devising Program Logistics

Amplification device support program logistics is simply how the system works. Chapter 3, "Defining and Marketing Support Programs," summarized the necessary skills needed for audiologists to manage support programs. They must be able to perform a systematic analysis of service-delivery sites to specify program needs. The process requires establishing program procedures and lines of communication between and among support program personnel.

1. *Audiologists determine who will serve as audiologic support personnel.*

2. *Audiologists must decide on program documentation.* Such documentation includes daily visual and listening check sheets for hearing aids (Appendix VI-D), cochlear implants (Appendix VI-E), FM systems (Appendix VI-F), and sound-field FM classroom amplification systems (Appendix VI-G). Daily check sheets serve to provide the documentation for:

- compliance with federal regulation,
- service provisions to children as specified in their Individualized Education Plans (IEPs),
- records of services provided for fiscal accountability, and
- records of special problems that require intervention.

From time-to-time, school districts are audited for their compliance with federal regulations. We have found that auditors often inspect records of hearing aid monitoring programs, particularly the actual hearing aid check sheets. In addition, these check sheets should be part of the children's permanent records, documenting services to be provided as specified in their IEPs. Furthermore, contract-for-service audiologists will find that these sheets are an excellent way to account for services provided when writing final reports to school administrators. Finally, each check sheet should contain a "Comments" section in which audiologic support personnel can make notes for special problems needing intervention. If children's hearing aids are chronically dirty, for example, parents may need to be instructed on the appropriate care of hearing aids.

3. *Establish procedures for situations needing immediate action by the audiologist.* For example, what are the procedures for reporting and repairing malfunctioning hearing aids, cochlear implants, FM systems, and sound-field FM amplification systems, or for handling equipment failures due to the need for cerumen management? The procedures should be as simple, effective, and quick as possible to repair necessary equipment. Audiologists must be accessible either through personal contact, telephone, or e-mail. As shown in Figure 6–3, being a good communicator is one of the human-relation skills necessary to manage audiologic support personnel in crisis situations. Audiologists in these positions must be vigilant in answering their phone messages and e-mail. Otherwise, problems can accumulate and become insurmountable.

4. *Establish program legitimacy in as many ways as possible.* For example, participation in a hearing aid monitoring program should be mentioned in children's IEPs and in the job descriptions of audiologic support personnel. English (1998) stated that if hearing aid monitoring statements are not written into children's IEPs, school districts are not required to provide these services. Thus, audiologists must actively seek to include components of the amplification device support program into children's IEPs for program viability. In addition, educational personnel's job descriptions should include participation as audiologic support personnel for program credibility. Public-school nurses may take

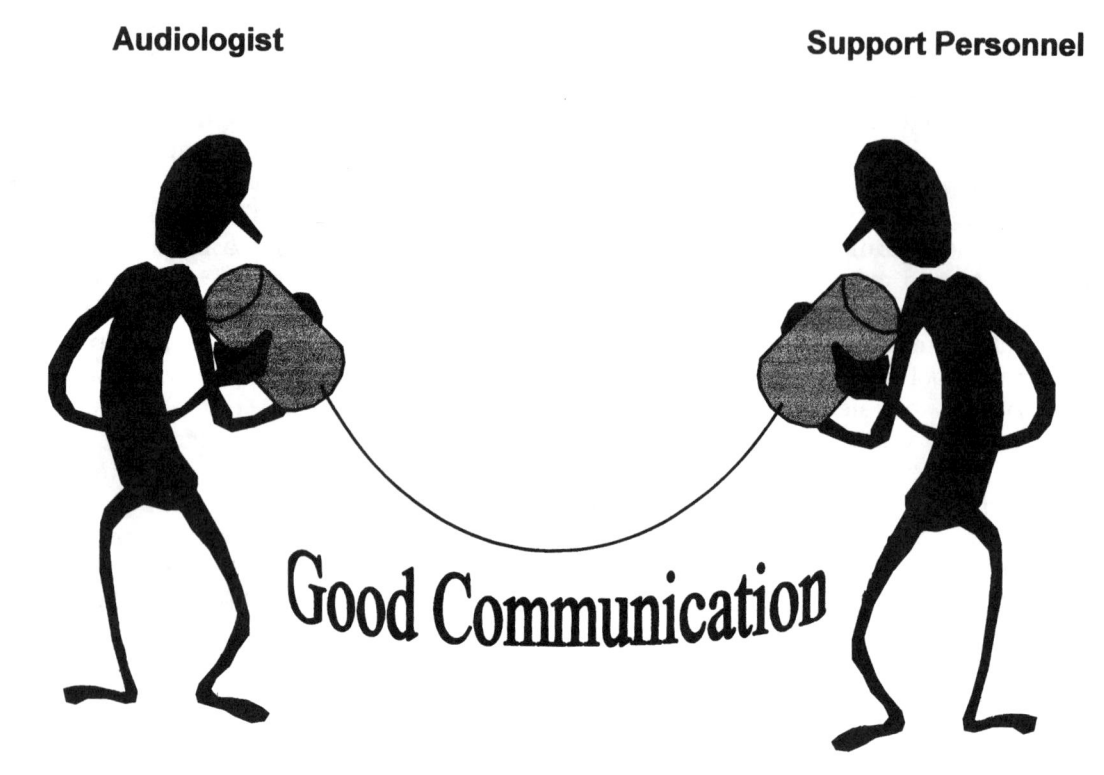

Figure 6–3. Good communication between audiologist and support personnel is a prerequisite for program success.

their role of performing daily visual and listening checks on children's hearing aids more seriously if it is written in their job descriptions.

Children's Role in Serving as Amplification Device Support Personnel

Ultimately, school-age children with hearing impairment and their families should be taught how to monitor hearing aids and other amplification devices. Elfenbein (1994) found that even though parents were aware of the need to monitor hearing aids, most did not have the equipment or the skills to do so. Parental motivation and follow through are very important. Similarly, students with hearing impairment are often overprotected, lacking the self-help and self-advocacy skills necessary for academic success (English, 1998). Thus, children with hearing impairment should be counseled about their hearing losses and taught self-help skills from an early age. Grunblatt and Daar (1994) developed a two-part educational program providing this information to children with hearing impairment. Part 1 is an educational program consisting of information on the following topics: (1) basic audiology, (2) hearing aid hygiene, (3) the FM system: how and why we use it, (4) know your audiogram, and (5) ask the audiologist. Each of the five educational classes lasts about 45 minutes and involves between 3 and 15 children who participate at their own level. In addition, classroom teachers emphasize lessons taught by audiologists through discussions and activities. Specific program protocols for Grunblatt and Daar appear in Appendix VI-H. Part 2 of the program consists of individualized counseling among students, school counselors, and the educational audiologist. Grunblatt and Darr (1994) believed that children with hearing impairment who are exposed to this information at an early age (i.e., 3 years old) will be better able to cope with their disability and be advocates for their own hearing health-care needs.

SUPPORT PROGRAMS IN CENTRAL AUDITORY PROCESSING DISORDERS (CAPD) SERVICE DELIVERY

One critical area for development of support programs is in central auditory processing disorders (CAPD) service delivery. Parents of children with CAPD can be frustrated in trying to find support for their children for several reasons.

1. *CAPD service delivery may seem like a luxury to most school administrators who have limited financial and human resources to serve students with disabilities.* School administrators, for example, may feel that resources should be used on students with measurable hearing loss.
2. *Many school systems may elect to contract for specific audiologic services that may not include CAPD service delivery.* Some contract-for-service audiologists may even envision support programs in CAPD service delivery, but find that they are paid only to conduct audiologic screenings, evaluations, evaluate and fit personal FM systems, and maintain hearing aids.
3. *Educational personnel, including audiologists, may not have the necessary knowledge or skills to develop stellar CAPD service-delivery models.* Educational audiologists must have a thorough working knowledge of the topic that can be obtained only through specialized training in the field (Bellis, 1996).

Parents of children with CAPD can become frustrated with the system. Consider Mrs. Stewart and her son Jay in the example below.

> *Mrs. Stewart was very concerned about her son Jay, a third grader who was falling behind his classmates—especially in reading and spelling. His teacher, Mrs. Jones, reported that Jay had difficulty following directions, often misunderstood what was being said, was easily distractible, and acted out in class. Mrs. Jones recommended that Jay have an audiologic evaluation conducted by Starr Audiologist, the contract-for-service audiologist for the district. The evaluation determined that Jay's hearing sensitivity was within normal limits. Starr explained to Mrs. Stewart that Jay was exhibiting characteristics similar to patients with CAPD. Mrs. Stewart was fascinated and voraciously read all the information provided by the audiologist. Starr told Mrs. Jones that she would check with the director of special education regarding the possibility of conducting a CAPD evaluation. Unfortunately, the assessment was not covered in the school district's contract with Starr, the only audiologist within 75 miles of the town, who knew very little about the diagnosis and management of CAPD. Mrs. Stewart was disappointed to learn that there was no system in place to help her son achieve his academic potential.*

Comprehensive CAPD service delivery involves five interrelated program components (Bellis, 1996): (1) training and educating key individuals, (2) establishing screening procedures, (3) acquiring resources for CAPD assessments, (4) implementing management goals, and (5) collecting and analyzing data to determine program efficacy.

Training and Educating Key Individuals

Training and educating key participants is the first step in CAPD service delivery. Table 6–3 shows the individuals and the required knowledge for their competent participation in the support program (Bellis, 1996).

First, audiologists must train themselves by seeking out the necessary knowledge base for CAPD service delivery. In addition, audiologists must have a vision for the overall support program, including the pertinent roles, prerequisite knowledge, and skills of key participants. Audiologists are responsible for educating and training all other participants. Chapter 5 discussed how to create effective inservice programs. With regard to multiskilling, the appropriate model to use is collateral multiskilling, in which audiologists train and educate other professionals to participate in support programs for CAPD service delivery. The formats of inservices should be informational (e.g., educational impact of CAPD, classroom management techniques, and so on) and a combination of informational and skill-based (e.g., CAPD test administration, scoring, and interpretation). Appendix VI-I contains "Misconceptions of School Personnel about CAPD"

Table 6-3. Professionals involved in support programs for CAPD service delivery: Required knowledge.

Team Member	Required Knowledge
Audiologist	■ Training and knowledge base necessary for comprehensive CAPD service delivery ■ Theoretical underpinnings and methods of practical application of scientific theory ■ Time management
Speech-language pathologist	■ Appropriate methods of diagnosing CAPD ■ CAPD management
Educator	■ Educational impact of CAPD ■ Classroom management suggestions
Educational psychologist	■ Neurophysiological bases of CAPD ■ Appropriate methods of diagnosing CAPD ■ Need for accurate measures of cognitive and psychoeducational abilities ■ Emotional impact of CAPD
Administrator	■ Prevalence of CAPD ■ Rationale for comprehensive CAPD services ■ Current recommendations for service delivery ■ Funding issues
Other professionals	■ The nature and impact of CAPD ■ Appropriate methods of diagnosing CAPD ■ The need for private practitioners to work closely with educational professionals
Parents	■ The nature of CAPD ■ Management suggestions ■ Prognosis for success

Source: From *Assessment and Management of Central Auditory Processing Disorders in the Educational Setting: From Science to Practice,* by T. J. Bellis, 1996, p. 241. San Diego, CA: Singular Publishing Group. Reprinted with permission.

(Hall & Mueller, 1997) to be used to plan inservices on this topic. However, audiologists must develop more sophisticated protocols for the specialized training required by speech-language pathologists, educational psychologists, administrators, and other professionals. The reader is referred to Bellis (1996), Johnson et al. (1997), and Masters, Stecker, and Katz (1998) for further information.

Screening Procedures

Bellis and Burke (1996) advocated a multidisciplinary team approach to identify children with CAPD for the purpose of gathering adequate information (e.g., educational, social, speech-language, cognitive, and medical characteristics) to formulate initial impressions of the auditory capabilities of children. The team consists of the following professionals and their respective roles (Bellis & Burke, 1996):

- Audiologist
  ⇒ manages and coordinates CAPD effort, and
  ⇒ performs audiologic evaluation to rule out peripheral hearing loss.
- Speech-language pathologist
  ⇒ determines child's receptive and expressive language abilities, and
  ⇒ determines written language and associated abilities.
- Educator provides information regarding child's listening and learning behaviors in the classroom.
- Psychologist determines child's cognitive skills and capacities for learning.
- Parents provide information regarding:
  ⇒ developmental milestones,
  ⇒ auditory behavior in the home, and
  ⇒ medical and academic history.
- Physician rules out presence of pathology that may affect learning abilities.

Resources for Comprehensive CAPD Assessment

Audiologists must possess both appropriate assessment tools and adequate knowledge, instrumentation, and time to conduct CAPD evaluations. Many of these tests require training and two-channel audiometers. Dichotic speech tests, for example, need two channels for the simultaneous presentation of two different signals to each ear. In addition, relatively few audiometers have the capability to perform masking level difference (MLD) testing. Morever, CAPD assessment is quite time-consuming. Bellis (1996) stated that not all educational audiologists need to be involved in CAPD service delivery, especially if there is a regional assessment center that will perform these evaluations for several school districts. In addition, local colleges and universities with speech and hearing clinics are excellent referral sources for comprehensive CAPD assessment.

Audiologists need to be aware of the existence of several specific test batteries for CAPD assessment. Johnson et al. (1997) provided a list of at least eight approaches, some of which are: Bellis (1996), Chermak (1992), Colorado Department of Education (1996), Ferre and Wilber (1986), Medwetsky (1994), Utah State University (Von Almen, Blair, & Spriet, 1990), Vanderbilt University Medical Center (Hall, Baer, Byrn, Wurm, Henry, Wilson, & Prentice, 1993), and Willeford (1977). Readers are referred to Johnson et al. (1997) for a synopsis of these approaches. Audiologists can select an existing test battery or develop their own. Selection of a specific test battery should reflect audiologists' theoretical approach to CAPD and provide direct suggestions for management.

Implementation of Management Goals

Johnson et al. (1997) stated that there are four areas for educational management of CAPD in children:

- classroom modifications,
- amplification,
- direct treatment, and
- compensatory strategies.

With regard to classroom modifications, audiologists can work with school administrators, teachers, and interior designers to improve the acoustic environments for children with CAPD. Audiologists should provide CAPD inservices to these individuals including how to create optimal learning environments. Educational personnel need to understand how classroom acoustics (i.e., reverberation and noise) can affect the concentration and attention of children with CAPD. *Reverberation* is the continuation of acoustic energy due to the reflections of that energy off the room's surfaces even though the source of that energy has been terminated (Nabelek & Nabelek, 1994). The index of severity for reverberation is called reverberation time, abbreviated by the capital letter "T." *Reverberation time* is the time that it takes for the sound pressure level of a sound to decrease 60 dB after its source has been terminated (Crandell & Smaldino, 1995). *It is recommended that the reverberation times in children's classrooms not exceed 0.4 seconds* (Crandell & Smaldino, 1995). Reverberation tends to prolong vowel energy in such a way that it masks or "smears" over the softer consonants that follow.

Noise is any unwanted sound and can be of three types: (1) external (i.e., outside of the school), (2) internal (i.e., inside the school), and (3) classroom (i.e., inside the classroom). The index of severity for noise is the *signal-to-noise ratio* (S/N), which is the relative intensity of the signal (i.e., teachers' voice) to that of the background noise. *The minimum signal-to-noise ratio for children's classrooms is + 15 dB* (i.e., meaning that the teacher's voice should be 15 dB more intense than the background noise) (Crandell & Smaldino, 1995). Audiologists can perform acoustic surveys of classrooms and report the results to teachers and school administrators. (Readers are referred to Berg [1993] and Crandell, Smaldino, and Flexer [1995] for step-by-step classroom acoustic survey protocols.) Educational audiologists, teachers, school administrators, and others can try to improve classroom acoustics through suggestions listed in Table 6–4 (Crandell & Smaldino, 1995).

Professional acoustic modification of classrooms can be expensive. Some relatively inexpensive measures can improve acoustic conditions, however (e.g., putting tennis balls on the bottom of children's chairs, mounting artwork on the classroom walls, covering blackboards when not in use, having children wear soft-soled shoes). If reverberation times and S/Ns cannot be improved to recommended levels, then the use of FM amplification should be considered.

Table 6–4. Suggestions for improving classroom acoustics.

EXTERNAL NOISE REDUCTION

- Place classrooms away from high noise sources (e.g., traffic, railroads, and construction sites).
- Ensure that external walls block out at least 45 to 50 dB of sound originating outside of the school.
- Ensure that there are no cracks or openings in exterior walls that can let noise in.
- Ensure that external wall windows are properly installed, are heavy weighted or double paned, and that they remain closed.
- Use landscaping strategies (e.g., hedges) as sound buffers.
- Use concrete barriers between school buildings and noise sources.

INTERNAL NOISE REDUCTION

- Relocate classes for children with hearing impairment to quiet areas of the building.
- Use fiberglass or lead sheets for acoustic isolation of classrooms separated by drop ceilings.
- Use double- or thick-walled constructions for interior walls.
- Use acoustical ceiling tile and carpeting in hallways.
- Use acoustically treated doors for classrooms.
- Line heating and cooling ducts serving more than one classroom with acoustically treated materials.
- Back blackboards with absorptive materials to reduce sound transmission from adjacent rooms.

REDUCTION OF CLASSROOM NOISE

- Locate children away from high-noise areas.
- Replace or acoustically treat malfunctioning air conditioning and heating units and ducts.
- Install thick wall-to-wall carpeting.
- Place rubber tips on students' chairs.
- Acoustically treat furniture.
- Hang thick curtains or acoustically treated venetian blinds over windows.
- Avoid open-plan classrooms.
- Use acoustically treated barriers that go from ceiling to floor between teaching areas.
- Maintain fluorescent lighting systems.
- Reduce computer noise by placing rubber pads or carpet remnants under units.
- Encourage children to wear soft-soled shoes.

REDUCTION OF REVERBERATION

- Cover reflective surfaces with absorptive materials.
- Use thick carpeting on the floor.
- Use curtains or thick draperies over windows.
- Position mobile blackboards at angles with walls and each other to reduce the possibility of "flutter" echo.
- Hang artwork on the walls.

Source: Adapted from "Acoustic Modifications in Classrooms," by C. C. Crandell and J. J. Smaldino, 1995. In C. C. Crandell, J. J. Smaldino, and C. Flexer (Eds.), *Sound Field FM Amplification: Theory and Practical Applications* (pp. 83–92). San Diego, CA: Singular Publishing Group.

With regard to the use of amplification systems, educational audiologists should first consider what type of amplification is most appropriate. Generally, two types of FM amplification systems are available; (1) personal FM systems, and (2) sound-field FM classroom amplification systems. *Personal FM systems*, as shown in Figure 6–4, are those in which the teacher wears a microphone and the student wears a receiver (Stein, 1998).

A note must be made about the recommended use of terminology by the "Guidelines for Fitting and Monitoring FM Systems" (ASHA, 1994). Those guidelines suggested using the term "self-contained" for FM systems with receivers that are coupled directly to children's ears and using the term "personal" for systems with receivers that are coupled to children's personal hearing aids. In this textbook, we will refer to both systems as personal FM systems to distinguish them from sound-field FM classroom amplification systems. *Sound-field FM classroom amplification systems*, as shown in Figure 6–5, consist of a transmitter, a receiver, and from one to four strategically placed loudspeakers within the classroom that amplify the teacher's voice (Stein, 1998).

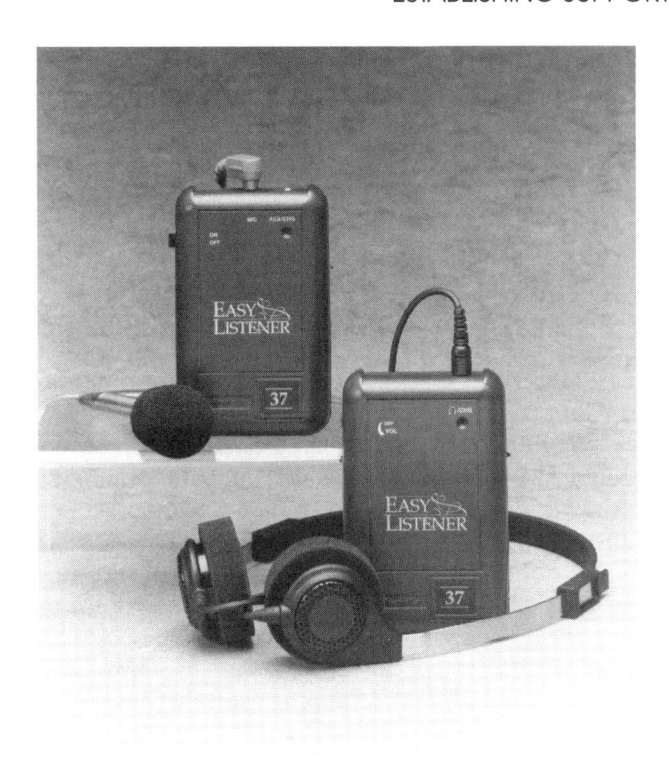

Figure 6–4. Personal FM system. (Photo courtesy of Phonic Ear Inc. 1998.)

Selection of the appropriate amplification systems requires a careful consideration of several variables. First, are there only a few students with CAPD in the school? If there are only one or two children, perhaps personal FM systems would be appropriate. Do children change classrooms frequently throughout the school day? If so, personal FM systems again may be more appropriate. If there are several children requiring "special" listening conditions in a self-contained classroom, then perhaps a sound-field FM classroom amplification system would be a more appropriate choice. Regardless of the equipment selected, communication with other educational personnel is critical for successful program implementation.

Reeh and Carlson (1997) suggested establishing a trial program for personal FM systems among children with CAPD. Such a program should consist of a referral process, a trial period, and a decision-making process. Reeh and Carlson's referral process consisted of: (1) audiologic evaluation of children with CAPD with a recommendation for FM use; (2) review of the appropriateness of recommendation by the edu-

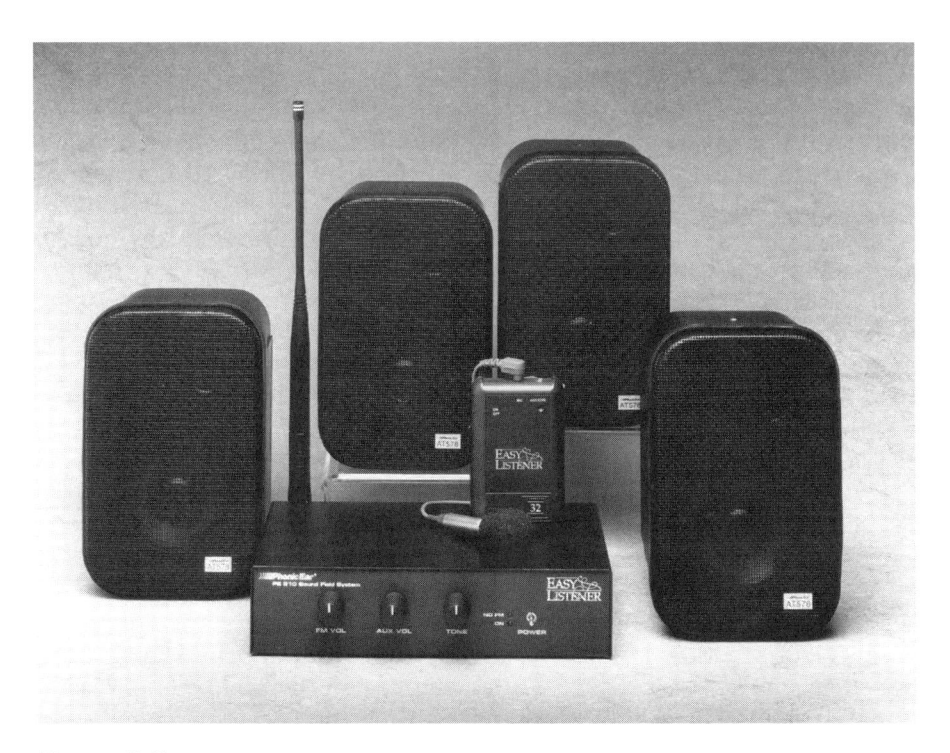

Figure 6–5. Sound-field FM classroom amplification system. (Photo courtesy of Phonic Ear Inc. 1998.)

cational audiologist; (3) assessment of the classroom environment; and (4) pretrial interviews with children, parents, and teachers. In reviewing the audiologic evaluation and other data, educational audiologists should be wary of making "blanket" recommendations for all children with CAPD to use personal FM systems. (For further discussion of this issue, see Bellis, 1996.)

Educational audiologists must assess the learning environment to order accessories to be used with children with FM systems. Assessment of the learning environment should include the classroom style (i.e., closed classroom, open-concept ideas, split-grade classrooms, and team teaching), the classroom design (i.e., portable classrooms, classroom space utilization, and classroom seating), and the learning style (i.e., didactic, interactive, small-group activities, and individual work) (Edwards, 1995). Team teaching requires inservice training on the care and use of the child's personal FM system for all teachers, for example. Similarly, if a variety of learning styles is used in the classroom, then a lavalier microphone should be used for didactic teaching along with a microphone that can be passed around for small discussion groups.

Educational audiologists should interview children, parents, and teachers before initiation of the trial period. Children with CAPD should be made aware that educational personnel are considering their use of a personal FM system. Some children have no idea what is going on, which may contribute to their ultimate refusal to use the device. Children with CAPD need to be asked about how they feel about using a personal FM system. Interviews with the parents and teachers not only provide valuable assistance in planning the trial period, but also provide an opportunity to share important information regarding the results of clinical testing. For example, educational audiologists should explain to parents and teachers how the test results relate to the children's behaviors. In addition, audiologists should seek teachers' and parents' input regarding children's characteristics. They should ask:

- Are these particular children forgetful or destructive?
- How do the children behave in the classroom?
- How are the children's emotional states? Do they have low self-esteem?
- Will personal FM systems cause more problems than they are worth?
- Are there any other handicapping conditions?

In addition to informal questions, teachers and parents should complete formal behavioral checklists, such as the *Fisher's Auditory Problems Checklist* (Fisher, 1976) or the *Screening Instrument for Targeting Educational Risk* (S.I.F.T.E.R.) (Anderson, 1989). Audiologists should carefully consider all information obtained during classroom visits and interviews. In some cases, the use of personal FM systems may not be the best solution for all children with CAPD, for those who seem like good candidates, a trial program should follow.

Trial periods begin with a delivery of the personal FM system to the child. Parents, teachers, and children should be instructed on its care and use. A letter should be sent to the special education office prior to the initiation of the trial period. Classroom teachers or their assistants should be designated as audiologic support personnel in the amplification device support programs. They should attend appropriate inservice training sessions and should be given daily check sheets to document the daily monitoring of children's personal FM units. The educational audiologist should call classroom teachers at least once a week during the first two weeks of the trial period to see if they have any questions, if the personal FM systems are working properly, and if children are accepting and wearing the devices.

Trial periods should last several weeks to assess the full effect of children's use of personal FM systems. Classroom teachers should complete the same behavioral checklists and conduct the same interviews as before the initiation of the trial period to determine the efficacy of personal FM system use. Audiologists should also perform functional listening evaluations of children both with and without the FM units involving sentence recognition manipulating variables such as modality (auditory only versus auditory visual), speaker-to-listener distance (close versus distant), and listening condition (quiet versus noisy) (Stein, 1998). Readers are referred to Johnson et al. (1997) for specifics on this procedure, which are summarized in Appendix VI-J.

At the conclusion of the trial period, educational audiologists should convene members of the CAPD support program to discuss the implications of children's ongoing use of personal FM systems. If trial periods are successful, the committee can then make final recommendations regarding the use of personal a FM system to the children's IEP teams regarding: settings, accessories, situations for use and non-use, and audiologic support personnel responsible for checking the devices. Some school districts may have limited funding for personal FM systems. Chapter 4, "Funding Support Programs," provided some suggestions for possible funding sources for equipment.

Sound-field FM amplification systems, described earlier, are a recommended amplification strategy when several children with CAPD are within a single classroom. Flexer (1995) provided a checklist of important points regarding sound-field FM amplification systems:

- Hearing and listening are the invisible cornerstones of children's education.
- Auditory discrimination is a prerequisite for rudimentary academic competencies that are necessary for success in school.
- Any type of hearing problem, if unmanaged, can have a negative impact on academic development.
- Even though the teachers' voices may be audible, it does not mean that they are intelligible for all students to understand every word being said.
- Information must be heard (i.e., data input) before it can be understood (i.e., data processing).
- Sound-field FM amplification systems are beneficial for all children in a classroom.

The efficacy of using sound-field FM amplification among children with CAPD has not been well-documented in the literature. Crandell et al. (1995) provided an excellent rational for using this technology among this population, however. Readers are advised to consult that source for further information.

With regard to direct treatment, the reader is referred to three timely textbooks on management of CAPD: Chermak and Musiek (1992), Bellis (1996), and Masters et al. (1998). Regarding the use of compensatory strategies for children with CAPD, Appendix VI-K contains the Vanderbilt Balance and Hearing Center's list of suggestions for parents and teachers, as well as strategies for use at home (Hall & Mueller, 1997). Bellis (1996) strongly urged, however, that clinicians resist the temptation to make general recommendations to classroom teachers and other educational personnel regarding management of CAPD. Moreover, she advised clinicians to avoid preprinted lists of "general" suggestions without first considering their appropriateness for the specific child in question.

Challenges Facing CAPD Service-Delivery Support Programs

Bellis (1996) stated that audiologists have two major challenges in CAPD service delivery: (1) time and (2) lack of training. First, with the current shortage of educational audiologists, most school-based clinicians find little time to meet the needs of children with CAPD single-handedly. Developing a CAPD service-delivery support program with a delegation of responsibilities to related educational personnel can allow audiologists to focus their time and attention on critical issues. In addition, two major factors have contributed to the lack of sufficient training for most audiologists to assess and manage CAPD competently. First, few training programs offer enough instruction on CAPD to allow graduates to provide services in this area (Bellis, 1996). Second, there is a lack of consensus regarding preferred practice in CAPD service delivery (Bellis, 1996). In fact, audiologists may find colleagues in the school setting who doubt the appropriate use of CAPD as a diagnostic label. After an exhaustive review of the literature, Cacace and McFarland (1998) concluded that empirical evidence supporting the modality-specific nature of CAPD was extremely limited, calling into question the validity of using CAPD as a diagnostic label. They further stated that there is no theory, no formal statistics on incidence or prevalence, and no standardized format for diagnosing this condition. Audiologists must be prepared to respond to such criticisms if CAPD service delivery is to be successful.

COUNSELING SUPPORT PROGRAMS

Family counseling is another key area for establishing support programs for children with hearing impairment and their families. Family counseling can involve parent, sibling, and peer support programs. The need for counseling support programs in educational settings will increase as mandated Universal Infant Hearing Screening Programs identify more and more children with hearing impairment. The advent of otoacoustic emission (OAEs) and automated auditory brainstem response (AABR) screening protocols enables audiologists to identify children with hearing loss within a few hours of birth. Early identification of hearing loss can be particularly useful in counseling parents with hereditary hearing loss who are especially anxious about their babies' hearing status. Figure 6–6A and 6–6B show such mothers who have been informed that their babies had passed the OAE screening, thereby alleviating their stress and anxiety. Early identification of hearing loss can lead to earlier acceptance and intervention at a much younger age for other parents.

Support programs are needed for parents because they often experience a roller coaster of emotions soon after being notified of their children's hearing loss (Van Hecke, 1994). Parents need to complete the appropriate stages of the grieving process (e.g., shock, denial, anger, depression, and so on) in order to accept their children's hearing losses. Parents may develop inappropriate coping strategies (e.g., insisting that the child "look normal," being unable to accept the child's hearing loss, being interested in invisible completely-in-the-canal [CIC] hearing aids) without intervention and support. Counseling is important for these parents because children's acceptance of their hearing loss largely depends on their families' attitudes (Loeb & Sarigiani, 1986; Thibodeau, 1994). Parents' shame may cause children to feel the same way, for example. Children may feel "less than perfect," resulting in low self-esteem. They may develop an unreasonable fear of being judged negatively or teased as a result of wearing hearing aids, which is also known as the "hearing aid effect" (Blood, Blood, & Danhauer, 1977).

Audiologists can assist families with their adjustment by trying to understand the reasons behind parents' feelings (Thibodeau, 1994). Audiologists should explore parents' feelings by requesting, "Tell me how you feel when someone notices your child's FM systems or hearing aids" (Thibodeau, 1994; Van Hecke, 1994). Assisting parents in verbalizing their negative feelings often

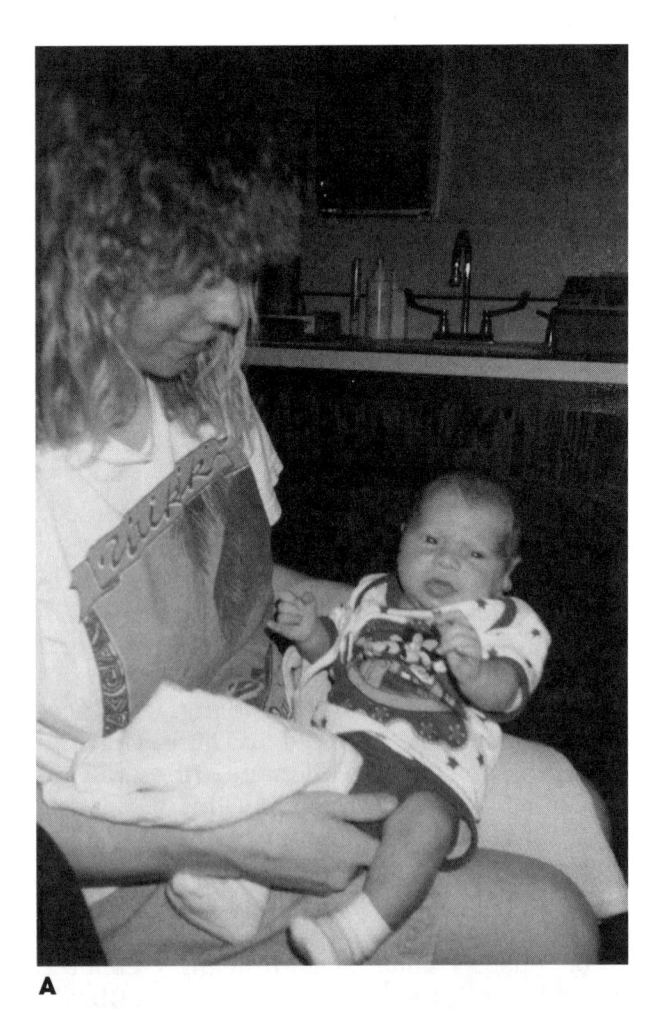

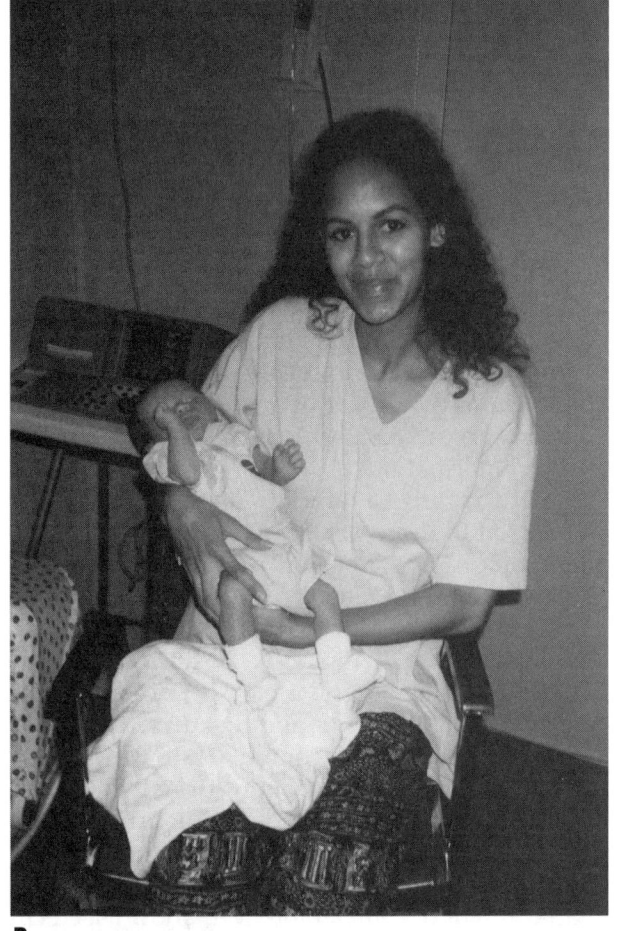

Figure 6–6. A mother with a severe hearing loss (A) and a deaf mother (B) are informed that their babies had passed otoacoustic emissions (OAE) screening.

helps them accept their children's hearing losses. Morever, siblings should also be included in counseling sessions because they may feel conflicting emotions toward their brother or sister with a hearing loss (Atkins, 1994). Appendix VI-L provides a list of suggestions regarding the siblings of children with hearing impairment (Atkins, 1994). Audiologists must recognize when parents need to be referred to mental-health professionals or would benefit from talking to other parents of children with hearing impairment, who can come close to understanding what they are feeling (Atkins, 1994). Parent support groups provide members with: (1) an assurance that they are not alone; (2) a sense of extended family; (3) comradery in navigating through educational, medical, and philosophical options; (4) companionship and understanding; (5) problem solving in a nonthreatening context; and (6) a sense of confidence in meeting the needs of their children (Atkins, 1994).

Support groups are best organized at the school level. A support group consisting of parents of children with hearing impairment at a particular elementary school can be very beneficial for a number of reasons. First, parents of children with hearing impairment of the same age have a lot in common (e.g., their children may have the same teacher, children may befriend each other, and so on). Second, these groups can be effective in lobbying for issues that could improve service delivery to their children in the school. Third, these groups may organize needed fundraisers (e.g., bake sales, walk-a-thons, and so on) for support programs.

Audiologists should serve as a catalyst for the establishment of these support groups. They can suggest that teachers and parents form a support group by sending letters such as the one shown in Appendix VI-M. The letter should describe what the support group is, possible functions it could serve, and dates for informational meetings for parents. At the meetings, audiologists should introduce themselves, review their roles and responsibilities, and discuss possibilities of forming a parent support group. Some parents may be enthusiastic, others may have no interest, and some may find it impossible to participate. Thus, audiologists must understand the possible obstacles to the these support groups at the outset: (1) practical issues related to attendance (e.g., distance, transportation, child care), (2) language and cultural barriers, (3) emotional issues (e.g., pride, disappointment, and impatience), (4) comparing one child's progress to that of someone else's child, (5) reluctance to face other stress-related matters (e.g., alcoholism, other substance abuse, child abuse, illness), and (6) only trusting the audiologist (Atkins, 1994).

If parents are interested in forming a group, they must understand that it is *their* group, not the audiologists'. Furthermore, they must address the following issues (Atkins, 1994):

- Is the purpose of the group clear to all participants?
- Should the meetings be educational, administrative, recreational, or emotionally supportive?
- Who should lead the group? Ideally, the leaders of support groups should be parents who have successfully navigated through the psychological adjustment and practical implications of having children with hearing impairment.

Leaders of the parent support group actually serve as audiologic support personnel who work closely with the audiologist and other educational personnel. Leaders should follow these rules (Trychin, 1994):

- Do not preach.
- Ask questions.
- Be prepared.
- Make sure that all group members understand what is being said and done.
- Try not to embarrass people.
- Do not let one or two parents monopolize the group.
- Have group members take turns.
- Do not get involved in arguments about what is right or wrong.
- Do not try to be an expert.
- Provide members with feedback regarding the communication that occurs in the group.

Effective group sessions often follow these rules (Trychin, 1994):

- No one bluffs.
- Only one person speaks at a time.
- The speaker must use the microphone.
- Group members treat each other gently and with respect.

Support groups for children and teens with hearing impairment may also be highly beneficial. *Adolescents may have a difficult time verbalizing their feelings about their hearing impair-*

ments and wearing noticeable hearing aids and FM systems. Teenagers have a need for both peer approval and independence from parents (Altman, 1996). In some cases, teenagers may reject amplification because of how their hearing aids look or the need to rebel against authority figures. Teenagers may view audiologists as another group of adults who cannot possibly understand where they are coming from. Thus, educational audiologists may try to organize support groups consisting of other students with hearing impairment or related disabilities.

Audiologists should try to create an open and supportive atmosphere in which teenagers feel comfortable sharing their thoughts and feelings. The same "ground rules" for parent support groups should apply to peer support groups. Furthermore, audiologists should gently initiate interaction amongst participants and then assume the role of moderator. Some adolescents may not feel comfortable with groups. Those students may be paired with an older peer or mentor with whom they feel comfortable talking to in a one-on-one interaction. Still, some students may be so shy that they only feel comfortable confiding in the audiologist. Audiologists must be very careful in how they communicate with these sensitive teenagers. Interrogating teenagers with a series of yes-no questions will elicit only shrugs and "I don't know" responses. Open-ended questions can encourage teenagers to verbalize their fears about hearing aid stigma. Altman (1996) suggested using the following strategies in counseling teenage patients about amplification:

- Establish rapport.
- Consider the adolescent as a consultant.
- Develop adolescents' problem-solving and decision-making skills.
- Watch for unaddressed family issues.
- Refer to other professionals when necessary.

Some adolescents may be so "cosmetically sensitive" about the visibility of their amplification devices that they refuse to wear them. Educational audiologists might investigate the fitting of less obtrusive hearing instruments, such as FM receivers that are packaged in behind-the-ear cases (e.g., Phonic Ear's "Free Ear"). *Educational audiologists might also suggest to children's personal audiologists that they consider using completely-in-the-canal (CICs) with their young patients.* Some audiologists may feel that because earmolds have to be replaced frequently due to growth of the pinna and ear canal (Johnson & Danhauer, 1997), CICs are inappropriate for children. Although the pinna continues to grow until about 9 years of age, the external auditory canal does not grow appreciably after about seven years of age (Northern & Downs, 1991). Many manufacturers are willing to remake CIC shells for children when necessary, especially if second-year insurance policies are purchased during the initial hearing aid fitting.

Some audiologists also may believe that CICs are too fragile to be used by children and teenagers due to their high activity levels and their tendency to be careless with items such as eyeglasses, orthodontic appliances, and so on. Because CICs have been found to be very comfortable and virtually invisible (Staab, 1995; Staab & Lybarger, 1994), students may be less likely to take them out than they would be with larger hearing aids. Furthermore, the placement of CICs deep into the ear canal may make them the most desirable of hearing instruments for children involved in high-activity sports, such as baseball, basketball, gymnastics, tennis, and track. Deep canal fittings may reduce the likelihood of injury to the pinnae in sports when compared to other styles of hearing aids. CIC hearing aids are protected by the cartilaginous portion of the pinna and the outer one-third of the ear canal. Ears fitted with other styles of hearing aids may be at risk for injury if the devices are forcefully lodged into outer ear structures. Figures 6–7A, 6–7B, and 6–7C show two young athletes who have opted for CIC hearing aids.

In addition to establishing support groups, audiologists can establish cost-efficient "Family Resource Centers" at key schools that house educational programs for students with hearing impairment. The resource center may be housed in any small room, or it may even be located in a corner of a classroom. The resource center may include books and periodicals concerning hearing loss, books about speechreading and auditory training, conversational strategies, sign language, legal issues, Deaf culture, assistive listening devices, medical issues, and educational options that can be available for checkout (Tye-Murray, Witt, Schum, Kelsay, & Schum, 1994). Appendix VI-N contains some resources for families on adjusting to hearing loss and the use of hearing aids (Thibodeau, 1994). Figure 6–8 shows a young mother who frequently uses the family resource center at the preschool program for children with hearing impairment.

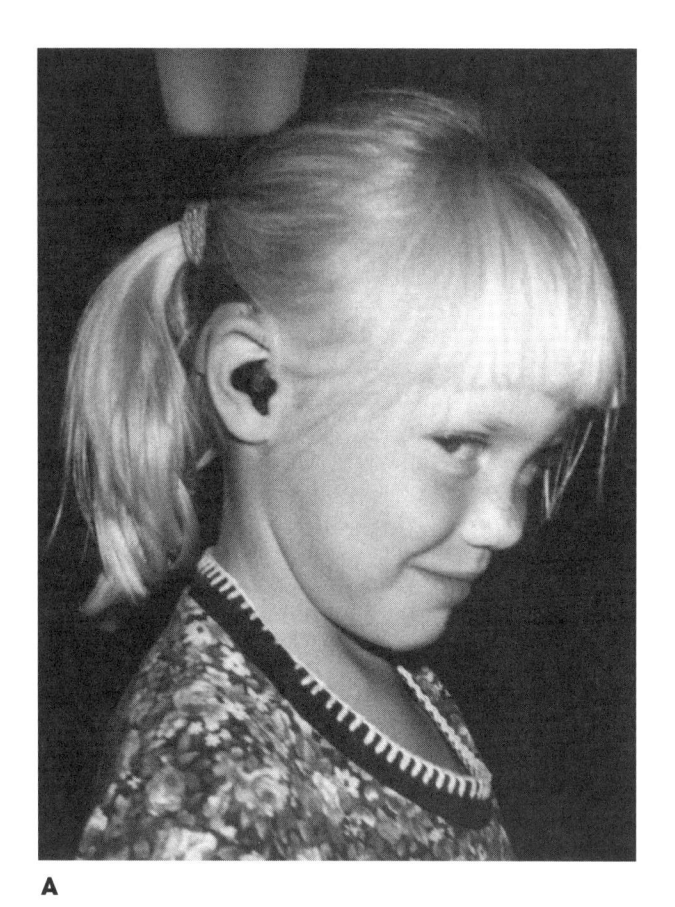

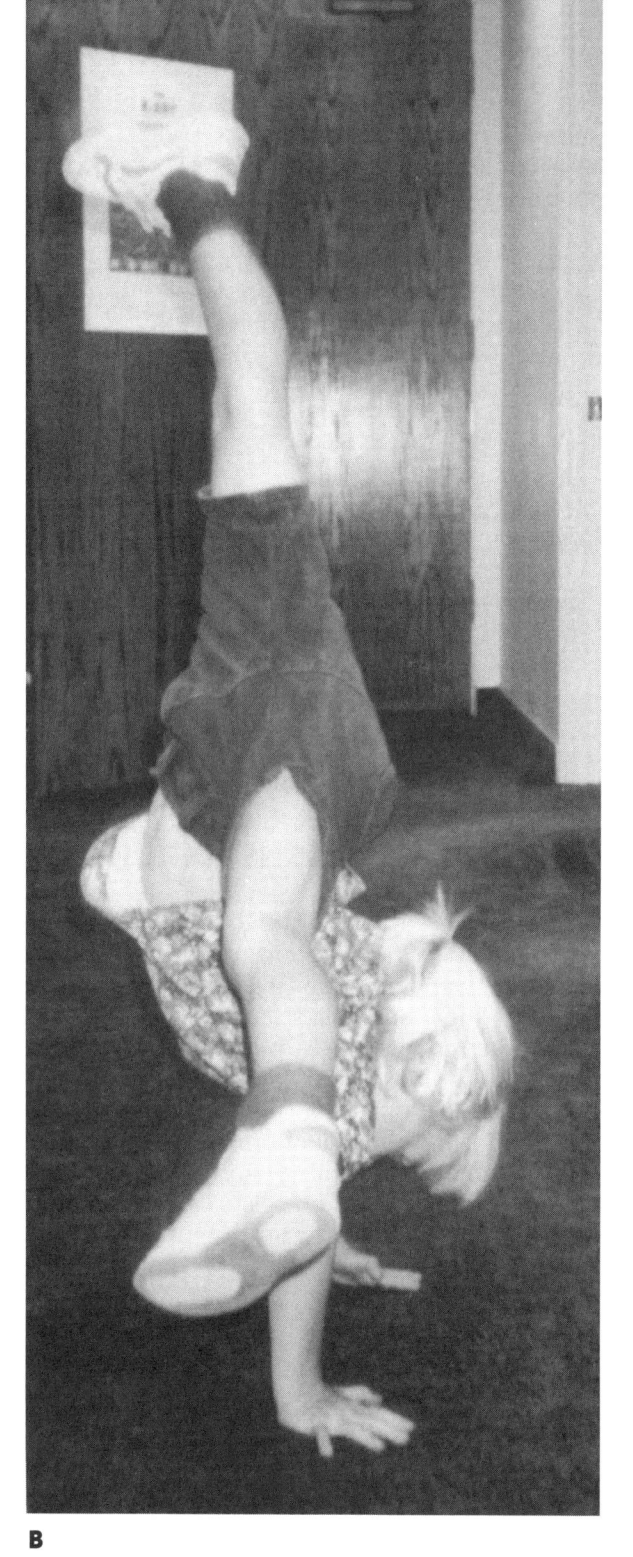

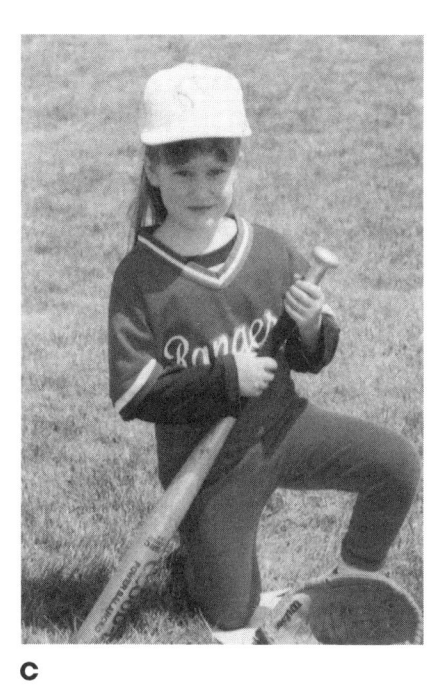

Figure 6–7. Two active girls who have opted for completely-in-the-canal (CIC) hearing aids. The child shown in (A) and (B) was delighted when she was able to go from her behind-the-ear (BTE) hearing aids shown in (A) to her present CICs as shown in (B). Although CICs may not be appropriate for all children, both of these young girls are now able to wear their CICs in active sports activities.

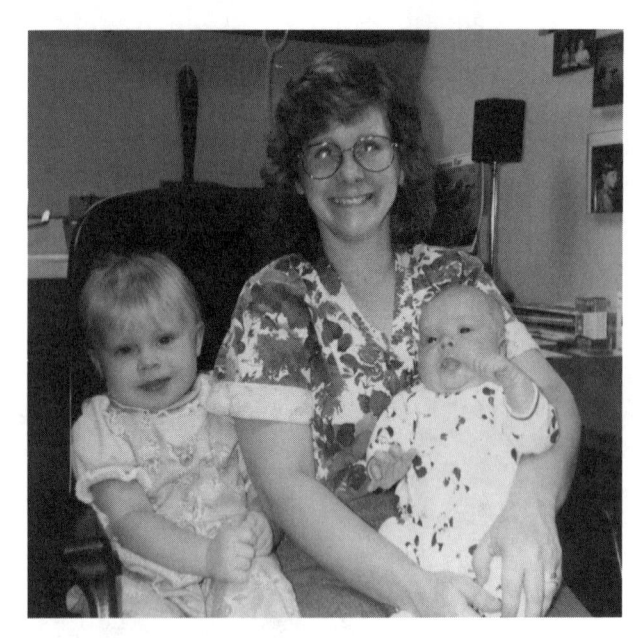

Figure 6–8. A young mother who uses the family resource center at a preschool for children with hearing impairment.

SUPPORT PROGRAMS IN POSTSECONDARY EDUCATIONAL INSTITUTIONS

Audiologists can assist high school students with hearing impairment and their parents make the transition from high school to postsecondary educational institutions. Hearing healthcare professionals must understand: (1) the laws protecting students with disabilities in postsecondary educational institutions and related organizations, (2) the role of programs for students with disabilities on college and university campuses, and (3) the audiologists' role in assisting students in transition and potential contributions to programs for students with disabilities.

Laws and Related Organizations Regarding Postsecondary Students with Disabilities

Postsecondary institutions must abide by the statutes of Section 504 of the Rehabilitation Act and the Americans with Disabilities Act (ADA) (1990). According to these laws, students with disabilities have an equal opportunity to pursue an education. Section 504 of the Rehabilitation Act of 1973 states that:

No otherwise qualified handicapped individual in the United States . . . shall, solely by reason of his handicap, be excluded from participation in, be denied the benefits of, or be subjected to discrimination under any program or activity receiving Federal financial assistance.

The term "qualified handicapped individual" needed elaboration, however. Thus, Congress passed the Rehabilitation Act Amendments of 1974 to clarify participant eligibility:

(a) Section 7(6) of the Act was amended by adding the following new sentence: "For purposes of Title IV and V of this Act, such terms mean any person who:
(A) has a physical or mental impairment which substantially limits one or more of such person's major life activities,
(B) has a record of such impairment, or is
(C) regarded as having such impairment.

The Americans with Disabilities Act (ADA) (1990) is a federal law that provides protection from discrimination for individuals on the basis of disability. The ADA extends protection for persons with disabilities to include employment in the private sector, transportation, public accommodations, services provided by state and local government, and telecommunications.

The Association of Higher Education on Disabilities (formerly the Association on Handicapped Student Service Programs in Postsecondary Education) is a nonprofit organization founded in 1978 and is comprised of persons from the United States, Canada, and other countries who are committed to promoting the full participation of students with disabilities in college and university life. The organization was established to strengthen the professionalism of individuals who are involved in providing services for students with disabilities and to improve the quality of those services. The mission of the organization is to provide unique leadership, focus, and expertise supported by a commitment to: communication, networking, professional development, training, research, and advocacy. Membership information and other ADA resources are provided in Appendix VI-O.

Programs for Postsecondary Students with Disabilities

Programs for students with disabilities can "level the playing field" for and greatly enhance the overall educational experience of students with disabilities. Auburn University has an outstanding Program for Students with Disabilities (PSD). This program works closely with Auburn University's 504/ADA Compliance Office. The PSD provides services to students who have met the academic and technical standards for admission or participation in the university's programs and activities, but who have a history of, or are regarded as having, a physical or mental impairment that limits activities (e.g., self-care, manual tasks, walking, seeing, hearing, speaking, breathing, learning, and/or working). Common types of disabilities include: blindness or low vision, deafness or impaired hearing, communication disorder, impaired mobility, cerebral palsy, seizure disorder, muscular dystrophy, multiple sclerosis, cancer, heart disease, HIV/AIDS, psychological difficulties, diabetes, learning disabilities, brain injury, addictive disease, and attention deficit disorder. The PSD support services include:

- screening of disability documentation,
- determination of appropriate accommodations,
- resource room with specialized equipment,
- communication with faculty regarding student needs,
- student-group participation, and
- referrals to other available campus resources.

The purpose of accommodations is to reduce the impact of students' disabilities on their ability to obtain an education. Appropriate accommodations include: alternative evaluation methods, changes in test format, class note takers, enlarged print or braille, extended time on exams, extra time on assignments, FM systems, interpreter services, modification of program requirements, permission to tape lectures, priority registration, removal of structural barriers, special parking permits, specialized computer equipment, text telephone (TT telephone), textbooks on tape, and use of a calculator or spellchecker. Health and safety issues for students with disabilities include: permission to eat, drink, or use the restroom as needed; procedures for assistance in an emergency; physical accessibility of the classroom, workstation, field trip, internship, and so on; precautions regarding the use of chemicals; and use of a service animal in all locations. Accommodations for students with hearing impairment include: captioned films and videos, class note taker, extended time on tests,

FM system (wireless microphone), good view of instructor, interpreter services, preferential seating, reassignment to another class (if the instructor is difficult to understand), and use of TDD for telephone calls.

The PSD serves not only Auburn University students, but also the faculty and staff. For example, the PSD facilitates communication between students with disabilities and their instructors. In addition, the PSD sponsors (along with the Auburn University Committee for Persons with Disabilities and the ADA/504 Compliance Office) timely workshops on disability issues in higher education. These workshops contain important information for admission counselors, academic advisors, teaching faculty, employment supervisors, and students.

The PSD also has support groups for students with disabilities:

- FOCUS on academics provides weekly meetings between individual students with disabilities and undergraduate or graduate-student counselors to discuss disability-related academic problems such as: communication with instructors, decision making, organization, self-advocacy, stress, study skills, support resources, and time management.
- TASK MASTERS is a weekly support group that addresses many of the same issues as FOCUS on academics, except that there is input and feedback from group members.
- Job Club is for students who are leaving school and entering the job market with questions about disability-related issues in the workplace such as: When do you tell a prospective employer about a disability? How do you request or obtain accommodations in the workplace? How do you obtain medical insurance for a pre-existing condition? Guest speakers with expertise in these areas often make presentations at the meetings.
- Health Club is a support group for students with chronic illnesses (e.g., HIV/AIDS, cancer, Crohn's disease, diabetes, heart disease, kidney disease, lupus, and so on). Guest speakers with various areas of expertise address the group.

Audiologists' Role in Assisting Students in Transition

Audiologists should consider Billy's story:

> *Like most of his peers, Billy, a high school senior, was looking forward to going to college in the fall. His parents were especially proud of him because he was diagnosed with a moderate-to-severe sensorineural hearing loss when he was 2 years old. Fortunately, Billy was fit with hearing aids and enrolled in the local university's preschool program for infants and toddlers with hearing impairment. To his parents' amazement, Billy started talking within months. With appropriate aural habilitation management, Billy was mainstreamed into a regular kindergarten class and excelled academically—in part because of the excellent services provided by the school district's educational audiologist. Unfortunately, routine audiologic evaluations revealed that Billy's hearing loss had become more severe. Nevertheless, through the use of a personal FM system and through accommodations made to his academic program as stated in his Individualized Education Program (IEP), Billy continued to excel in the classroom and in several team sports. His personal audiologist was especially pleased when she successfully fit Billy with bilateral completely-in-the-canal (CIC) hearing aids in the 11th grade. Billy's confidence soared. Not only was he the star quarterback, but he and his date were voted the prom king and queen! In January of his senior year, Billy received a football scholarship to State University.*
>
> *It was a bittersweet moment on that late August morning as Billy backed his car out of the driveway on his way to State University. Billy's mother bravely held back the tears as she waved good-bye. Billy's father was so proud. Both parents could hardly believe that their son, who was a late talker with a severe hearing impairment, was off to college. After a two-hour drive, Billy checked into the dormitory and reported to football practice. Billy enjoyed orientation week and even pledged a fraternity. He felt as if he had a "fresh start." With his CIC hearing aids, no one knew of his hearing loss. For once, he was just like everyone else. With late night fraternity parties and other activities, Billy often overslept, making him late for early morning football practice and his Tuesday and Thursday honors psychology class. He often managed to slip into class and take a seat in the back without the professor noticing, but he became frustrated. He couldn't hear the professor, who often spoke to the class with his back turned as he wrote on the blackboard. In addition, Billy had a difficult time concentrating, with the other students chatting and passing notes. By midsemester, Billy was having difficulty in all four of his classes. Billy had "Ds" on two midterm exams. Coach was disappointed in Billy. In addition, he believed that Billy had a "bad attitude" because at times he didn't seem to listen on the football field. Coach scheduled a meeting with Billy and the athletic academic counselor to discuss his poor academic performance. When asked why he was having so much difficulty, Billy softly explained, "Coach, I didn't want anybody to know, but I have a hearing loss."*

Unfortunately, Billy's story is all too common for postsecondary students with hearing impairment who manage to "beat the odds" by qualifying for admission to colleges and universities but fail to fulfill their academic potential for a variety of reasons. *College students with hearing impairment have a relatively high dropout rate of 71% compared to only 47% for students without disabilities* (English, 1998). Like Billy, some students with hearing impairment may view college as an opportunity for a fresh start and a chance to be "just another face in the crowd." Although this is understandable, students' denial of their disabilities can prove disastrous to their academic careers. In addition, many teenagers with hearing impairment have been overprotected and poorly informed about the role of self-advocacy (English, 1998).

English (1998) stated that research has shown that high school students with hearing impairment often:

- do not know their legal rights,
- do not know who is responsible for protecting those rights in a work or college setting, and
- are not aware that they are eligible for financial and technical assistance.

Students and their parents may not grasp the dynamics of the transition of support services from high school to postsecondary educational institutions. As stated earlier, high school students' with hearing impairment have "protected status" under the Individuals with Disabilities Education Act (ADA) (1990), which guarantees a free and appropriate public education (FAPE) in the least restrictive environment (LRE), through use of a variety of technical and instructional supports. In postsecondary educational institutions, however, students' and their parents do not realize that the "safety net" of the IDEA (English, 1998) has been removed. They must take a proactive approach to secure the necessary accommodations that will ensure an equal opportunity to receive an education.

Fortunately, a recent amendment of the IDEA (i.e., Section 300.45, 34 Code of Federal Regulations) stated that for students age 16 years and older, Individualized Education Plans (IEPs) must include a statement of the needed transition services, including a designation of each participating agency's responsibilities, linkages, or both (English, 1998). Transition planning should include students' development of the self-advocacy skills to identify, seek out, and obtain the assistance needed to succeed in the postsecondary environment (English, 1998). Educational audiologists can encourage high school seniors with hearing impairment and their parents who are applying for admission to postsecondary educational institutions to inquire about programs for students with disabilities. In fact, educational audiologists should explain these issues to high school guidance counselors who advise these students.

Appendix VI-P provides an example of a letter that educational audiologists can send to high school seniors with hearing impairment and their parents. In the letter, educational audiologists should express their congratulations to parents regarding their children's graduation from high school. In addition, they should inform parents about the Section 504 of the Rehabilitation Act of 1973, the ADA, and the necessary steps for ensuring that appropriate accommodations will be made for their children by postsecondary educational institutions. Students and their parents should:

- investigate colleges and universities regarding the existence of programs for students with disabilities;
- inquire about specific program components for students with hearing impairment by asking questions such as:
  ⇒ Does the program provide appropriate accommodations?
  ⇒ Does the institution have a speech and hearing clinic on campus that can handle students' hearing health-care needs?
  ⇒ If not, is there an audiologist in town that could provide those services?;
- send documentation of their disability to the appropriate offices on campus because current documentation is required;
- make an appointment with a disability specialist from the program for students with disabilities to apply for services as soon as possible (programs for students with disabilities may require advance notification for some accommodations, such as oral interpreters);
- contact the local Department of Vocational Rehabilitation Services to determine eligibility for any benefits under federal programs; and
- not hesitate to contact the program for students with disabilities at any time, if they have any questions.

In summary, educational audiologists should play a key role in facilitating students' transition from high school to postsecondary educational institutions, thereby increasing the likelihood of continued academic achievement.

Audiologists' Role in Programs for Students with Disabilities

Audiologists' potential role in programs for students with disabilities varies depending on their relationship with the postsecondary educational institution. Audiologists who are employees of the college or university's speech and hearing clinic may possibly provide the following services for the program for students with disabilities:

- Hearing screenings
- Audiologic evaluations
- Hearing aid evaluations, fitting, and deliveries
- Hearing aid repair
- Coordination of ALD Program
- Coordination of support program for students with hearing impairment
- Presentation of inservices to faculty, staff, and students (e.g., hearing health care, effective communication, and so on)
- Consultation regarding improving classroom acoustics

The relationship between the university speech and hearing clinic and the program for students with disabilities can be formal or informal. Formal relationships are those that are clearly designated in university policies and job descriptions. Informal relationships are those alliances that are formed on a case-by-case basis. Regardless of the type of relationship, an open, two-way channel of communication between the speech and hearing clinic and the program for students with disabilities is needed to meet the needs of students with hearing impairment.

Audiologists in private practice near colleges and universities without speech and hearing clinics may market their practices to programs for students with disabilities through letters of introduction. Audiologists in private practice could offer to develop a support program within the program for students with disabilities. Private-practice audiologists could perform those functions listed above for the college- or university-based audiologist. Although not directly located on-site, the private-practice audiologist can make a direct impact on meeting the hearing health-care needs of students with hearing impairment. Students can check their hearing instruments at the Hearing Aid Check Station set up by the audiologist within the program for students with disabilities, for example. The Hearing Aid Check Station should be equipped with hearing aid stethoscopes, battery testers, extra batteries for purchase, forced-air bulbs, wax picks, alcohol pads, and so on. Audiologists can create a Web site that is accessible 24 hours a day for busy students who need to ask questions, seek advice, or request an appointment for audiologic services.

SUMMARY

This chapter has discussed the development of support programs in educational settings. The current realities of audiologic service delivery in the public schools necessitate developing cost-efficient support programs in key areas. Support programs for educational settings can either be formal or informal. The types and number of supports programs can vary from school district to school district and depend on the service-delivery model in place. Specifically, we have reviewed development of informal support programs and formal support programs for amplification devices, CAPD service delivery, family counseling, and postsecondary educational settings. Audiologists who provide educational-based services can take pride in the fact that in addition to assisting students with their hearing losses (and their families), they are also making an important impact on their personal development. Thus, providing support programs in educational settings can be highly rewarding for audiologists, and can be a stimulating component to a private practice.

LEARNING ACTIVITIES

- Investigate local school districts' use of educational audiology service-delivery models.
- Develop a resource notebook containing useful information regarding local, state, and national support organizations for parents of children with hearing impairment.
- Develop a list of Web sites pertinent to educational audiology.
- Determine the adequacy of support programs for students with hearing impairment at local postsecondary educational institutions.

REFERENCES

Altman, E. (1996). Meeting the needs of adolescents with impaired hearing. In F.N. Martin & J.G. Clark (Eds.), *Hearing care for children* (pp. 197–210). Needham Heights, MA: Allyn & Bacon.

American Academy of Audiology. (1997). Position statement and guidelines of the consensus panel on support personnel in audiology. *Audiology Today, 9*(3), 27–28.

American Speech-Language-Hearing Association. (1985). Guidelines for identification audiometry. *Asha, 27*, 49–52.

American Speech-Language-Hearing Association. (1989). Audiologic screening of newborn infants at risk for hearing impairment. *Asha, 31*, 89–92.

American Speech-Language-Hearing Association. (1990). Guidelines for screening for hearing impairment and middle-ear disorders. *Asha, 32*(Suppl. 2), 17–24.

American Speech-Language-Hearing Association. (1991a). Amplification as a remediation technique for children with normal peripheral hearing. *Asha, 33*(Suppl. 3), 22–24.

American Speech-Language-Hearing Association. (1991b). Guidelines for the audiologic assessment of children from birth through 36 months of age. *Asha, 33*(Suppl. 5), 37–43.

American Speech-Language-Hearing Association. (1991c). The use of FM amplification instruments for infants and preschool children with hearing impairment. *Asha, 33*(Suppl. 5), 1–2.

American Speech-Language-Hearing Association. (1993). Guidelines for audiology services in schools. *Asha, 35*(Suppl. 10), 24–32.

American Speech-Language-Hearing Association. (1994, March). Guidelines for fitting and monitoring FM systems. *Asha, 36*(Suppl. 12), 1–9.

American Speech-Language-Hearing Association. (1995). Acoustics in educational settings. *Asha, 37*(Suppl. 14), 15–19.

Americans with Disabilities Act of 1990, Public Law 101-336, 42, U.S.C. 12101 et seq.: *U.S. Statutes at Large, 104*, 327–378 (1991).

Anderson, K. (1989). *Screening instrument for targeting educational risk (S.I.F.T.E.R.)*. Tampa, FL: Educational Audiology Association.

Atkins, D. V. (1994). Counseling children with hearing loss and their families. In J.G. Clark & F.N. Martin (Eds.), *Effective counseling in audiology: Perspectives and practice* (pp. 116–146). Englewood Cliffs, NJ: Prentice-Hall Inc.

Bellis, T. J. (1996). *Assessment and management of central auditory processing disorders in the educational setting: From science to practice*. San Diego, CA: Singular Publishing Group.

Bellis, T. J., & Burke, J. (1996). Screening. In T. J. Bellis (Ed.), *Assessment and management of central auditory processing disorders in the educational setting: From science to practice* (pp. 91–112). San Diego, CA: Singular Publishing Group.

Berg, F. (1993). *Acoustics and sound systems in schools*. San Diego, CA: Singular Publishing Group.

Bess, F., Sinclair, J., & Riggs, D. (1984). Group amplification in schools for the hearing-impaired. *Ear and Hearing, 5*, 138–143.

Blood, G. W., Blood, I., & Danhauer, J. L. (1977). The hearing aid effect. *Hearing Instruments, 28*(6), 12.

Cacace, A.T., & McFarland, D.J. (1998). Central auditory processing disorder in school-aged children: A critical review. *Journal of Speech, Language, and Hearing Research, 41*, 355-373.

Chermak, G. D. (1992, July). *Beyond diagnosis: Strategies and techniques for management of central auditory processing disorders across the lifespan*. Presentation given at the Institute for Management of the Communicatively Handicapped, Logan, UT.

Chermak, G. D., & Musiek, F. E. (1992). Managing central auditory processing disorders in children and youth. *American Journal of Audiology: A Journal of Clinical Practice, 1*(3), 61–65.

Colorado Department of Education. (1996). *Central auditory processing disorders: A team approach to screening, assessment, and intervention practices*. Denver, CO: Author.

Cornelisse, L. E., Seewald, R. C., & Jamieson, D. G. (1994). Wide-dynamic-range compression hearing aids: The DSL [i/o] approach. *The Hearing Journal, 47*(10), 23–26.

Crandell, C. C., & Smaldino, J. J. (1995). Acoustical modifications in classrooms. In C. C. Crandell, J. J. Smaldino, & C. Flexer (Eds.), *Sound-field FM amplification: Theory and practical applications* (pp. 83–92). San Diego, CA: Singular Publishing Group.

Crandell, C. C., Smaldino, J. J., & Flexer, C. (1995). *Sound-field FM amplification: Theory and practical applications*. San Diego, CA: Singular Publishing Group.

Education for all Handicapped Children Act of 1975, Public Law 94-142, 20, U.S.C. 1401-1461: *U.S. Statutes at Large, 89*, 773–779 (1975).

Education of the Handicapped Act Amendments of 1986, Public Law 99-457, 20, U.S.C. 1400 et seq.: *U.S. Statutes at Large, 100*, 1145–1177 (1986).

Edwards, C. (1995). Identifying and managing the learning environment. In C. C. Crandell, J. J. Smaldino, & C. Flexer (Eds.), *Sound-field FM amplification: Theory and practical applications* (pp. 93–106). San Diego, CA: Singular Publishing Group.

Elfenbein, J. L. (1994). Monitoring preschoolers' hearing aids: Issues in program design and implementation. *American Journal of Audiology: A Journal of Clinical Practice, 3*(2), 65–69.

English, K. (1998). What happens when I graduate from high school? Transition planning and self-advocacy skills for deaf and hard-of-hearing teens. *Perspectives* [On-line], *2*(3), Available Internet Address: www.perspect.htm@audiology.org (Educational Audiology Specialty Resources at the American Academy of Audiology Web site).

Ferre, J., & Wilber, L. (1986). Normal and learning disabled children's central auditory processing skills: An experimental test battery. *Ear and Hearing, 7*, 336–343.

Fisher, L. I. (1976). *Fisher Auditory Problems Checklist*. Cedar Rapids, IA: Grant Woods Education Agency.

Flexer, C. (1995). Rationale for the use of sound-field FM amplification systems in classrooms. In C. C. Crandell, J. J. Smaldino, & C. Flexer (Eds.), *Sound-field FM amplification: Theory and practical applications* (pp. 3–16). San Diego, CA: Singular Publishing Group.

Gaeth, J., & Lounsbury, E. (1966). Hearing aids and children in elementary schools. *Journal of Speech and Hearing Disorders, 31*, 283–289.

Grunblatt, H., & Darr, L. (1994). A support program: Audiological counseling. *Language, Speech, and Hearing Services in Schools, 25,* 112–114.

Hall, J. W., Baer, J. E., Byrn, A., Wurm, F. C., Henry, M. M., Wilson, D. S., & Prentice, C. H. (1993). Audiologic assessment and management of central auditory processing disorder (CAPD). *Seminars in Hearing, 14*(3), 254–264.

Hall, J. W., & Mueller, H. G. (1997). *Audiologists' desk reference: Volume 1: Diagnostic audiology, principles, and practices.* San Diego, CA: Singular Publishing Group.

Individuals with Disabilities Education Act of 1990 (IDEA), Public Law 101-476, 20, U.S.C. 1400 et seq.: U.S. Statutes at Large, 104, 1103-1151 (1990).

Johnson, C. D., Benson, P. V., & Seaton, J. B. (1997). *Educational audiology handbook.* San Diego, CA: Singular Publishing Group.

Johnson, C. E. (1999). Dimensions of multiskilling: Considerations for educational audiology. *Language, Speech, and Hearing Services in Schools, 30,* 4–10.

Johnson, C. E., Clark-Lewis, S., & Griffin, D. (1998). Experience, attitudes, and competencies of audiologic support personnel in a rehabilitation hospital. *American Journal of Audiology: A Journal of Clinical Practice, 7*(2), 26–31.

Johnson, C. E., & Danhauer, J. L. (1997). CIC instruments: Cosmetic issues. In M. Chasin (Ed.), *CIC handbook* (pp. 151–167). San Diego, CA: Singular Publishing Group.

Kemker, F., McConnell, F., Logan, S., & Green, B. (1979). A field study of children's hearing aids in a school environment. *Language, Speech, and Hearing Services in Schools, 10,* 47–53.

Loeb, R., & Sarigiani, P. (1986). The impact of hearing impairment on self-perceptions of children. *Volta Review, 88,* 89–100.

Masters, M. G., Stecker, N. J., & Katz, J. (1998). *Central auditory processing disorders: Mostly management.* Needham Heights, MA: Allyn & Bacon.

Maxon, A. B., & Brackett, D. (1981). Mainstreaming hearing-impaired children. *Audio Journal for Continuing Education, 6,* 10.

Medwetsky, L. (1994). Educational audiology. In J. Katz (Ed.), *Handbook of clinical audiology* (4th ed., pp. 503–520). Baltimore, MD: Williams & Wilkins Co.

Mueller, H. G., & Hall, J. W. (1998). *Audiologists' desk reference: Volume II: Audiologic management, rehabilitation, and terminology.* San Diego, CA: Singular Publishing Group.

Musket, C. H. (1995). Maintenance of personal hearing aids. In R. J. Roeser & M. P. Downs (Eds.), *Auditory disorders in school children: The law, identification, remediation* (3rd ed., pp. 201–218). New York: Thieme Medical Publishers, Inc.

Nabelek, A. K., & Nabelek, I. V. (1994). Room acoustics and speech perception. In J. Katz (Ed.), *Handbook of clinical audiology* (4th ed., pp. 624–637). Baltimore, MD: Williams & Wilkins Co.

Northern, J. L., & Downs, M. P. (1991). *Hearing in children* (4th ed.). Baltimore, MD: Williams & Wilkins Co.

Reeh, H.L., & Carlson, D.L. (1997). *Development of an ALD trial program for the CAPD student.* Instructional course presented at the 9th Annual Convention of the American Academy of Audiology, Ft. Lauderdale, FL.

Rehabilitation Act of 1973, Section 504, 29, U.S.C. 794, *U.S. Statutes at Large,* 87, 335–394 (1973).

Reichman, J., & Healey, W. C. (1989). Amplification monitoring and maintenance in schools. *Asha, 31*(10), 43–46.

Runnels, C. A. (1994). Support personnel. In C. Peters-Johnson, S. Karr, & J. Langsam (Eds.), *Communication, creativity, collaboration: Current challenges for school supervisors and administrators* (pp. 75–78). Rockville, MD: American Speech-Language-Hearing Association.

Smedley, T., & Plapinger, D. (1988). The nonfunctioning hearing aid: A case of double jeopardy. *Volta Review, 90*(2), 77–84.

Staab, W. J. (1995). Deep canal hearing aids. In B. Ballachanda (Ed.), *The human ear canal* (pp. 155–180). San Diego, CA: Singular Publishing Group.

Staab, W. J. & Lybarger, S. L. (1994). Characteristics and use of hearing aids. In J. Katz (Ed.), *Handbook of clinical audiology* (4th ed., pp. 657–722). Baltimore, MD: Williams & Wilkins Co.

Stein, R. L. (1998). Application of FM technology. In M. G. Masters, N. A. Stecker & J. Katz (Eds.), *Central auditory processing disorders: Mostly management* (pp. 89–102). Boston: Allyn & Bacon.

The Pediatric Working Group of the Conference on Amplification for Children with Auditory Deficits. (1996). Amplification for infants and children with hearing loss. *American Journal of Audiology: A Journal of Clinical Practice, 5*(1), 53–68.

Thibodeau, L. M. (1994). Counseling for pediatric amplification. In J. G. Clark & F. N. Martin (Eds.), *Effective counseling in audiology: Perspectives and practice* (pp. 147–183). Englewood Cliffs, NJ: Prentice-Hall Inc.

Trychin, S. (1994). Helping people cope with hearing loss. In J.G. Clark & F.N. Martin (Eds.), *Effective counseling in audiology: Perspectives and practice* (pp. 247–277). Englewood Cliffs, NJ: Prentice-Hall Inc.

Tye-Murray, N., Witt, S., Schum, L., Kelsay, D., & Schum, D. J. (1994). Feasible aural rehabilitation services for busy clinical settings. *American Journal of Audiology: A Journal of Clinical Practice, 3*(3), 33–37.

U.S. Department of Education. (1994). *Sixteenth annual report to congress on the implementation of the individuals with disabilities education act* (p. A-212). Washington, DC: U.S. Government Printing Office.

Van Hecke, M. L. (1994). Emotional responses to hearing loss. In J. G. Clark & F. N. Martin (Eds.), *Effective counseling in audiology: Perspectives and practice* (pp. 92–115). Englewood Cliffs, NJ: Prentice-Hall Inc.

Von Almen, P., Blair, J., & Spriet, S. (1990). Central auditory assessment. *Educational Audiology Newsletter, 7*(2), 10–11.

Werven, G. (1993). Support personnel: An issue for our times. *American Journal of Speech-Language Pathology: A Journal of Clinical Practice, 2*(2), 9–12.

Willeford, J. (1977). Assessing central auditory behavior in children: A test battery approach. In R. Keith (Ed.), *Central auditory dysfunction* (pp. 43–72). New York: Grune & Stratton.

APPENDIX VI-A

Letter to Classroom Teachers

XYZ INDEPENDENT SCHOOL DISTRICT
"For their future..."

August 20, 1999

Ms. Ima Teacher
Carver Elementary School
1122 Prosperity Way
Quality of Life City, CA 94545

Dear Ms. Teacher,

I would like to introduce myself. My name is Starr Audiologist. I have been contracted to provide audiologic services to the XYZ Independent School District for the 1999-2000 school year. One area for service provision is maintaining the amplification devices in the self-contained classrooms for children with hearing impairment.

On Friday, September 10th, I will be visiting Carver Elementary School. I would like to schedule an appointment to visit your classroom and talk with you regarding any special needs or concerns that you may have. I would appreciate if you could contact students' parents to remind them to send their children's hearing aids to school on that day, regardless of their condition.

I will be calling you this week. Please think of a time that would be convenient for you on Friday the 11th. I look forward to working with you. If you have any questions, please feel free to call me at 555-1122 or write me via e-mail at *EarstoYou@aol.com*.

Sincerely,

Starr Audiologist, Ph.D.
Certificate of Clinical Competence in Audiology (CCC-A)
Fellow of the American Academy of Audiology (FAAA)

APPENDIX VI-B

Classroom Amplification Device Inventory Sheet

XYZ INDEPENDENT SCHOOL DISTRICT
"For their future..."

AMPLIFICATION DEVICE INVENTORY SHEET

Teacher _____ Room# _____ School _____

Personal Hearing Aids

Name	Ear Fit	Make/Model #	Serial #	Functioning?
	Right Left Right Left Right Left Right Left Right Left Right Left Right Left Right Left Right Left Right Left Right Left Right Left			

Group/Personal FM Systems

Transmitters

Name	Make/Model #	Serial #	Comments

Receivers

Name	Make/Model #	Serial #	Coupled to Aid?	Comments

Cochlear Implants/Sound-Field FM Amplification Systems?

APPENDIX VI-C

Parent Letter and Informed-Consent Form

XYZ INDEPENDENT SCHOOL DISTRICT
"For their future..."

September 20, 1999

Ms. Ima Parent
1000 Rose Avenue
Quality of Life City, CA 94545

Dear Ms. Parent,

I would like to introduce myself. My name is Starr Audiologist. I have been contracted to provide audiologic services to the XYZ Independent School District for the 1999-2000 school year. One area for service provision is maintaining the amplification devices in the self-contained classrooms for children with hearing impairment. As part of this service, children's hearing aids will be checked everyday for proper functioning either by trained classroom teachers, assistants, or myself. In addition, on-site repairs will be made, as necessary. Parents will be notified if hearing aids need to be sent to the manufacturer for repair.

Attached, please find an informed-consent form for your child's participation in this program. Please fill out this form and return it via the self-addressed, self-stamped envelope. In addition, please provide information regarding status of hearing aid warranties, personal audiologists, and any pertinent billing information. I look forward to working with you in meeting the hearing health-care needs of your child. If you have any questions, please call me at 555-1122 or write to me via e-mail *EarstoYou@aol.com.*

Sincerely,

Starr Audiologist, Ph.D.
Certificate of Clinical Competence in Audiology (CCC-A)
Fellow of the American Academy of Audiology (FAAA)

Informed-Consent Form

XYZ INDEPENDENT SCHOOL DISTRICT
"For their future..."

INFORMED-CONSENT FORM

I, _____ agree/do not agree (Circle one) to have my child, _____ participate in the hearing aid monitoring program for the 1999–2000 school year.

If I agree to have my child participate, I understand either the audiologist, the classroom teacher, or other trained educational personnel will check my child's hearing aids on a daily basis. I also understand that this individual will perform basic troubleshooting procedures, as necessary. I understand that I will be notified if my child's hearing aids need repair.

Signature: _____

Address: _____

_____

My child has their own audiologist: Yes   No

If yes, his/her address and phone number is:

_____

_____

_____

Is your child's personal hearing aid under warranty?   Yes   No

Insurance or Medicaid Information (including billing numbers):

APPENDIX VI-D

Hearing Aid Check Sheet

XYZ INDEPENDENT SCHOOL DISTRICT
"For their future..."

HEARING AID CHECK SHEET

Name:_____

Teacher/Room:_____

Hearing Aid Make/Model/Serial #:_____

Place a CHECK in the box if OK.

Item to Check	Date							
Visual • Case clean & uncracked • Well-fitting earmold • External control set correctly • Sound bore clear of wax • Tubing undamaged • Battery positioned correctly • Battery contacts uncorroded • Battery charged • Free of moisture		☐ ☐ ☐ ☐ ☐ ☐ ☐ ☐ ☐	☐ ☐ ☐ ☐ ☐ ☐ ☐ ☐ ☐	☐ ☐ ☐ ☐ ☐ ☐ ☐ ☐ ☐	☐ ☐ ☐ ☐ ☐ ☐ ☐ ☐ ☐	☐ ☐ ☐ ☐ ☐ ☐ ☐ ☐ ☐	☐ ☐ ☐ ☐ ☐ ☐ ☐ ☐ ☐	☐ ☐ ☐ ☐ ☐ ☐ ☐ ☐ ☐
Listening • No feedback when on child • Adequate volume • Good sound quality • Volume wheel moves smoothly • No unusual sounds		☐ ☐ ☐ ☐ ☐	☐ ☐ ☐ ☐ ☐	☐ ☐ ☐ ☐ ☐	☐ ☐ ☐ ☐ ☐	☐ ☐ ☐ ☐ ☐	☐ ☐ ☐ ☐ ☐	☐ ☐ ☐ ☐ ☐

Comments:

APPENDIX VI-E

Cochlear Implant Check Sheet

XYZ INDEPENDENT SCHOOL DISTRICT
"For their future..."

COCHLEAR IMPLANT CHECK SHEET

Name:_____

Teacher/Room:_____

Hearing Aid Make/Model/Serial #:_____

Place a CHECK in the box if OK.

Item to Check	Date							
Visual • Parts intact • Battery contacts clean • Battery adequately charged (Turn function switch to "T" [test] and the "M" [microphone] light should glow) • Speech processor and coil functioning (Hold signal check next to the transmitting coil and the signal light should glow) **Listening** • Signal transmitted (Switch function knob to "N" [normal], turn sensitivity control knob at child's usual setting and speak into microphone, watching for "M" light to flash) • Ling Five Sound Test w/ Child **Precautions** • Speech processor worn securely • Cords tucked under clothing • Precautions for rain • Removed for sports • Spare batteries/cords on hand • Covered if worn on front		☐ ☐ ☐ ☐ ☐ ☐ ☐ ☐ ☐ ☐ ☐ ☐	☐ ☐ ☐ ☐ ☐ ☐ ☐ ☐ ☐ ☐ ☐ ☐	☐ ☐ ☐ ☐ ☐ ☐ ☐ ☐ ☐ ☐ ☐ ☐	☐ ☐ ☐ ☐ ☐ ☐ ☐ ☐ ☐ ☐ ☐ ☐	☐ ☐ ☐ ☐ ☐ ☐ ☐ ☐ ☐ ☐ ☐ ☐	☐ ☐ ☐ ☐ ☐ ☐ ☐ ☐ ☐ ☐ ☐ ☐	☐ ☐ ☐ ☐ ☐ ☐ ☐ ☐ ☐ ☐ ☐ ☐

Comments:

APPENDIX VI-F

Personal FM System Check Sheet

XYZ INDEPENDENT SCHOOL DISTRICT
"For their future..."

PERSONAL FM SYSTEM CHECK SHEET

Name:_____

Teacher/Room:_____

Hearing Aid Make/Model/Serial #:_____

Place a CHECK in the box if OK.

Item to Check	Date							
Transmitter (T) to Receiver (R) without children. • Parts intact • Transmitter/receiver crystals match • Battery charged • Adequate quality of sound (Ling Five Sound Test through environmental microphones) • No static/intermittency when receiver cord shaken		☐ ☐ ☐ ☐ ☐	☐ ☐ ☐ ☐ ☐	☐ ☐ ☐ ☐ ☐	☐ ☐ ☐ ☐ ☐	☐ ☐ ☐ ☐ ☐	☐ ☐ ☐ ☐ ☐	☐ ☐ ☐ ☐ ☐
Place transmitter near sound source (tape recorder with music) • Adequate sound quality (FM only) • No static/intermittency when mic/antenna cord shaken		☐ ☐	☐ ☐	☐ ☐	☐ ☐	☐ ☐	☐ ☐	☐ ☐
Receiver (R) Transmission to Ear with Children. (If child's aid is coupled to R, check aid first). • Clean earmold bores • Adequate quality of sound to children (environmental mic) • No feedback on child		☐ ☐ ☐	☐ ☐ ☐	☐ ☐ ☐	☐ ☐ ☐	☐ ☐ ☐	☐ ☐ ☐	☐ ☐ ☐
Place transmitter near sound source (tape recorder with music) • Adequate quality of sound to children (FM-only) • No feedback on child.		☐ ☐	☐ ☐	☐ ☐	☐ ☐	☐ ☐	☐ ☐	☐ ☐

Comments:

APPENDIX VI-G

Sound-Field FM Amplification System Check Sheet

XYZ INDEPENDENT SCHOOL DISTRICT
"For their future..."

SOUND-FIELD FM AMPLIFICATION SYSTEM CHECK SHEET

Name:_____

Teacher/Room:_____

Hearing Aid Make/Model/Serial #:_____

Place a CHECK in the box if OK.

Item to Check	Date							
Visual Check								
• Parts intact		☐	☐	☐	☐	☐	☐	☐
• Mic/transmitter to receiver/amplifier crystals match		☐	☐	☐	☐	☐	☐	☐
• Mic/transmitter battery charged		☐	☐	☐	☐	☐	☐	☐
Listening Check								
• Adequate quality of sound through each loudspeaker		☐	☐	☐	☐	☐	☐	☐
• No static/intermittency when mic/antenna cord shaken		☐	☐	☐	☐	☐	☐	☐
• No static/intermittency when receiver/amplifier to loudspeaker cords shaken		☐	☐	☐	☐	☐	☐	☐
• No feedback with complete teacher mobility		☐	☐	☐	☐	☐	☐	☐

Comments:

APPENDIX VI-H

Protocol for Children's Educational Program on Hearing Loss[1]

Topic 1: Basic Audiology

Goal: Inform students about the causes of hearing loss and related issues.

Outline:
- Sound
- How we hear
- Parts of the ear and their functions
- The audiometer
- How hearing is tested
- Causes of hearing loss

Suggestions:
- 3 to 4 year olds: visit audiology test booth with teacher and devise group play audiometry activities
- 5 to 6 year olds: look in each other's ears with otoscopes
- 7 to 10 year olds: show real ossicles to children
- 11 to 15 year olds: assign roles of audiologist and patient and have students obtain thresholds on each other

Topic 2: Hearing Aid Hygiene

Goal: Promote good hearing aid hygiene and basic understanding of the various parts of the hearing aids.

Outline:
- Putting on the hearing aid
- Parts and functions of the hearing aid
- Testing batteries and troubleshooting
- Cleaning earmolds
- Proper storage of hearing aids when not in use

Suggestions:
- 3 to 5 year olds: teach them to put hearing aids on by themselves
- 6 to 7 year olds:
- Teach basic troubleshooting
- Teach how to clean earmolds
- Teach facts about hearing aids (e.g., cost)
- Acknowledge realistic expectations for hearing aids

Topic 3: The FM System: How and Why We Use It

Goal: Help children understand the FM system and its importance in classroom instruction.

---

[1] Adapted from "A Support Program: Audiological Counseling," by H. Grunblatt and L. Darr, 1994. *Language, Speech, and Hearing Services in Schools, 25,* 112–114.

Outline:
➢ Appropriate and inappropriate behavior while using the FM unit
➢ How to turn on the FM unit
➢ How to set the volume controls
➢ How and when to set FM versus hearing aid on the FM unit
➢ Benefits of the FM system
➢ FM units versus hearing aids for classroom instruction

Suggestions:
➢ Teach teachers:
  ✔ Proper settings
  ✔ Proper levels
  ✔ Proper controls
➢ Teach students appropriate behaviors with units:
  ✔ Avoid chewing on cords
  ✔ Don't throw units
  ✔ Don't separate cords from units
➢ 3 to 5 year olds: teach them to put the units on
➢ 6 to 9 year olds:
  ✔ Teach appropriate behaviors through picture handouts
  ✔ Provide "hands-on" manipulation of controls
  ✔ Teach how to set controls for various situations (e.g., class, hallways, bathrooms, speech treatment rooms, and so on)
➢ 12 to 15 year olds: demonstrate advantage of wearing FM systems in various listening conditions (e.g., noise and reverberation) to encourage their use

Topic 4: Know Your Audiogram

Goal: Help children plot their own audiograms and understand symbols as they relate to their hearing losses.

Outline:
➢ Pitch/frequency
➢ Loudness/decibels
➢ Plotting an audiogram
➢ Range of hearing loss
➢ Students' personal audiograms
➢ Unaided and aided audiograms

Suggestions:
➢ Not for children under 11 years old
➢ Over 11 years old: teach students how to understand the audiogram (e.g., degree/configuration, comparison with normal hearing, and unaided versus aided audiograms)

Topic 5: Ask the Audiologist

Goal: Address students' concerning any topic related to their hearing loss.

Outline:
➢ Why do I have a hearing loss?
➢ Will I hear in the future?
➢ How much do hearing aids cost?

APPENDIX VI-I

Misconceptions of Educational Personnel About CAPD[1]

(Gleaned, and in some cases quoted, from tape recordings of M-team meetings and transcriptions of due process hearings.)

➤ "One of the reasons that we've [school personnel] been more cautious about that [implementing ALD use with CAPD children] is that it's kind of like doing drug trials in that to the extent to which you don't want to prescribe something that has been limitly [sic] researched. And the ALDs have not been widely researched."

➤ "Audiologists say that ALDs just simply make their job easier. But again, that's something that they say intuitively and not from a research base."

➤ "If he were to go [for CAPD assessment] he's probably going to come back as positive for central auditory processing because, number one, he has attention deficit disorder and the research shows us that kids who have ADDs typically come back as positive for auditory processing as well."

➤ "I don't really agree with [the parents request for a CAPD assessment] . . . I have recommended those for other kids and I'm so sure that this kid has characteristics of CAPD that it would be superfluous information. We already have indicators for CAPD . . . I'm convinced that [the CAPD assessment] will come back positive."

➤ "One of the things that he [the audiologist] recommends for every kid is an ALD."

➤ "The cost for a CAPD assessment ranges from $500 to as high as $3000."

➤ "ALDs are very expensive. We can't afford to fit 10 to 30% of the children in any given class with an ALD."

➤ "No matter how the CAPD assessment comes out, it won't affect the kind of program that is going to be provided."

➤ "An audiologist is not an educator. An audiologist hasn't had the training or classroom experience which would qualify him or her to make recommendations about the educational management of a child with CAPD."

➤ "All of the tests used in assessment of CAPD are quite new and experimental. This is really a controversial issue among audiologists."

➤ "We could go ahead and complete the CAPD assessment, but what do you do if the child is shown to have CAPD?"

[1] From *Audiologist's Desk Reference: Volume 1: Diagnostic Audiology, Principles, and Practices*, by J. W. Hall & G. W. Mueller, III, 1997, pp. 547–548. San Diego, CA: Singular Publishing Group. Reprinted with permission.

APPENDIX VI-J

The Functional Listening Evaluation

Cheryl DeConde Johnson
Weld County School District 6, Greeley, Co

Peggy Von Almen
Utah State University

Purpose of The Functional Listening Evaluation:

The purpose of this evaluation is to determine how a student's listening abilities are affected by noise, distance, and visual input. It is designed to simulate the student's listening ability in a situation that is more representative of his or her actual listening environment than the sound booth. This protocol is based on a listening paradigm suggested by Ying (1990), and by Ross, Bracken, and Maxon (1992).

Materials Needed: Cassette Tape Recorder
Sound Level Meter (can be purchased inexpensively from Radio Shack)
Noise Tape (Multi-Talker Babble-can be purchased from Auditec)
Tripod or stand to hold sound level meter (optional)
Sentence/Word Lists for scoring
Tape measure or yard stick
Masking tape or marker (optional)

Environment for Testing:

Use the student's classroom during a time when it is empty; if this is not possible choose a room that most closely simulates the size, ambient noise level, and floor and wall surfaces of the student's classroom.

Physical Set-up of Test Environment:

Close: Noise and examiner are 3 feet in front of the student (see Diagram A).
Distant: Noise remains 3 feet in front of the student; examiner moves back to a distance of 15 feet from the student (see Diagram B).

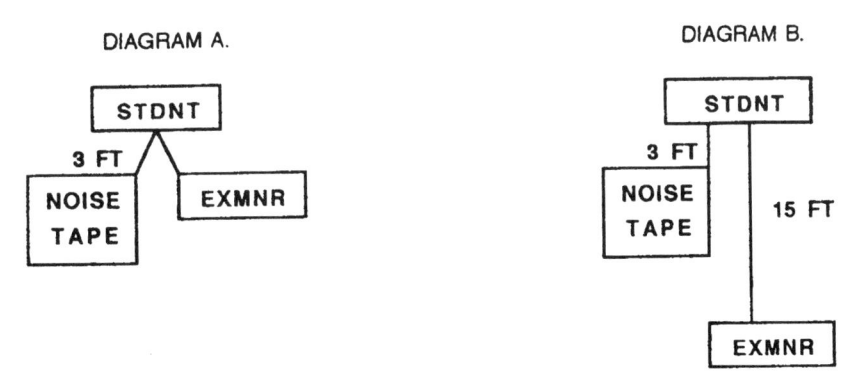

DIAGRAM A.

```
      [STDNT]
     3 FT /
[NOISE]  [EXMNR]
[TAPE ]
```

DIAGRAM B.

```
      [STDNT]
     3 FT |
[NOISE]   |
[TAPE ]  15 FT
          |
       [EXMNR]
```

For ease these distances can be marked with masking tape on the floor; be sure that the markers are from the student's ear to the examiner's mouth.

Types of Evaluation Materials:

Whenever possible sentence material should be used since it is more like speech encountered in the classroom. However, due to age and limited language and memory abilities of some students, it may be necessary to use single words. In selecting either sentence or word materials caution should be used to ensure that the vocabulary and sentence structure is appropriate for the student's language ability. When the student has poor speech intelligibility, it may be necessary to use materials which allow picture-pointing responses.

Possible Sentence Materials:	BLAIR Sentences	WIPI Sentences
	SPIN Sentences (older students)	BKB Sentences
	PSI Sentences	
Possible Word Lists:	PB-K	NU-CHIPS
	WIPI	

In most cases there will not be enough lists for the entire protocol (8 lists are needed). When selecting lists to repeat, try to use lists which were more difficult for the student.

Presentation Levels:

Speech: Monitor with sound level meter so that speech averages 75dBA at 1 foot from the examiner's mouth.

Noise: Set with sound level meter so that noise, which is 3 feet from the student, averages 60 dBA at the student's ear.

This will result in a signal-to-noise ratio of +3 dB in the close condition. The signal-to-noise ratio in the distant condition will vary depending upon the acoustics of the room, but it will be approximately -5 dB.

Presentation Protocol:

The evaluation should be conducted in the student's typical hearing mode. If hearing aids are usually worn at school, they should also be worn during the evaluation. This protocol can also be used to demonstrate the improved listening ability with FM amplification.

Eight sentence or word lists should be presented in the following order, as indicated by the numbers on the scoring matrix:

1.	AUDITORY-VISUAL	CLOSE	QUIET
2.	AUDITORY	CLOSE	QUIET
3.	AUDITORY-VISUAL	CLOSE	NOISE
4.	AUDITORY	CLOSE	NOISE
5.	AUDITORY-VISUAL	DISTANT	NOISE
6.	AUDITORY	DISTANT	NOISE
7.	AUDITORY	DISTANT	QUIET
8.	AUDITORY-VISUAL	DISTANT	QUIET

This order was selected to present easier tasks at the beginning and end of the protocol.

The examiner should present the speech materials at a normal, but not slow, rate. The student should repeat the test stimuli or point to the appropriate picture, as dictated by the material used.

It will take approximately 30 minutes to set up and administer the test protocol if sentences are used as the stimulus. If words are used, the protocol will take about 20 minutes.

ESTABLISHING SUPPORT PROGRAMS IN EDUCATIONAL SETTINGS 193

FUNCTIONAL LISTENING EVALUATION

NAME: _____ DATE: _____

EXAMINER: _____ AGE/DOB: _____

AUDIOMETRIC RESULTS

HEARING SENSITIVITY: PURE TONE AVE: RIGHT EAR _____ LEFT EAR _____

WORD RECOGNITION: RIGHT EAR ____% @ ____dBHL LEFT EAR ____% @ ____dBHL

SOUND FIELD: ___AIDED ___UNAIDED
QUIET ____% @ ____dBHL
NOISE ____% @ ____dBHL @ ____S/N

FUNCTIONAL LISTENING EVALUATION CONDITIONS

AMPLIFICATION: ___NONE ___HEARING AIDS ___FM ___SOUND FIELD
___OTHER

CLASSROOM AMBIENT NOISE LEVEL: _____ dBA

ASSESSMENT MATERIAL: _____ SENTENCES _____ WORDS

MODIFICATIONS IN PROTOCOL:

INTERPRETATION MATRIX

	NOISE QUIET	NOISE
CLOSE-AUD	2	4
CLOSE-AUD/VISUAL	1	3
DISTANT-AUD	7	6
DISTANT-AUD/VISUAL	8	5

Average of above scores: ____% ____%
QUIET NOISE

	DISTANCE CLOSE	DISTANT
QUIET-AUD	2	7
QUIET-AUD/VISUAL	1	8
NOISE-AUD	4	6
NOISE-AUD/VISUAL	3	5

____% ____%
CLOSE DISTANT

	VISUAL INPUT AUD-VIS	AUD
CLOSE-QUIET	1	2
CLOSE-NOISE	3	4
DISTANT-NOISE	5	6
DISTANT-QUIET	8	7

____% ____%
AUD-VIS AUD

INTERPRETATION AND RECOMMENDATIONS

FUNCTIONAL LISTENING MATRIX

	CLOSE/QUIET	CLOSE/NOISE	DISTANT/QUIET	DISTANT/NOISE
AUDITORY/VISUAL	1	3	8	5
AUDITORY	2	4	7	6

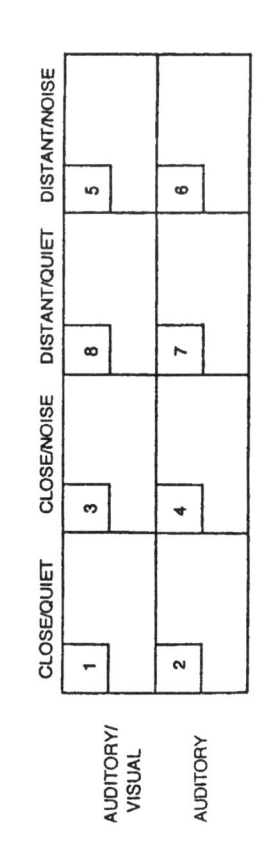

CHERYL DECONDE JOHNSON
WELD COUNTY SCHOOL DISTRICT 6, GREELEY, CO

PEGGY VON ALMEN
UTAH STATE UNIVERSITY

Scoring:

Scoring should be done using the protocol established for the selected test materials. All scores should be reported in percent correct.

Variations in Protocol:

This protocol is based on the listening situation in a typical classroom. For an individual student, it may be useful to modify this protocol to account for variations in the level and source of noise, classroom size, typical listening distances for the student, or other factors. In order to accommodate these variations, the following modifications should be considered:

1. Placement of noise/tape recorder.
2. Distance of examiner from student for the distant condition.
3. Level of noise.
4. Order of presentation.

Any modifications of the typical protocol should be noted on the test form.

Interpretation:

In order to interpret the effects of noise, distance, and visual input for the individual student, the conditions can be compared on the Interpretation Matrix. These scores can be used to determine educational modifications which would be beneficial for the student. They can also be shared with the student's parents and teachers to help them understand their student's listening abilities and needs.

Scores may be affected by different speakers, rate of speaking, attention of the listener, or status of amplification. As long as variables are kept constant throughout the evaluation, comparisons can be made.

References:

Ross, M., Brackett, D., & Maxon, A. (1991). *Assessment and management of mainstreamed hearing-impaired children.* Chapter 5: Communication Assessment (pp. 113–127). Austin, TX: Pro-Ed.

Ying, E. (1990). Speech and language assessment: Communication evaluation. In M. Rose (Ed.), *Hearing-impaired children in the mainstream* (pp. 45–80). Parkton, MD: York Press.

APPENDIX VI-K

Suggestions for Parents, Teachers, and Other Persons Close to Children With CAPD[1]

CHARACTERISTICS OF CHILDREN WITH AUDITORY PROCESSING PROBLEMS

Definition: A person with auditory processing problems has difficulty in the reception and interpretation of auditory information in the absence of a hearing loss.

When one begins to look at a list of the symptoms of an auditory processing problem, often the results look very similar to the symptoms of peripheral hearing loss (a loss of hearing caused by a problem in the ear itself). The list itself will be very similar because in both cases the person with the problem cannot make sense out of what he or she is hearing. The person with the auditory processing problem may hear the sounds loud enough, but not understand the message, and therefore act like he or she cannot hear. The following list gives some things to look for in these children, but understand that children with these symptoms need a regular hearing test to determine if their hearing is normal. It is possible that a child with a central auditory processing problem will demonstrate only some of these symptoms or perhaps none of these symptoms. These are areas that a teacher or parent could begin to look at to obtain some information about the child's listening behavior.

➢ Does the child have difficulty in the areas of reading and spelling?

➢ Does the child "pay attention only when he or she wants to," or have difficulty responding to part of the message?

➢ Does the child appear puzzled by some auditory information and say "huh" or "what" often?

➢ Does the child have difficulty staying on task and completing an assignment or project?

➢ Does the child look around for visual cues from other children before beginning an assignment?

➢ Does the child appear to tune out what is in the environment and become lost in "his or her own little world"?

➢ Does the child have upper respiratory problems such as allergies, sinus, colds, adenoid problems, or mouth breathing?

➢ Does the child have a history of fluctuating hearing loss or ear infections?

➢ Has the child had earaches, feelings of pressure in the ears, discharge from the ears, or complained of noises in the ears?

➢ Does the child ever seem confused about where sounds are coming from and have trouble locating them quickly?

➢ Does the child have difficulty telling the difference between words that sound similar, such as cone/comb or lath/laugh?

---

[1] From *Audiologist's Desk Reference: Volume I: Diagnostic Audiology, Principles, and Practices,* by J. W. Hall, III, and H. G. Mueller, III, 1997, pp. 550–551. San Diego, CA: Singular Publishing Group. Reprinted with permission.

- Does the child demonstrate unusual expressions or body postures while listening, such as facial expressions, turning or tilting of the head, or turning the body?
- Does the child respond fairly well in quiet situations, but have great difficulty listening in noisy situations such as with the TV on or in a noisy crowd or classroom?
- Does the child have difficulty remembering what is heard such as names, stories, numbers, multiple directions?
- Does the child have trouble saying certain sounds correctly or have reduced language abilities or know the meaning of words as well as the other children of his or her age group?
- Can the child learn children's songs and TV jingles easily?
- Does the child pay attention to sounds in the environment? Is there curiosity about sound and attempts to imitate sounds?
- Can the child associate certain sounds correctly with the source, such as a moo sound with a picture of a cow?
- Does the child often confuse directions or words and think something else was said?
- Does the child have difficulty keeping information heard in the correct sequence?
- Does the child respond to very simple instructions, but not to more complex instructions?
- Does the child tend to use the same words or phrases over and over instead of responding appropriately to changing verbal information?
- Is the child very visually alert, as demonstrated by watching the speakers faces very closely or by watching what others are doing?
- Does the child have difficulty associating letters of the alphabet with the sounds being made?
- Does the child show behaviors that are inappropriate (i.e., aggression, withdrawal, or impulsiveness)?
- Is the child slow to respond to auditory information, as if it takes longer to think through the information?
- Is the child easily distracted and appear to have a short attention span?
- Does the child do poorer on tests that require verbal language understanding than on tests where something is actually done with the hands?
- Does the child have trouble working independently?
- Does the child perform very inconsistently, well at times, and very poorly on the same task at other times?

The list could go on and on, but these characteristics can give you a place to start. Many of these symptoms are seen at times in a lot of children without central auditory processing problems. If, however, your child or student is having some or many of these symptoms much of the time and is not progressing as you expect, a closer look at the problem is warranted.

COMMON SENSE SUGGESTIONS FOR PARENTS OF CHILDREN WITH CAPD[2]

May be limited to a single sheet, and laminated for posting on the refrigerator, and other handy places. Parents often report that simply knowing what their child's problem is, and the increased appreciation of their child's problems, has made a big difference to the entire family, including of course their child.

- A child with auditory processing problems seems to hear inconsistently. If your child seems to hear some things, but not others, do not assume he or she is purposely ignoring you.

- You will have greater success in communicating with your child if there are no other activities (other children or adults laughing or talking, television or radio playing, dishwasher or vacuum cleaner running, etc.) competing with you.

- During communication, learn to control your child's environment by providing a quiet setting. Take the child to a quiet room, shut off the TV, ask others to be quiet for a moment, etc.

- Delay important conversation until a quiet time can be found.

- Make a point of finding "quiet conversation periods" on a regular basis during the course of each day.

- Simplify your language level if your child does not seem to understand.

- Try slowing down your rate of speech if your child continues to have trouble understanding. One way to accomplish this is to pause between utterances, especially after your child has finished talking and before you respond.

- If you have to repeat something for your child, try saying it in a different way (different words, different type sentence).

- Do not try to have discussions when you and your child are in separate rooms.

- When conversing, allow the child adequate time to respond.

- Your child may need time to rest and recuperate after school. Allow time for relaxation before asking him or her to do chores, homework, and so on.

- Read aloud to your child and discuss what you have read.

- Praise any accomplishment (academic or otherwise) that represents even small improvements over previous levels. It is not helpful to compare his or her performance to other children.

---

[2] From *Audiologist's Desk Reference: Volume I: Diagnostic Audiology, Principles, and Practices*, by J. W. Hall, III, and H. G. Mueller, III, 1997, p. 552. San Diego, CA: Singular Publishing Group. Reprinted with permission.

SUGGESTIONS FOR TEACHERS OF CHILDREN WITH CAPD[3]

Students with central auditory processing problems will respond to changes their environment and teaching program in a variety of ways. Some of these suggestions will help some students but of no benefit to others. Some students will appear to be helped by most suggestions; others will be very difficult to help, no matter what is tried. The best suggestion is to try these ideas and carefully observe the student to see what works. The goal is to help the student become more comfortable and learn better in his or her educational environment. Parents, administrators, and educational staff can work together as a team in determining what appears to be in the best interest of a particular student.

- **Reduce Distractions:** Avoid extraneous noises and visual distractions, especially when giving instructions and teaching new concepts. Before giving instructions, stand close to the student and call the student's name or touch his or her shoulder to make sure you have his or her attention. Use of the student's name during teaching time will also help hold his or her attention. Traditional classrooms are generally less distracting than open-style classrooms. Reduce motor activities during verbal presentation (i.e., in P.E., avoid giving complicated directions during calisthenics; avoid explanations while student is drawing or coloring).

- **Preferential Seating:** Provide seating away from known auditory and visual distractions such as open windows, pencil sharpeners, doorways, air conditioners, computers, and learning centers. You may have to experiment to find the best location for each student.

- **Delivery Style:** Avoid multiple commands. Presenting instructions in the simplest form possible. Gestures that enhance the message may be helpful, but extraneous gestures and excessive movement while delivering the message may be distracting. Speaking at a slower than normal rate will improve auditory comprehension skills. Speak clearly and at a comfortably loud level, using words within the student's vocabulary. Research has shown that background noise is often equal to or louder than the teacher's voice.

- **Instructional Transitions:** By reviewing past material before beginning new lessons, the teacher will give the student a feeling of success. In addition, the student will be better prepared to assimilate new information. Preassigned readings and home assignments will also help when introducing new concepts and topics. Try to use "pretuning" techniques to focus the student's attention on the subject coming up. Words such as "Listen," "Ready," and "Remember this one" seem to be effective for signaling an important message.

- **Attenuate Distractions:** Sound-attenuating ear muffs and earplugs may help the student tune out distractions during seatwork. If several pairs of earmuffs are made available to the class, the student with auditory processing difficulties will not feel singled out.

- **Visual Aids:** Visual aids, including overheads, opaque projectors, and computers may be utilized to supplement the teacher's oral presentations as well as to provide an alternative mode to the auditory channel. Combining the visual and auditory modes of learning may benefit all students in the classroom. Written instructions may be provided in conjunction with verbal instructions to aid the student in following directions.

- **Auditory Exhaustion:** Students with auditory processing problems tend to fatigue or exhaust more easily due to the external distractions of the classroom. Teachers may want to consider special adaptations to allow for this fatigue. These might include avoiding demanding auditory tasks when the student is already fatigued. This might be accomplished by presenting auditory tasks early in the day or by alternating lessons requiring a higher amount of auditory

---

[3] From *Audiologist's Desk Reference: Volume I: Diagnostic Audiology, Principles, and Practices*, by J. W. Hall, III, and H. G. Mueller, III, 1997, pp. 553–554. San Diego, CA: Singular Publishing Group. Reprinted with permission.

processing with less demanding study periods. Physical activity can be used for reduction of the stress. Keeping such a child in from recess should be used with caution.

- **Check Comprehension:** The teacher should watch for signs of inattention, decreased concentration or understanding. Instructions may need to be repeated and/or simplified for the student. To check for understanding, the student should be asked to repeat the instructions in his or her own words. Besides being a good check, this will also improve his or her listening habits since the student knows he or she will be expected to do this occasionally. To help with reading comprehension, the student may be allowed to subvocalize while reading until such time as this in unnecessary.

- **Be Supportive:** Many students with auditory processing problems experience a lack of self-confidence or diminished self-worth due to comparisons made by self or others concerning their performance versus classmates. Demanding performance that is comparable to other students is not recommended. Professionals working with the student should reinforce all work performed successfully to help alleviate this problem.

- **Buddy System:** A buddy system can be started by having one student, who appears to be strong in auditory processing, help the student who is having difficulty. Various methods may be tried to find what seems to be the most beneficial. Assistance may include note-taking, assistance with instructions, small group projects, and tutoring.

- **Classroom Adaptations:** Class lessons or instructions can be recorded so the child can hear the material again at a later time. Mild amplification might be used to assist the student in attending to the teacher. This should be done with caution, and only with the assistance and supervision of an audiologist. The classroom may be sound treated to reduce background noise by adding drapes, carpets, and sound-absorbing materials. The teacher may wish to structure the classroom in a more traditional format to reduce background distractions. Written directions and assignments should be given, along with verbal instructions. The student should be encouraged to ask for repetition of instructions, if needed. When repeating instructions, rephrase and reword the instructions. Verbal information should be presented in a brief, concise, and clear fashion. Another compensatory practice would be teaching the student good note-taking skills. Small group and individual instruction is very helpful whenever possible.

APPENDIX VI-L

Suggestions Regarding Siblings of Children With Hearing Impairment[1]

➤ Let your children know you are available to talk and listen to them.

➤ Be open and share your feelings with your children to help them feel safe in discussing their feelings with you.

➤ Children need permission to express their feelings and thoughts without threat of feeling judged. You may need to be creative in eliciting these thoughts.

➤ Admit that you do not have all the answers.

➤ Avoid making comparisons among siblings and praise them for helping one another and for helping in the family.

➤ Demand the same behavior in the child who has a hearing impairment that you demand from your other children.

➤ Responsibilities and chores should be equally divided according to ability and age.

➤ Help siblings to develop their own identity and pursue their own interests.

➤ Reassure all siblings of their importance in the family by asking for their input and advice in family discussions. Value them.

➤ Emphasize the positive interactions that you observe among siblings.

➤ Periodically provide your hearing child with correct age-appropriate information about hearing loss, language, listening, and hearing aids so that they will have the information when questioned by friends or strangers.

➤ Role-play situations to provide siblings with specific responses they can give when they are asked specific questions.

➤ Allow siblings to watch and to participate in activities designed to help the child with a hearing loss.

➤ Reserve time in your schedule to spend with each child alone; let this be consistent and something the child and you can count on.

➤ If a decision must be made that inconveniences the hearing siblings in favor of the child who has a hearing impairment, discuss it openly before it happens.

➤ Make sure that your hearing children know that they are not responsible for their sibling's hearing loss.

➤ Invite the siblings' friends to your home or on outings to see how the child with a hearing impairment functions within your family.

[1] From "Counseling Children With Hearing Loss and Their Families, " by D. V. Atkins, 1994, p. 145. In J. G. Clark and F. N. Martin (Eds.), *Effective Counseling in Audiology: Perspectives and Practice* (pp. 116–146). Englewood Cliffs, NJ: Prentice-Hall. Reprinted with permission.

- Notice if your hearing children are making up for what they perceive as your disappointment in having a child with a hearing impairment.

- All brothers and sisters have difficulties relating to each other from time to time.

- Attempt to keep the lives of all children somewhat separate with regard to toys, friends, special programs so that the individuality of each child can be ensured.

APPENDIX VI-M

Letter to Parents Regarding Support Group

XYZ INDEPENDENT SCHOOL DISTRICT
"For their future..."

To: The Parents of Children in the Hearing-Impaired
Program at Carver Elementary
Date: September 9, 1999
From: Starr Audiologist, CCC-A, FAAA
RE: Establishment of a Parent Support Group

Two informational meetings will be held this month for parents interested in establishing a parent support group. Such a support group can serve many important functions for the families associated with the Hearing-Impaired Program at Carver Elementary. For one thing, it can help parents and families cope with hearing loss. In addition, support groups in the past have organized "Mothers' Day Out" programs and have served as a strong advocate group for the educational programs at Carver. If interested, please attend one of the following meetings. Child care will be available.

Date: Tuesday evening, September 14, 1999
Time: 6:00 p.m.
Place: Carver Elementary Library

Date: Thursday evening, September 16, 1999
Time: 6:00 p.m.
Place: Carver Elementary

APPENDIX VI-N

Materials for Families of Children With Hearing Loss[1]

Literature Dealing with Hearing Loss and Hearing Aids: Toward Acceptance

Preschool and Elementary

A Button in Her Ear (1976) by Ada Litchfield
Niles, IL: Albert Whitman & Company

Anna's Silent World (1977) by Bernard Wolf
Philadelphia, PA: J.P. Lippincott Company

Claire and Emma (1976) by Diana Peter
New York: John Day Company

Ear Gear (1986) by Carole B. Simko
Washington DC: Gallaudet University Press

Hearing Aids for You and the Zoo (1984) by
Richard Stoker & Janine Gaydos
Alexander Graham Bell Association for the Deaf
3417 Volta Place, NW
Washington, DC 20007-2778
(202) 337-5220 (TDD/Voice)

Lisa and Her Soundless World (1984) by
Edna Levine
New York: Human Sciences Press

My Friend Leslie: The Story of a Handicapped Child (1993) by Maxine Rosenberg
New York: Lothrop, Lee, & Shepard Books

Tim and his Hearing Aid (1975) by Ronnie, Eleanor, & Jean Porter
Alexander Graham Bell Association for the Deaf
See address above.

We Can! (1980) by Robin R. Star
Alexander Graham Bell Association for the Deaf
See address above.

Adolescents

Chelsea: The Story of a Signal Dog (1992) by Paul Ogden
Boston: Time Warner Co.

How the Student with Hearing Loss Can Succeed in College: A Handbook for Families & Professionals (1990) by Carol Flexer, Denise Wray, & Ron Leavitt
Alexander Graham Bell Association for the Deaf
See address above.

Silent Night (1990) by Sue Thomas and S. Rickley Christian
Alexander Graham Bell Association for the Deaf
See address above.

What's That Pig Outdoors: A Memoir of Deafness (1991) by Henry Kisor
Alexander Graham Bell Association for the Deaf
See address above.

Resources for Families

A Difference in the Family, Living with a Disabled Child (1981) by Helen Featherstone
New York: Penguin Books

Amy: The Story of a Deaf Child (1985) by Lou Ann Walker
New York: Lodestar Books, E.P. Dutton

Broken Ears, Wounded Hearts (1983) by George Harris
Washington, DC: Gallaudet University Press

Hearing Aids: A User's Guide (1991) by Wayne Staab
512 East Canterbury Lane
Phoenix, AZ 85022

---

[1] From "Counseling for Pediatric Amplification," by L. M. Thibodeau, 1994, pp. 178–179. In J. G. Clark and F. N. Martin (Eds.), *Effective Counseling in Audiology: Perspectives and Practice* (pp. 147–183). Englewood Cliffs, NJ: Prentice-Hall. Reprinted with permission.

Hearing Aids: Who Needs Them? (1991) by
David Pascoe
St. Louis, MO: Big Bend Books

When Your Child Is Deaf: A Guide for Parents (1991) by David M. Luterman & Mark Ross
Alexander Graham Bell Association for the Deaf
See address above.

APPENDIX VI-O

ADA Resources for High School Seniors With Hearing Impairment and Their Families

Association of Higher Education on Disabilities
P.O. Box 21192
Columbus, OH 43221
(614) 488-4972 (V/TDD)

HEATH Resource Center
One Dupont Circle
Suite 800
Washington, DC 20036
(800)-54-HEATH (V/TDD)

Job Accommodation Network
809 Allen Hall
Morgantown, WV 26506
(800) 526-7234

Trace Research Center (Computer Technology)
Waisman Center
1500 Highland Avenue
Madison, WI 53705
(608) 262-6966 (V)
(608) 263-5408 (TDD)

APPENDIX VI-P

Letters to High School Seniors With Hearing Impairment and Their Families

XYZ INDEPENDENT SCHOOL DISTRICT
"For their future..."

October 8, 1999

To the Family of Billy McCloud
1234 Hope Way
Quality of Life City, CA 94545

Dear McCloud Family,

Congratulations on Billy's impending graduation from high school! It has been a pleasure working with you in meeting Billy's hearing health-care needs during the past several years. This is an exciting time in your lives as Billy anticipates further study at the college or university of his choice.

There are several issues that I would like to discuss with you as Billy prepares his admissions applications. During Billy's enrollment at Northwest High School, his hearing health-care needs were met as mandated by the Individuals with Disabilities Education Act (IDEA). However, at postsecondary institutions, Billy's access to an education is guaranteed by Section 504 of the Rehabilitation Act of 1973 and the Americans with Disabilities Act. However, it is Billy's responsibility to register with the program for students with disabilities at the institution.

Billy should contact the program for students with disabilities at each postsecondary institution that he applies to. He should inquire about the specific accommodations available for students with hearing impairment. I would be happy to discuss these issues with you in person. If you would like to schedule an appointment with me to discuss these issues, please feel free to call me at 555-1122 or write me via e-mail at *EarstoYou@aol.com*.

Sincerely,

Starr Audiologist, Ph.D.
Certificate of Clinical Competence in Audiology (CCC-A)
Fellow of the American Academy of Audiology (FAAA)

CHAPTER 7

Establishing Support Programs in Rehabilitation Hospitals

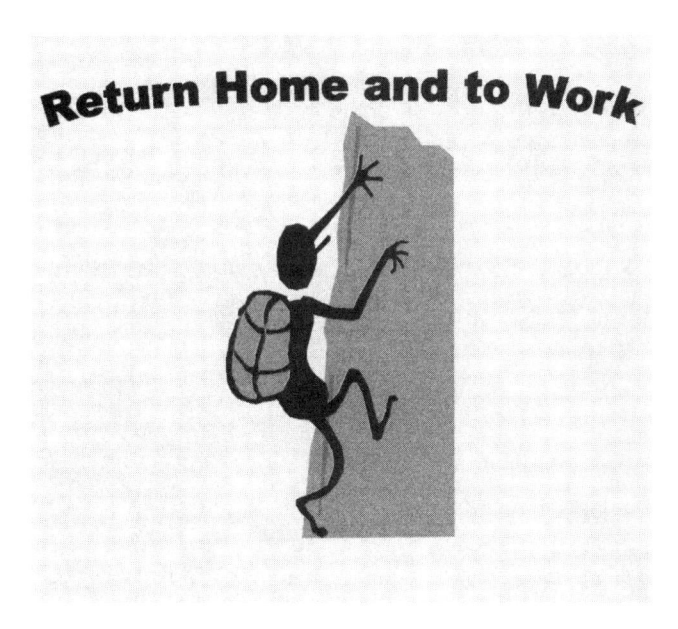

Figure 7-1. The goal of the rehabilitation hospital is to assist patients overcome their disabilities.

INTRODUCTION

Communication is a critical element in the rehabilitation of traumatically injured adults. *Patients cannot benefit from their rehabilitation program unless they can communicate with hospital staff.* Unfortunately, most rehabilitation hospitals do not employ a full-time audiologist or even identify or manage the hearing health-care needs of patients with hearing impairment. Thus, rehabilitation hospitals often contract for services with an audiologist who may be on-site only one day a week or less. Johnson, Clark-Lewis, and Griffin (1998) found that rehabilitation-hospital staff estimated that about one-fourth of their patients are hearing aid wearers. Audiologists must devise cost-efficient support programs for rehabilitation-hospital patients with hearing impairment through the use of multiskilling and support personnel.

Speech-language pathologists commonly have academic and clinical training to prepare them for participation as audiologic support personnel. Speech-language pathology departments typically administer hearing screenings for rehabilitation-hospital patients. Rehabilitation-hospital patients with hearing impairment may never have a need to venture into the speech-language pathology department, however, and their hearing losses may continue to go undetected and unmanaged. Patients who are old enough to break a hip, are old enough to have a hearing loss, but not necessarily a speech or language problem! Thus, patients' hearing loss should be a hospital-wide concern, not just that of the speech-language pathology department.

The exclusive use of speech-language pathologists as audiologic support personnel is not enough to meet the hearing health-care needs of rehabilitation-hospital patients with hearing loss (Johnson et al., 1998). Morever, recent limitations in Medicare reimbursement for speech-language pathology services may decrease the importance of aural rehabilitation for stroke patients in urgent need of aphasia therapy, for example. Including nursing, occupational-therapy (OT), and physical-therapy (OT) staff in a hospital-wide aural rehabilitation support program may facilitate the goal of returning these patients home and to work. The purpose of this chapter is to enable readers to establish effective support programs for patients with hearing impairment in rehabilitation hospitals.

LEARNING OBJECTIVES

This chapter will enable the reader to:

- Understand service delivery in the rehabilitation industry
- Understand the effect of hearing loss on the rehabilitation process
- Describe the potential role of the audiologist in a rehabilitation hospital
- Describe the major components of a support program for rehabilitation-hospital patients with hearing loss

---

THE REHABILITATION INDUSTRY FOR THE NEXT MILLENIUM: THE HEALTHSOUTH MODEL
(HealthSouth, 1998)

Managed care has resulted in the formation of large corporations in an attempt to control the increasing costs of health care. The rehabilitation industry has also followed this model. The HealthSouth corporation was formed in 1984 and restructured the rehabilitation industry in less than 10 years. HealthSouth understands the industry and has a vision for the future. Its system has been designed to move patients through a logical health-care system that offers highly technical, less invasive procedures.

Without trying to sound like an advertisement for HealthSouth, we are focusing on it here because its model offers some good examples of service provision within the corporate rehabilitation arena. We would like to emphasize here that HealthSouth is in no way currently connected with the authors. HealthSouth has developed an integrated-services model that is a continuum of high-quality diagnostic, surgical, and rehabilitation procedures that are strategically combined to achieve excellent patient outcomes in the most cost-efficient manner possible. The HealthSouth Integrated Services Model was not designed to provide more services, but a comprehensive, integrated treatment system. Established diagnostic, surgery, outpatient, and inpatient facilities work together to provide high-quality, cost-effective services.

Currently, HealthSouth has nearly 1,000 diagnostic center facilities. Technology, staff ability, and commitment are emphasized at these centers. The organization ensures that all diagnostic facilities have the latest equipment and technology and staff that are adequately trained. In 1995, HealthSouth became the nation's largest provider of outpatient surgical services with 126 locations throughout the country. These centers were established to offer certain surgical procedures to be performed on a same-day basis, although some facilities are equipped to handle patient overnight stays. Some of the services provided in these outpatient surgical centers include gastroenterology, general surgery, gynecology, lithotripsy, ophthalmology, oral surgery, orthopedics, pain management, plastic surgery, podiatry, and urology. In addition to outpatient surgical centers, HealthSouth has more than 700 outpatient facilities in nearly every state. Highly skilled therapists and trainers provide expert, cost-effective outpatient sports medicine and rehabilitative care at these facilities. HealthSouth's outpatient division has accumulated a database of more than one million cases, which is one of the largest in the rehabilitation industry. Services provided in these outpatient centers include aquatic therapy, audiological screenings, biofeedback, driving assessments, family education, foot and ankle treatment, functional capacity evaluations, general orthopedics, hand therapy, headache treatment, injury prevention, neurology, neuropsychology, occupational therapy, pain management, physical therapy, speech therapy, spine rehabilitation, sports therapy, urinary therapy, vision therapy, and work hardening.

Audiologists typically do not provide services in these diagnostic centers or in outpatient surgical or rehabilitative facilities, but in rehabilitation hospitals. By the mid-1990s, HealthSouth operated more than 90 freestanding rehabilitation hospitals and inpatient rehabilitation units in acute-care hospitals in the United States. During the 1990s, HealthSouth formed partnerships with leading medical universities in the country, such as the University of Missouri, the University of Virginia, Vanderbilt University, and the University of Alabama at Birmingham. HealthSouth has established some innovative service-delivery procedures within these rehabilitation hospitals and units.

HealthSouth uses a visionary process of aiding patient progress through critical pathways that were first designed to facilitate schedule maintenance shutdowns of chemical plants in the 1950s. Today, they are used to redefine the way health-care facilities provide services under managed care. Critical pathways are proven patient-care guidelines that clearly define progressive strategic treatments, measurable milestones, inpatient progress, and expected outcomes. HealthSouth reports that they have 20 pathways for product lines, including stroke, brain injury, spinal-cord injury, neurology, general rehabilitation, amputee, orthopedics, pain management, and ventilation. Critical pathways are designed to:

- reduce length of stay,
- improve efficiency and effectiveness of patient care,
- be patient-outcome driven instead of clinician driven,
- reduce costs,
- increase interdisciplinary interaction,
- improve patient outcomes,
- integrate plans of care,
- assist with case management,
- streamline documentation and eliminate redundancy,
- allow more time for direct patient care,
- allow for concurrent quality reviews, and
- move patients quickly through the inpatient aspects of the continuum to home and outpatient programs.

Table 7–1 lists the inpatient rehabilitation programs, and Table 7–2 lists the outpatient programs offered at inpatient facilities.

TYPICAL AUDIOLOGIC SERVICE DELIVERY MODEL IN A REHABILITATION HOSPITAL

Few rehabilitation hospitals employ audiologists on a full-time basis unless they are full-time employees of an acute-care facility that has an independent rehabilitation unit. The most common service-delivery model is for an audiologist to be a contract-for-service employee of the rehabilitation hospital who provides services once a week. Contract-for-service audiologists often have a more difficult time establishing support programs for rehabilitation-hospital patients with hearing impairment because they are often viewed as "outsiders." The relationship between the audiologists and their immediate supervisors is an important one. Supervisors are the persons who will "sell" the idea of establishing support programs to rehabilitation-hospital administrators and enlist the cooperation of other departments in allowing their staff to serve as audiologic support personnel.

Establishing support programs for patients with hearing impairment requires the use of multiskilling and support personnel. Recall that multiskilling is the training of one professional to perform tasks that are typically assigned to those in other disciplines (Foto, 1996). Chapter 2 defined the different models of multiskilling. Managing audiologists typically use collateral and collateral-subordinate multiskilling models

Table 7-1. HealthSouth inpatient rehabilitation programs.

■ Alternative ventilation	■ Oncology
■ Amputee	■ Orthopedic
■ Arthritis	■ Pain management
■ Assessment	■ Pediatrics
■ Brain injury	■ Pediatric brain injury
■ Burn	■ Prognostic
■ Cardiac	■ Pulmonary
■ Chronic pain with chemical dependency	■ Short-stay orthopedics
■ Coma stimulation	■ Skilled nursing
■ Community re-entry	■ Spinal cord
■ Dialysis	■ Step down
■ Fast track	■ Stoke
■ General rehabilitation	■ Subacute
■ Joint replacement	■ Ten-day stroke evaluation
■ Mild brain injury	■ Transitional
■ Modified rehabilitation	■ Ventilator
■ Multiple sclerosis	■ Ventilator weaning
■ Neurobehavioral	■ Wound care
■ Neuropsychological	■ Young stroke

Source: From HealthSouth, 1998. Available: www.healthsouth.com.

in support programs for rehabilitation-hospital patients with hearing loss. Audiologists often must rely on registered nurses (i.e., collateral multiskilling) or their assistants (i.e., collateral-subordinate multiskilling) to check patients' hearing aids, for example. Johnson et al. (1998) found that these professionals need extensive inservice instruction to function as audiologic support personnel. Unfortunately, as discussed in Chapter 5, rehabilitation-hospital staff may resent being told what to do by an "outsider." Once these individuals realize the compounding effects of physical disability and hearing loss, however, they may be more than eager to participate as audiologic support personnel.

EFFECTS OF DISABILITY AND HEARING LOSS

Patients are admitted to an inpatient rehabilitation hospital or unit from an acute-care facility after their traumatic condition has stabilized. Rehabilitation-hospital patients who have endured a physical loss of function from an accident or stroke may feel overwhelmed and experience some emotional reactions to their disability. Dr. Selenick (HealthSouth, 1998) interviewed Hal Hoines, director of HealthSouth Riosa, who explained that sadness, fear, and denial are typical reactions to disability. Sadness may express itself as misdirected anger, irritability, sleep disturbance, loss of appetite, apathy, and loss of self-esteem, for example. Moreover, fearful patients may be overwhelmed and uncertain about the future. They may ask: Will I be able to take care of myself? Will I be able to earn a living? Who will take care of my family? Will I ever be normal again? Can I deal with this? Patients may become so depressed and hopeless that they may experience physical symptoms, such as heart palpitations, sweating, tremor, shortness of breath, and a sense of panic. Some patients, on the other hand, may be in denial and proceed through rehabilitation without acknowledging the longstanding implications of their disability.

Dr. Hoines reported that most patients adjust to their disability and go on to lead satisfying lives. Nonetheless, successful personal adjustment to disability requires early psychological intervention. He believes, however, that doctors often wait too long to make a referral for psychological intervention. At his facility, rehabilitation counselors or psychologists see all patients within 24 hours of admission. Dr. Hoines believes that mental health-care professionals who serve in this capacity must understand the nature of disability and possess the necessary experience to handle these cases.

Rehabilitation-hospital patients may experience even greater emotional discomfort if they have a hearing loss. Sensorineural hearing loss causes increased feelings of isolation, depres-

Table 7-2. HealthSouth outpatient programs at inpatient facilities.

■ Adaptive driving	■ Ortho-impairment
■ Amputee	■ Ortho-upper extremities
■ Aquatics	■ Orthopedics
■ Arthritis	■ Orthotics and prosthetics
■ Asthma	■ Pain blocks
■ Audiology	■ Pain management
■ Back program	■ Parkinson's disease
■ Back to school	■ Pediatric day treatment
■ Balance and gait	■ Pediatrics
■ Brace and limb clinic	■ Post-offer physicals
■ Brain injury day	■ Postpolio
■ Breast recovery	■ Pre-operative evaluations
■ Burn	■ Psychiatric evaluations
■ Cardiac rehabilitation	■ Pulmonary
■ Cerebral palsy	■ Pulmonary day
■ Chronic headaches	■ Return to work
■ Comprehensive rehabilitation	■ School therapy
■ Day hospital	■ Seating and positioning
■ Day treatment	■ Skin care
■ Fibromyalgia	■ Speech
■ Follow-up spinal cord clinic	■ Spinal-cord injury
■ Foot clinic	■ Spinal-cord clinic
■ Functional capacity assessment	■ Spine rehabilitation
■ Functional restoration	■ Sports medicine
■ Gait lab	■ Stroke
■ General rehabilitation	■ Stroke day program
■ Hand clinic	■ Total knee
■ Industrial rehabilitation	■ Urodynamics
■ Joint/hip replacement	■ Urology
■ Limb preservation	■ Vestibular program
■ Lymphedema	■ Vision therapy
■ Mild traumatic brain injury	■ Vocational rehabilitation
■ Modified pain	■ Wheelchair seating
■ Multiple sclerosis	■ Women's programs
■ Muscular dystrophy clinic	■ Work hardening/work start
■ Neurology	■ Work injury
■ Neuropsychiatric testing	■ Work perfect
■ Neuropsychiatry clinic	■ Wound care
■ Neuropsychology	■ Young stroke day treatment
■ Oncology	■ Young stroke

Source: From HealthSouth, 1998. Available: www.healthsouth.com.

sion, loneliness, frustration, and disappointment due to a decreased ability to communicate (Crandell, 1998). Hearing loss can have negative results in several key areas of patients' lives:

- Behavior (e.g., escape/avoidance, withdrawal/isolation, denial/avoidance, and negative behaviors)
- Emotions (e.g., anger, depression, anxiety, guilt, loss of self-esteem, and embarrassment)
- Thoughts (e.g., worry and inattention or poor concentration)
- Relationships (e.g., loss of intimacy, dependency, and loss of assertiveness) (Wayner & Abrahamson, 1996).

Furthermore, Crandell (1998) reported that hearing impairment has a negative effect on patients' overall health because individuals with hearing loss have a higher incidence of heart arhythmias, ischemic heart disease, hypertension, and osteoarthritis. In addition, the greater the degree of hearing loss, the greater the reduction in health status, activity level, interpersonal relationships, enjoyment of life, and physical mobility.

Undetected or unmanaged hearing loss can interfere with the delivery of medical and psychological services (Garstecki & Erler, 1998). Hearing loss can impede the recovery of rehabilitation-hospital patients in several ways. First, the negative emotional impact of patients' disability and hearing loss may interact synergistically, compounding their psychological problems. For example, a socially isolated and withdrawn 65-year-old retiree with hearing loss may not be able to cope with a stroke that results in his inability to communicate verbally with friends and family. Second, hearing loss makes it difficult for patients to communicate with rehabilitation-hospital staff. For example, Johnson et al. (1998) found that the majority of nursing, OT, and PT staff surveyed believed that rehabilitation-hospital patients with hearing impairment are more difficult to work with than patients with normal hearing. Furthermore, the majority of these rehabilitation-staff members felt that it was important for patients' hearing aids to be functioning during their hospital stay. Clearly, support programs for rehabilitation-hospital patients with hearing impairment may improve their morale, communication with staff, and facilitate their recovery process. Unfortunately, when coping with a recent trauma, many patients and their families either forget to use their hearing aids or elect not to wear them during their hospital stay for fear of losing these expensive devices. These points were exemplified for a recent rehabilitation-hospital patient. Griffin, Clark-Lewis, and Johnson (1997) told Vivian's story (see below).

Unfortunately, hearing aids in rehabilitation hospitals do have a habit of playing "hide and seek," disappearing, going through the laundry, being worn into the shower, or swimming in denture cups. These occurrences show the desperate need for both support programs for rehabilitation-hospital patients with hearing impairment and for inservices particularly directed at nurse's assistants (i.e., collateral-subordinate multiskilling).

Before her stroke, Vivian was a food-service supervisor in a retirement center. The residents there missed her sunny disposition and the interest she always showed in them. The same qualities were evident during Vivian's stay at a rehabilitation hospital. Despite her physical limitations, including limited speech production and no use of her right side, Vivian always had a smile for the staff and showed a genuine interest in other patients.

The only problem was that after a week in the hospital, Vivian was not showing much progress in her therapies. Always pleasant and apparently accepting of her therapists' suggestions, the nursing staff noticed that Vivian often seemed to lack the follow-through they expected from her level of comprehension, motivation, and cheerful disposition. Was she covering up a depression with her outward cheerfulness? Was there some reason why she really didn't want to get better? The staff was puzzled and began to wonder if her outward behavior was merely a cover-up.

A routine hearing screening and subsequent audiologic evaluation revealed the source of the problem. Before becoming a food-service supervisor, Vivian spent a number of years operating cleaning equipment in a laundry. As a result, she had developed a noise-induced hearing loss. Before beginning her work as a food supervisor in the retirement home, she was fitted with hearing aids that restored most of her hearing and enabled her to communicate effectively with her coworkers and residents of the retirement center. Unfortunately, all of this changed when Vivian had her stroke. No longer able to put her hearing aid in her right ear or change its tiny battery, Vivian relegated her hearing aids to their box, and her husband placed them in a drawer by her bed. With all of the worry of Vivian's stroke and stay at an acute-care hospital, Vivian and her husband didn't even think to bring her hearing aids to the rehabilitation hospital. When another family member noted that Vivian was not using her hearing aids, her husband expressed a concern that her hearing aids might get lost at the hospital. Vivian tried to get by on her sunny disposition and ability to lipread, but she was missing a lot. It had a negative impact on her therapies. She thought she understood most of what her therapists were saying to her, but she was not sure.

SUPPORT PROGRAMS FOR REHABILITATION-HOSPITAL PATIENTS WITH HEARING IMPAIRMENT

Successful support programs for rehabilitation-hospital patients with hearing impairment contain the following components:

- Continuity of management of the patients' hearing health-care needs (from preadmission to discharge)
- Effective hearing screening programs
- Availability of complete audiologic evaluations
- Hearing aid evaluations and fittings
- Hearing aid monitoring programs
- Comprehensive inservice programs for staff
- Assistive listening device (ALD) programs and communication accessibility
- Short-term aural rehabilitation

Continuity of Management of Patients' Hearing Health-Care Needs

The rehabilitation process begins prior to admission to the rehabilitation hospital. Most traumatically injured patients are admitted to an inpatient rehabilitation facility from an acute-care hospital after their health status has been stabilized. Patients and their families should be visited in the acute-care facility by a nurse liaison to assist in patients' transition to the rehabilitation hospital (Griffin et al., 1997; Johnson et al., 1998). During this visit, the nurse discusses important matters regarding the patients' admission to the rehabilitation hospital. The nurse liaison asks patients and their families about their hearing status and the use of hearing aids. Patients who believe they have a hearing loss should be noted by the nurse liaison who will ensure that a hearing screening is scheduled. Patients confirming the existence of a hearing loss and use of hearing aids are scheduled for an audiologic evaluation and hearing aid check. In addition, the nurse liaison reminds patients to bring along important personal items necessary for their rehabilitation program (e.g., workout clothes, sneakers, and their hearing aids).

Upon admission, patients with confirmed hearing loss should complete an informed-consent form to participate in the support program for patients with hearing impairment. By signing an informed-consent form similar to the one appearing in Appendix VII-A, patients agree to: (1) staff notification of hearing loss, (2) hearing aid monitoring, (3) audiologic services, and (4) participation in the ALD program. Patients can agree to participate in any or all aspects of the program. Although some patients may be sensitive about their hearing loss, those consenting to staff notification will have signs like those appearing in Appendix VII-B placed over their beds declaring their communication needs. Thus, staff need to know to: (1) use appropriate communication tips and strategies, (2) assist patients with inserting and removing their hearing aids, (3) check patients' hearing aids, and (4) obtain an ALD for patients' use during the day. In this way, patients' hearing health-care needs should be met during their hospital stay.

Effective Hearing Screening Programs

Effective hearing screening programs are an important part of support programs for rehabilitation-hospital patients with hearing impairment. All patients should have a hearing screening as part of their routine entrance evaluations. Otoacoustic emissions (OAEs) are an ideal screening measure requiring little or no cooperation from the patient, and minimal time to administer (Danhauer, 1997). In addition, OAE testing produces important information about the peripheral auditory system, has a relatively low cost-to-patient ratio, and can be administered by appropriately trained audiologic support personnel (Danhauer, 1997). OAE screening programs are an ideal place to use audiologic support personnel compatible with the guidelines set forth in the "Position Statement and Guidelines of the Consensus Panel on Support Personnel in Audiology" (AAA, 1997), which appears in Chapter 2, Appendix II-B.

Otoacoustic emissions also provide high reliability (e.g., copositivity and conegativity) and validity (e.g., high sensitivity and high specificity). Reliability is the consistency of measurement and validity is the truth in measurement. Screening measures can be reliable without being valid, but cannot be valid unless they are first reliable. With regard to reliability measures, copositivity is the extent to which two tests agree in identifying persons with a disorder, and conegativity is the agreement in identifying those without a disorder (Roeser, 1995). Validity measures include sensitivity, which refers to the proportion of patients with hearing impairment who are correctly identified by a screening test, and specificity, which is the proportion of patients with normal hearing who were correctly dismissed by the screening tool. Importance of reliability and validity data for program viability is discussed in Chapter 9, "Sustaining Stellar Support Programs: Outcome Measures."

Audiologists must market OAE screening programs to administrators carefully. These screening programs can be attractive to rehabilitation-hospital administrators for several reasons. First, OAEs can be conducted in a fraction of the time required to complete a routine pure-tone air-conduction screening. Second, nonprofessional audiologic support personnel can conduct OAE screenings allowing other professional staff (e.g., speech-language pathologists) to be more productive with their time. Third, reimbursement is often available for OAE testing, especially with the appropriate OAE RVS codes: (1) screening code (92587), or (2) in-depth diagnosis (92588) (Danhauer, 1997). Fourth, OAE testing equipment is available in small laptop computers and even hand-held screening devices that can be taken to patients' rooms for testing. Because OAEs can be reliably and validly obtained in moderately noisy rooms, OAE testing is ideal for busy hospitals. Fifth, the incorporation of OAE testing into routine patient care is innovative and consistent with the principles of managed care discussed in Chapter 1. Sixth, and most important, OAEs are nonbehavioral measures requiring no response from the patient who may be in a comatose state or unable to respond due to a recent trauma.

The biggest obstacle to incorporating OAE screening programs in rehabilitation hospitals is the initial start-up equipment costs. Systems range from $6,000 to $12,000 in addition to the costs of a computer and printer (Danhauer, 1997). Exact dollar quotations for equipment are difficult to estimate because prices often fluctuate with changes in technology (e.g., In 1999, OAE screeners were available for as low as $4,500), but we have included them to make this information as useful as possible. These costs may seem prohibitive to rehabilitation-hospital administrators, especially if the purchase request is made from a contract-for-service employee. Thus, audiologists must carefully plan their marketing strategy to rehabilitation-hospital administrators and remember some key points. First, they must market the idea to their immediate supervisors (e.g., director of the speech-language pathology department) before contacting administrators. Support must be obtained at this level if there is to be any chance for success. Second, audiologists should plan a short presentation to rehabilitation-hospital administrators about the OAE screening program. The presentation should be clear, organized, and last no longer than about 20 minutes. Appendix VII-C contains an "OAE Fact Sheet" (Danhauer, 1997) that can be used as both a handout and as overheads for the presentation. If administrators believe that the start-up funds for the equipment are too great, audiologists should consider the option of renting the equipment for about $200 a month (Danhauer, 1997). Fourth, if given the opportunity to start a trial OAE screening program, audiologists must make the most of it through proper documentation and cost/benefit analysis. They should keep accurate records with regard to the number of patients screened, audiologic support personnel involved, total time required for testing, revenue generated, and increases in referrals as evidence of program viability. The performance of hearing screening programs using OAE testing should be compared to previous screening methods. Data should be organized and presented to administrators in the most advantageous way possible.

Audiologists should also note that OAEs are not direct tests of hearing, but reflect the status of the peripheral auditory system. OAEs will not be present for patients with losses poorer than 30 to 50 dB HL. Furthermore, OAEs may be compromised for patients with certain outer or middle ear disorders (e.g., many that occur in patients who have experienced recent head trauma). Nevertheless, OAE screenings are still highly informative and will result in proper referrals for audiologic or medical follow-up, which is the point of the screening in the first place.

Implementing an OAE screening program requires audiologists to make several decisions: Should distortion product otoacoustic emissions (DPOAE) or transient-evoked otoacoustic emissions (TEOAE) be used? What type of equipment should be used? Who should do the screenings? How should these individuals be trained? Which screening protocols should be used? A complete discussion of the type of OAEs to use is beyond the scope of this chapter. The reader is referred to more complete discussions of this topic in the literature. Danhauer

(1997) recommended TEOAE measurements because they are highly sensitive to hearing losses poorer than about 30 dB HL. Although not supported by the literature, DPOAEs may increase the cut-off to about 50 dB HL when the primary frequencies (i.e., F1 and F2) are set at 70 dB SPL (Danhauer, 1997).

There are numerous manufacturers of OAE equipment. Audiologists should do market research by visiting exhibits at national conventions, as well as talking to local manufacturers' representatives and professional colleagues prior to deciding on a particular unit. Audiologists should not feel that they need to make a decision at the outset but should evaluate several units on a trial basis. Appendix VII-D contains a list of current OAE equipment manufacturers. Audiologists need to determine who will conduct the screening by selecting one or more multiskilling models. Inservice protocols to train support personnel to conduct OAE screenings must be developed. Appendix VII-E contains a combination informational and skill-based inservice protocol for this purpose. The topics for this inservice should include the purposes of hearing screenings, definition of OAEs, brief description of equipment, preparations for conducting OAEs, OAE protocols, troubleshooting equipment, documentation, and patient follow-up. In addition, a significant portion of the inservice should be supervised practicum. Participants should attend the "What is hearing loss and how does it affect communication?" inservice, which appears in Appendix V-E prior to attending the inservice on OAE screenings. Figure 7–2 shows a patient's hearing being screened using OAEs.

Other more traditional hearing screening methods include pure-tone air-conduction testing (see Appendix VII-F for a sample screening form) and self-report hearing-handicap inventories. Bess (1995) suggested two screening tools that can be used in hospital settings. He suggested using the *Hearing Handicap Inventory for the Elderly—Screening Version* (HHIE-S) (Ventry & Weinstein, 1982), which is a quick, simple, inexpensive, and self-administered inventory consisting of 10 items that probe social and emotional complications associated with hearing loss. The HHIE-S is composed of items from the *Hearing Handicap Inventory for the Elderly* (HHIE) (Ventry & Weinstein, 1982) that is intended for use with elderly people living independently or with their children. Appendix VII-G lists the 10 items on the HHIE-S, each with three possible responses of "no," "sometimes," and "yes." "No" responses earn 0 points, "sometimes" responses earn 2 points, and "yes" responses earn 4 points. Patients can earn from 0 to 40 points on the HHIE-S. The higher the HHIE-S score, the greater the self-perceived hearing handicap of the patient. Bess (1995)

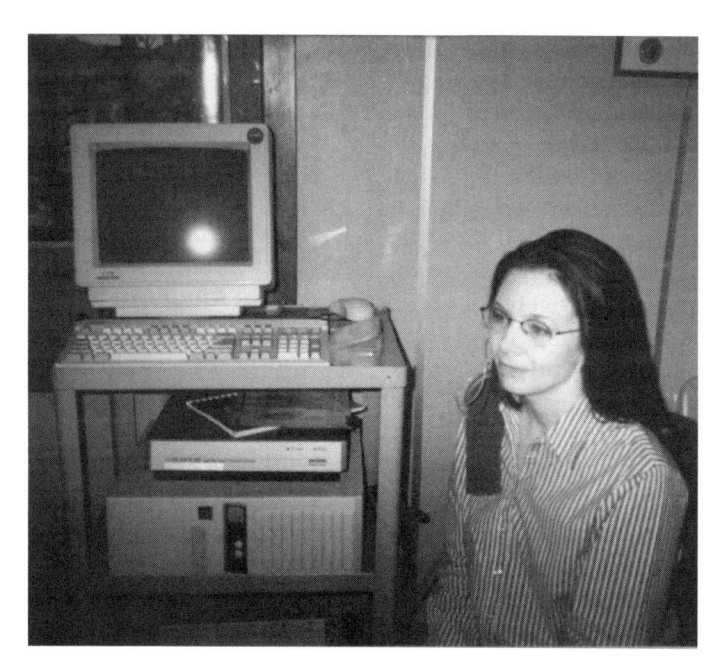

Figure 7–2. Screening using otoacoustic emissions.

found that the HHIE-S had a sensitivity of 72% and a specificity of 77%, with high test-retest reliability. Bess and his colleagues found that elderly patients with HHIE-S scores of 0 to 8 have only a 13% probability of having a hearing loss, whereas those with scores of 26 to 40 have an 84% probability of a significant hearing loss. The HHIE-S has a form for adults under 65 years of age called the *Hearing Handicap Inventory for Adults—Screening Version* (HHIA-S) (Newman, Weinstein, Jacobson, & Hug, 1991) that can also be used as a screening tool in a rehabilitation hospital. Appendix VII-H contains the HHIA-S. These self-assessments of hearing handicap pre- and post-rehabilitation can be used as efficacy measures of support programs. Outcome measures are discussed in Chapter 9, "Sustaining Stellar Support Programs." Patients who test positive on the hearing screening should be rescreened. Patients failing twice should be scheduled for complete audiologic evaluations. An example of a letter to patients and their families is included in Appendix VII-I.

Complete Audiologic Evaluations for Patients with Confirmed Hearing Loss and Those Failing Hearing Screenings

Upon hospital admission, patients who have confirmed hearing loss or already have hearing aids should be scheduled for an audiologic evaluation and hearing aid check. Audiologists must ask these patients if they have a personal audiologist and whether their hearing aids are under warranty in case the devices are found to be nonfunctional. In addition, patients who fail the hearing screening should be scheduled for a full audiologic evaluation. Contract-for-service audiologists may have a difficult time if they do not have adequate facilities or equipment onsite. They may have to make arrangements with the rehabilitation hospital to transport patients to their offices for audiologic evaluations. Transporting patients may be not only expensive, but difficult for those with mobility problems. Thus, large rehabilitation hospitals should possess adequate facilities and equipment to maintain a viable support program for patients with hearing impairment. Necessary facilities and equipment include: an office, a computer, a sound-treated test booth, an audiometer with sound-field testing capabilities, an immittance meter, an OAE system, an ABR system, a video-otoscope, a portable hearing aid analyzer/probe-tube microphone measurement system, and other equipment and supplies necessary to fit and service hearing aids. Equipment and materials needed for hearing aid evaluations and fittings are discussed in the next section. Patients should be counseled as to the nature, degree, and configuration of hearing loss, as well as options for rehabilitation. Ideally, newly diagnosed patients can be evaluated for and fit with hearing aids as part of their overall rehabilitation programs.

Hearing Aid Evaluation and Fitting Program

With all of the new hearing aid technologies that are available to the consumer, audiologists must be adequately prepared to fit their patients with hearing aids equipped with the latest features. Matching "high-tech" hearing aid features to rehabilitation-hospital patients can be a difficult task. It may be impossible unless the hearing health-care professionals' hearing aid evaluation, selection, and fitting protocols are complete and up-to-date. Mueller (1996) reported that a complete protocol includes: (1) self-assessment inventories, (2) measures of audibility, (3) suprathreshold measurements, (3) prescriptive methods, and (4) verification procedures. Table 7–3 lists the specific components in each area needed for a complete and up-to-date fitting protocol.

Mueller (1996) stated that self-assessment inventories are important for two reasons. First, they serve as a benchmark to measure post-fit benefit. Second, these inventories provide patients' perceptions of their degree of hearing handicap. Patients' lack of perceived hearing handicap may be a contraindication for hearing aid candidacy. Mueller recommended both the *Hearing Handicap Inventory for the Elderly* (HHIE) (Ventry & Weinstein, 1982) and the *Abbreviated Profile of Hearing Aid Benefit* (APHAB) (Cox & Alexander, 1995). The HHIE-S and HHIA-S were mentioned above. The APHAB is part of the Independent Hearing Aid Fitting Forum (IHAFF) (IHAFF, 1994) and consists of 24 questions, answered on a seven-point continuum from "always" to "never," with a numerical value assigned to each answer so that a percent can be calculated for four subscales: (1) ease of communication, (2) background noise, (3) reverberation, and (4) aversiveness (Mueller, 1996). The

Table 7-3. Specific components for an up-to-date hearing aid fitting protocol.

Self-Assessment Inventories

- Hearing Handicap Inventory for the Elderly (HHIE) (Ventry & Weinstein, 1982)
- Abbreviated Profile of Hearing Aid Benefit (APHAB) (Cox & Alexander, 1995)
- Client Oriented Scale of Improvement (COSI) (Dillon, James, & Ginis, 1997)

Audibility Measures

- Mueller and Killion's Method (Mueller & Killion, 1990)
- Humes' Method (Humes, 1991)
- Pavlovic's Method (Pavlovic, 1991)

Suprathreshold Measures and Prescriptive Methods

- Desired Sensation Level (i/o) (Cornilesse, Seewald, & Jamieson, 1997)
- FIG-6 (Killion & Fikret-Pasa, 1993)
- Visualization of Input/Output Locator Algorithm (VIOLA) (IHAFF, 1994)

Verification Methods

- Post-Fitting Self-Assessment Inventories
- Real-Ear Probe Tube Microphone Measurements (Real-Ear Insertion Response (REIRs))* and Real-Ear Aided Responses (REARs)*)
- Loudness Scaling*
- Aided Speech Measures*

*At patients' user volume-control-wheel setting.
Source: Adapted from "Hearing Aids and People: Strategies for a Successful Match," by H. G. Mueller, 1996, *The Hearing Journal, 49*(4), 13–28. Reprinted with permission.

APHAB is a useful clinical tool for measuring the outcome of hearing aid fittings, comparing alternative fittings, and tracking the success of a fitting over time (Cox & Alexander, 1995). Most importantly, the APHAB has been used as an excellent measure of both need for and benefit from "high-tech" hearing aids, such as digital signal processing (Arlinger, Billermark, Oberg, Lunner, & Hellgren, 1998) and multimemory hearing aids (Fabry, 1996). Another method of measuring self-assessment of hearing handicap is the *Client Oriented Scale of Improvement* (COSI) (Dillon, James, & Ginis, 1997). With this scale, the patient writes the self-report questionnaire by nominating and prioritizing up to five difficult listening situations.

Mueller (1996) believed that measures of audibility are important for: (1) determining hearing aid candidacy, (2) counseling, and (3) use as a benchmark for unaided versus aided benefit comparisons. At least three paper and pencil methods exist for calculating the audibility index (AI): (1) Mueller and Killion's Method (1990), (2) Humes' Method (1991), and (3) Pavlovic's Method (1991) (Killion, Mueller, Pavlovic, & Humes, 1993). The most widely used is Mueller and Killion's (1990) Count-the-Dot Audibility Index. Mueller (1996) stressed the importance of not confusing audibility with speech recognition scores. Audibility is the percent of the speech message that is audible, not necessarily understandable.

Mueller (1996) stated that obtaining patients' loudness discomfort levels (LDLs) simply is not adequate for determining amplification characteristics for the wide range of possible input levels for hearing aids. Mueller suggested evaluating patients' unaided loudness growth functions using pure-tone stimuli. In particular, elderly patients need structure, good instructions, and appropriate response formats to provide both reliable and valid estimations of loudness (Holmes, 1995; Mueller, 1996). Useful loudness perception assessment has the following elements: (1) measurement of a loudness growth function, (2) standard instructions, (3) ascending levels, (4) frequency-specific stimuli, (5) ability to perform either manual or computer-driven testing, (6) acceptable test-retest reliability within a reasonable time frame, and (7) generation of data in 2-cc coupler level for direct comparison to hearing aid performance specifications (Cox, 1995). The Contour Test is a loudness test that meets all seven criteria listed above, determines the level at which warbled tones fit into the seven loudness categories developed by Hawkins, Walden, Montgomery, and Prosek (1987), and has software that administers and scores the test (Cox, 1995). The seven categories of loudness developed by Hawkins et al. (1987) are: (1) very soft; (2) soft; (3) comfortable, but slightly soft; (4) comfortable; (5) comfortable, but slightly loud; (6) loud, but OK; and (7) uncomfortably loud. Although the details of the test are not provided here, Cox (1995) suggested obtaining loudness data at two frequencies for each fitted ear. These data are valuable in setting the various parameters for compression and the need for multichannel hearing aids.

Mueller (1996) stated that the National Acoustics Lab-Revised (NAL-R) (Byrne & Dillon, 1986) prescriptive method is currently the most widely used method in the United States. It provides frequency-specific hearing aid gain that will place average speech at patients' most comfortable listening level (MCL). Mueller (1996) advised that the NAL prescriptive method is adequate for selecting hearing aid gain for average speech inputs (i.e., 65 dB SPL) or for fitting linear gain throughout the speech frequencies. To obtain targets for soft, medium, and loud speech, however, other methods should be considered. These methods include: (1) the Desired Sensation Level [i/o] method (DSL [i/o]) (Cornelisse, Seewald, & Jamieson, 1994), (2) FIG-6 (Killion & Fikret-Pasa, 1993), or (3) Visualization of Input/Output Locator Algorithm (VIOLA) (IHAFF, 1994). The DSL [i/o] method is recommended for wide dynamic range compression (WDRC) hearing aids and for those with very low compression kneepoints (Mueller, 1996). The FIG-6 method is a computer-based program to fit nonlinear hearing aids that have WDRC, such as those with K-AMP processing. The computer program uses patients' audiometric thresholds to provide three gain and frequency-response targets, one for each of three input levels of low-level sounds (i.e., 40 dB SPL), moderate-level sounds (i.e., 65 dB SPL), and high-level sounds (i.e., 95 dB SPL) (Gitles & Niquette, 1995). The VIOLA is a component of the IHAFF suite that is a hearing aid fitting and verification protocol for nonlinear hearing aids consisting of three computer programs (Ricketts & Van Vliet, 1994). By using the warble-tone loudness data from two or more frequencies obtained with the Contour Test, VIOLA assists in the selection of the best gain, maximum output, and compression characteristics (Mueller, 1996; Ricketts & Van Vliet, 1994). Once the amplification characteristics have been selected, verification measures must be completed.

Mueller (1996) stated that verification involves repeating some previously made measures in the preselection and selection process plus some additional ones. The same self-assessment inventories can be administered to new hearing aid owners after a suitable period of acclimatization of six to eight weeks (Gatehouse, 1992; Gatehouse & Killion, 1993). Unfortunately, many rehabilitation-hospital patients will be discharged before acclimitization. Discharged patients may have to return to the inpatient facility for outpatient audiology services. Similarly, measures of aided audibility can be made in three ways by obtaining: (1) aided sound-field thresholds; (2) real-ear insertion responses (REIRs) and adding the insertion gain at each frequency to unaided pure-tone thresholds; and (3) real-ear aided responses (REARs) (using a speech-shaped, low-input signal) and comparing the findings to patients' unaided ear canal SPL thresholds (Mueller, 1996). Mueller (1996) stated that these measures should be completed at the patients' user volume-control-wheel setting and with the hearing aid not in compression. In addition to real-ear probe tube microphone measurements, other verification measures include loudness scaling, and aided speech measures (Mueller, 1996) not to be discussed here. Appendix VII-J contains the list of sources to obtain the necessary materials mentioned above.

New hearing aid users should be given instructions describing the care, maintenance, use, and appropriate expectations of hearing aids. Appendix VII-K contains the handouts for the hearing aid delivery. Each patient should be required to demonstrate basic hearing aid skills. In addition to basic insertion and removal and battery use, for example, patients are shown how to perform visual and listening checks on their hearing aids using appropriate equipment. Audiologists should carefully observe each patient and determine the level of assistance each will need to manage the hearing aids according to the categories described in the next section.

Some rehabilitation-hospital patients may be paralyzed from a stroke or head injury and may need to incorporate hearing aid use and maintenance into their OT and PT rehabilitation plans. Thus, members of these departments must have some knowledge of the sequence of motor skills involving insertion and removal, as well as care of hearing aids. Appendix VII-L contains an informational sheet for OT and PT staff that presents the sequence of steps for each of these tasks. Furthermore, partially paralyzed patients who are current CIC wearers or who are fit with these styles of hearing aids at the rehabilitation hospital may have difficulty inserting these aids into their ears. Appendix VII-M contains a visualization and imagery technique for CIC insertion by Danhauer and Danhauer (1997) that may be helpful for the OT and PT staff.

Hearing Aid Monitoring Program

All patients who own hearing aids and all those fit with aids during their hospital stay should participate in the hearing aid monitoring program upon consent. The program is to ensure that all patients' hearing aids function during their hospital stay. Hearing aids should undergo a complete visual and listening check each morning completed by the patient, a staff member, or both based on the level of assistance needed. The continuum for the degree of assistance required for maintaining hearing aids used in the "Guidelines for Audiology Service Delivery in Nursing Homes" (ASHA, 1997) is useful for rehabilitation hospitals even though reasons for patients' incapacitation may be different. There are four levels of assistance required, which are summarized below:

- **Independent:** Patients are responsible for care and maintenance of hearing aids on a day-to-day basis. Patients can manipulate hearing aid controls and change batteries on their own. A hearing aid check station is available on each floor for these residents to use each morning prior to beginning daily therapies. The hearing aid check station can be a desk or a table in a community use area. It should contain two hearing aid stethoscopes, two battery testers, two forced-air bulbs, numerous wax picks, alcohol pads, and so on. Patients are responsible for reporting any problems with, loss of, or damage to their hearing aids to the nursing staff or to the audiologist.
- **Partial Assistance:** Patients are responsible for care and maintenance of hearing aids on a day-to-day basis, although they need assistance with these tasks. Nursing staff works closely with OT and PT departments on patients' rehabilitation goals regarding self-care skills, including hearing aid care and maintenance. Patients are encouraged to complete tasks as independently as possible with assistance as needed from nursing staff.
- **Full Assistance:** Hearing aids are held by nursing staff, which is responsible for putting hearing aids on patients each morning. The nursing staff is responsible for routine visual and listening checks and for removing the batteries from the hearing aids before the patient goes to sleep at night. The nursing station on each floor should also have portable hearing aid check kits to take to the rooms of patients' with severe mobility problems. The nursing staff is responsible for reporting hearing aid loss or damage to the audiologist.
- **Supervised-Use:** Nursing staff takes total responsibility for hearing aids. Patients only use hearing aids in the presence of 1:1 supervision by staff or family members. The nursing staff is responsible for daily visual and listening checks and for removing hearing aid batteries after use. The nursing staff is responsible for reporting any hearing aid loss or damage to the audiologist.

Most likely, few if any rehabilitation-hospital patients will require supervised use of hearing aids. A hearing aid status list should be posted in each nursing unit for a quick and easy reference (ASHA, 1997). The hearing aid status list should contain the following information (ASHA, 1997):

- Patients' name and room number
- Hearing aid make, model, and serial number
- Ear(s) fitted
- Hearing aid battery size
- Level of assistance needed
- Any other comments (e.g., tasks to work on, volume-control wheel setting)

Appendix VII-N contains an example of a "Patients' Hearing Aid Status List." The list should be modified each week to account for patient turnover. Information appearing on this list should also be in patients' charts and in the audiologist's office. A copy of the "Chart Note: Patient's Hearing Aid Status" that goes into patients' charts appears in Appendix VII-O. In addition to the above information, this form contains information regarding patients' personal audiologist (if applicable), warranty, and billing information (e.g., audiology network). Furthermore, a hearing aid check sheet should be given to patients at the independent level of hearing aid care to document daily completion of this task. Appendix VII-P is an example of a "Hearing Aid Check Sheet." Keeping these sheets in a three-ring binder or on a clipboard near the hearing aid check station can decrease the likelihood of loss and neglect. Nurses will also use the sheets to check the hearing aids of patients needing assistance. The hearing aid check sheets will be used for important outcome measures that will be described in Chapter 9. Appendix VII-Q contains a daily log documenting hearing aid use for patients requiring supervised use of hearing aids (ASHA, 1997).

The audiologist should be contacted when basic troubleshooting cannot alleviate problems with hearing aids. Presently, e-mail is the quickest and most reliable way to contact contract-for-service audiologists, especially if their practices are several miles from the rehabilitation hospital. For example, phone messages can get buried on audiologists' desks and "snail mail" is far too inefficient. E-mail messages must contain pertinent information, such as the patients' name, make, model, serial number, ear fitted, the problem with the hearing aid, specific attempts at troubleshooting, and outcomes. This information allows the audiologist to analyze the facts and possibly solve the problem on the spot. If patients' hearing aids require repair, they should be sent to the manufacturer as soon as possible via express mail. In addition, loaner hearing aids or alternate communication devices such as ALDs should be provided to patients in the interim.

Assistive Listening Device Program and Communication Accessibility

Recall that the Americans with Disabilities Act (ADA) is a federal law (Public Law 101-336) passed in 1990 to provide protection from discrimination based on an individual's disability. There are five major sections or titles to this law: I. Employment, II. Public Services and Transportation, III. Public Accommodations and Commercial Facilities, IV. Telecommunications, and V. Miscellaneous Provisions. Audiologists managing support programs for rehabilitation-hospital patients with hearing impairment should acquire expertise in ADA regulations and assume a leadership role in the interpretation of this law with regard to communication accessibility. They should also become actively involved in the demonstration, evaluation, and installation of recommended equipment (Leavitt, 1996). Recommendations regarding ADA compliance made by a contract-for-service audiologist may not be well received by rehabilitation-hospital administrators. Again, discussing the presentation of recommendations for compliance with one's immediate supervisor may increase the likelihood for success.

Communication accessibility under the ADA is taking action to ensure that rehabilitation-hospital patients with communication disabilities have access to goods, services, and facilities and are not treated differently than any other patients (ASHA, 1995). The ADA requirements for effective communication are to provide any necessary auxiliary communication aids and services and to make aurally delivered information available to patients with hearing and/or speech impairments (ASHA, 1995). Specifically, the ADA (1990) requires providing:

- telecommunication devices for the deaf (TDD) and an accessible telephone or alternative service (if telephone service is provided to customers/patients on more than an incidental basis),
- means for two-way communication in emergency situations that does not require hearing or speech for communication,
- closed-caption decoders (if patient rooms are equipped with televisions),
- removing structural communication barriers (if they are inexpensively and easily removed),
- alternative service when barriers are not easily removed, and
- following accessibility standards (ASHA, 1995).

Audiologists can assist the rehabilitation hospital and ensure cost-effective ADA compliance by doing the following (ASHA, 1995):

- performing a facility-accessibility audit including identification of any barriers to communication;
- determining overall and individual auxiliary aids and services needs;
- developing a plan to remove barriers and obtain assistive devices;
- performing an ongoing audit and maintenance of accessibility features;
- modifying discriminatory policies, practices, and procedures; and
- consulting and obtaining assistance from rehabilitation professionals, disability organizations, consumers, and federal agencies.

Appendix VII-R contains a "Facility Communication Accessibility Checklist" that can assist audiologists in determining which areas need improvement. One of the most important tasks is to determine needs in auxiliary aids and services. Necessary auxiliary communication aids and services are determined from a consideration of the expressed preference of the individual with the disability, and the level and type of communication exchange (ASHA, 1995). Selection of appropriate aids and services (low-tech and high-tech) is based on facility resources and patients' communication needs (ASHA, 1995). Examples of communication aids and services are presented in Table 7–4 (ASHA, 1995).

Specifically, the types of auxiliary aids ordered for hospitals have included: text telephones for emergency rooms and receptionists; phone amplifiers; door-knock alerting devices; vibrating alarm clocks; telecaption decoders; personal hardwire amplification systems; and FM, infrared, or loop systems for conference rooms (Leavitt, 1996). Selection of appropriate assistive technology for patients involves three steps (Rothstein & Everson, 1994):

- conducting a functional assessment of the patients' abilities (physical/cognitive abilities and personal preferences),
- evaluating the patients' environment (tasks wanted or needed to be performed), and
- searching for proper technologies to match the circumstances.

Appendix VII-S contains a "Listening Questionnaire" (Sandridge, 1995) that can assist in determining patients' needs for auxiliary aids

Table 7–4. Examples of communication aids and services.

In Assembly Areas, Meetings, and Conversations

- Assistive listening devices and systems (ALDs)
- Communication boards (word, symbols)
- Qualified interpreters (oral, cued speech, and sign language)
- Real-time captioning
- Written communication exchange and transcripts
- Computer-assisted note taking
- Lighting on speaker's face
- Preferential seating for good listening and viewing position
- Electrical outlet near accessible seating
- Videotext displays

In Telecommunications

- Hearing aid compatible telephones
- Volume-control telephone handsets
- Amplified telephone mouthpieces
- Telecommunication device for the deaf (TDD) or text telephone
- Facsimile machines that use visual symbols
- Computer/modem
- Interactive computer software with videotext
- TDD/telephone relay systems

In Buildings

- Alerting, signaling, warning, and announcement systems using amplified auditory signals
- Visual signals (flashing strobes)
- Vibrotactile (touch) devices
- Videotext displays

In Prepared (non-live) Materials

- Written materials in alternate formats (e.g., symbols, pictures)
- Aurally delivered materials in alternate formats (e.g., captioned videotapes, written transcript, sign interpreter)
- Notification of accessibility options (e.g., alternative formats)

Source: From "Communication and the ADA (Effective Communication and Accessibility)," by American Speech-Language-Hearing Association, 1995, p. 2. Rockville, MD: Author. Reprinted with permission.

and services. In addition, Appendix VII-T contains "Considerations for Purchasing Auxiliary Devices" (Rothstein & Everson, 1994). Once equipment has been purchased, appropriate staff members should be contacted for inservice training on the equipment. ALDs do not have to be expensive. Figure 7–3 shows a rehabilitation-hospital patient who successfully uses an inexpensive ALD.

Leavitt (1996) suggested that the audiologist should oversee not only equipment selection, but installation and instruction on the proper operation of the systems especially with regard to interfacing devices for ALDs such as neckloops, silhouette conductors, audio-input cords, and so on. Leavitt (1996) also recommended that the audiologist oversee the installation of and provide training in the use of the hospitals' text telephones, telecaption decoders, and related devices. Furthermore, even the most well-designed ALD program can falter if the audiologist is not available to turn on devices, replace batteries, assist patients with telephone use, and so on. Once again, the use of multiskilled audiologic support personnel can be invaluable here.

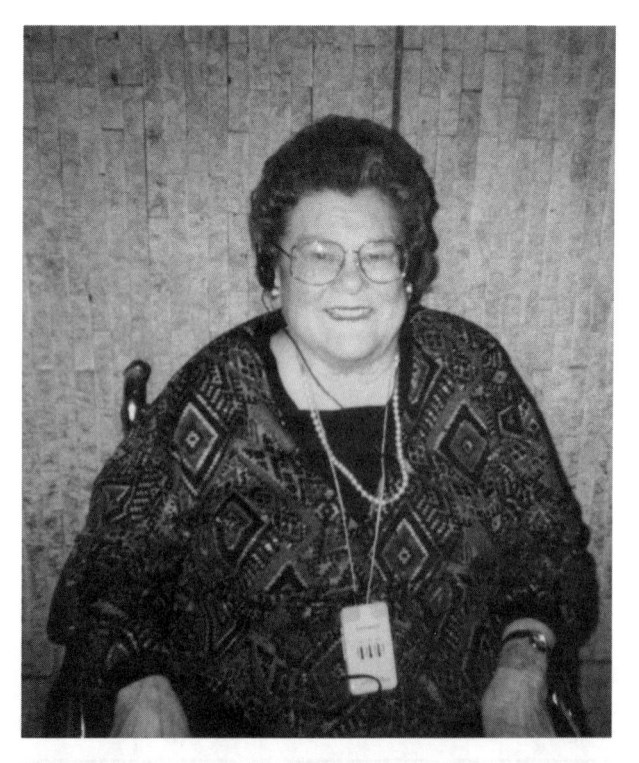

Figure 7–3. Rehabilitation-hospital patient successfully using an inexpensive assistive listening device.

Short-Term Aural Rehabilitation

The average length of stay at rehabilitation hospitals rarely exceeds 2 months. Thus, patients with hearing impairment frequently need short-term aural rehabilitation focusing on effective communication and speechreading that can be provided by speech-language pathologists or the audiologist. Patients and their families may need some suggestions for effective communication strategies, such as the use of "clear speech" (Schum, 1997). Clear speech has been found to be effective in enhancing speech intelligibility. Appendix VII-U is a handout that can be given to patients and their families (Abel, 1998). They may also be counseled on the benefits of speechreading to facilitate communication. Appendix VII-V contains appropriate handouts for this purpose. Aural rehabilitation can continue on an outpatient basis for discharged patients if needed.

SUMMARY

This chapter has discussed the establishment of support programs for patients with hearing impairment in rehabilitation hospitals. Traumatically injured adults are transferred from acute-care to rehabilitation hospitals. It is often at this point that hearing loss can be identified, diagnosed, and managed for the first time. Although rehabilitation-hospital patients' residency is relatively short, their hearing health-care needs may be met through support programs so they can optimally benefit from their intervention programs. Service delivery in the rehabilitation industry and components of support programs were discussed, and useful information has been provided.

REFERENCES

Abel, S. H. (1998). Clear speech handout. Auburn, AL: Author.

American Academy of Audiology. (1997). Position statement and guidelines of the consensus panel on support personnel in audiology. *Audiology Today, 9*(3), 27–28.

American Speech-Language-Hearing Association. (1995). Communication and the ADA (effective communication and accessibility). Rockville, MD: Author

American Speech-Language-Hearing Association. (1997, Spring). Guidelines for audiology service delivery in nursing homes. *Asha, 39*(Suppl. 17), 15–29.

Americans with Disabilities Act of 1990, Public Law 101–336, 42, U.S.C. 12101 *et seq*: *U.S. Statutes at Large, 104*, 327–378 (1991).

Arlinger, S., Billermark, E., Oberg, M., Lunner, T., & Hellgren, J. (1998). Clinical trial of a digital hearing aid. *Scandinavian Audiology, 27*(1), 51–61.

Bess, F. H. (1995). Page ten: Applications of the hearing handicap inventory for the elderly—screening version (HHIE-S). *The Hearing Journal, 48*(6), 10, 51–55.

Byrne, D., & Dillon, H. (1986). The National Acoustic Laboratories' (NAL) new procedure for selecting gain and frequency response of a hearing aid. *Ear and Hearing, 7*, 257–265.

Chartrand, M. S. (1998). Growing your practice/business with strategic philanthropy. *The Hearing Review, 5*(7), 35–36.

Cherry, R., & Rubenstein, A. (1988). Speechreading instruction for adults: Issues and approaches. *The Volta Review, 90*(5), 289–306.

Cornelisse, L. E., Seewald, R. C., & Jamieson, D. G. (1994). Wide-dynamic-range compression hearing aids: The DSL[i/o] approach. *The Hearing Journal, 47*(10), 23–26.

Cox, R. M. (1995). Page ten: Using loudness data for hearing aid selection: The IHAFF approach. *The Hearing Journal, 48*(2), 10, 39–41, 43–44.

Cox, R. M., & Alexander, G. C. (1995). The abbreviated profile of hearing aid benefit. *Ear and Hearing, 16*, 176–183.

Crandell, C. C. (1998). Hearing aids: Their effects on functional health status. *The Hearing Journal, 51*(2), 22, 24, 27–28, 30, 32.

Danhauer, J. L. (1997). How otoacoustic emissions can change your audiology practice. *The Hearing Journal, 50*(4), 62, 64, 66, 68–69.

Danhauer, J. L., & Danhauer, K. J. (1997). Solving CIC hearing aid insertion and comfort problems. In M. Chasin (Ed.), *CIC handbook* (pp. 169–191). San Diego, CA: Singular Publishing Group.

Dillon, H., James, A., & Ginis, J. (1997). Client oriented scale of improvement (COSI) and its relationship to several other measures of benefit and satisfaction provided by hearing aids. *Journal of the American Academy of Audiology, 8*, 27–43.

Fabry, D. A. (1996). Page ten: Clinical applications of multimemory hearing aids. *The Hearing Journal, 49*(8), 10, 53.

Foto, M. (1996). Multiskilling: Who, how, when, and why? *The American Journal of Occupational Therapy, 50*, 1.

Garstecki, D. C., & Erler, S. F. (1998). Hearing loss, control, and demographic factors influencing hearing aid use among older adults. *Journal of Speech, Language, and Hearing Research, 41*, 527–537.

Gatehouse, S. (1992). The time course and magnitude of peripheral acclimatization to frequency responses: Evidence from monaural fitting of hearing aids. *Journal of the Acoustical Society of America, 92*, 1258–1268.

Gatehouse, S., & Killion, M. C. (1993). HABRAT: Hearing aid brain rewiring accommodation time. *Hearing Instruments, 44*(10), 29–30, 32.

Gitles, T. C., & Niquette, P. T. (1995). Fig 6 in ten. *The Hearing Review, 2*(10), 28, 30.

Griffin, D. J., Clark-Lewis, S., & Johnson, C. (1997). Rehabilitating patients with hearing impairments. *Outcomes: A Publication of HealthSouth Corporation, 2*(4), 20–21.

Hawkins, D. B., Walden, B. E., Montgomery, A., & Prosek, R. A. (1987). Description and validation of an LDL procedure designed to select SSPL-90. *Ear and Hearing, 8*, 162–169.

HealthSouth. (1998). Available Internet: www.healthsouth.com.

Holmes, A. E. (1995). Hearing aids and the older adult. In P. B. Kricos & S. A. Lesner (Eds.), *Hearing care for the older adult: Audiologic rehabilitation* (pp. 59–74). Boston, MA: Butterworth-Heinemann.

Humes, L. E. (1991). Understanding the speech problems of the hearing impaired. *Journal of the American Academy of Audiology, 2*, 59–69.

Johnson, C. E., Clark-Lewis, S., & Griffin, D. (1998). Experience, attitudes, and competencies of audiologic support personnel in a rehabilitation hospital. *American Journal of Audiology: A Journal of Clinical Practice, 7*(2), 26–31.

Independent Hearing Aid Fitting Forum (IHAFF). (1994). *The unveiling of a comprehensive hearing aid fitting protocol for the 21st century.* Presented at the Jackson Hole Rendezvous, Jackson Hole, WY.

Killion, M. C., & Fikret-Pasa, S. (1993). The three types of sensorineural hearing loss: Loudness and intelligibility considerations. *The Hearing Journal, 46*(11), 31–36.

Killion, M. C., Mueller, H. G., Pavlovic, C. V., & Humes, L. E. (1993). A is for audibility. *The Hearing Journal, 46*(4), 15.

Leavitt, R. (1996). Working together to facilitate communication for hearing-impaired people in hospitals. *The Hearing Review, 3*(6), 16, 19–20.

Mueller, H. G. (1996). Hearing aids and people: Strategies for a successful match. *The Hearing Journal, 49*(4), 13–15, 19, 22–23, 26–28.

Mueller, H. G., & Killion, M. C. (1990). An easy method for calculating the articulation index. *The Hearing Journal, 43*(9), 14–17.

Newman, C. W., Weinstein, B. E., Jacobson, G. P., & Hug, G. A. (1991). Test-retest reliability of the Hearing Handicap Inventory for Adults. *Ear and Hearing, 12*, 355–357.

Pavlovic, C. V. (1991). Speech recognition and five articulation indexes. *Hearing Instruments, 42*(9), 20–24.

Ricketts, T. A., & Van Vliet, D. (1994). Updating our fitting strategies given new technology. *American Journal of Audiology: A Journal of Clinical Practice, 5*(2), 29–35.

Roeser, R. J. (1995). Screening for hearing loss and middle ear disorders in the schools. In R. J. Roeser

& M. P. Downs (Eds.), *Auditory disorders in school children: The law, identification, and remediation* (3rd ed., pp. 76–100). New York: Thieme.

Rothstein, R., &, Everson, J. M. (1994). Assistive technology for individuals with sensory impairments. In F. F. Flippo, K. J. Inge, & J. M. Barcus (Eds.), *Assistive technology: A resource for school, work, and community* (pp. 105–132). Baltimore, MD: Paul H. Brookes.

Sandridge, S. A. (1995). Beyond hearing aids: Use of auxiliary aids. In P. B. Kricos & S. A. Lesner (Eds.), *Hearing care for the older adult: Audiologic rehabilitation* (pp. 127–166). Boston, MA: Butterworth-Heinemann.

Schum, D. J. (1997). Beyond hearing aids: Clear speech training as an intervention strategy. *The Hearing Journal, 50*(10), 36–38, 40.

Tye-Murray, N. (1998). *Foundations of aural rehabilitation: Children, adults, and their family members.* San Diego, CA: Singular Publishing Group.

Ventry, I. M., & Weinstein, B. E. (1982). The hearing inventory for the elderly: A new tool. *Ear and Hearing, 3,* 128–134.

Walker, G., & Dillon, H. (1982). *Compression in hearing aids: An analysis, a review, and some recommendations (NAL report 90).* Sydney: Australian Government Printing Service.

Wayner, D., & Abrahamson, J. (1996). How to gain a larger slice of the "communication pie." *The Hearing Review, 3*(9), 32–34.

APPENDIX VII-A

Informed Consent for Participation in Support Program

XYZ REHABILITATION HOSPITAL
On the road to your recovery...

INFORMED CONSENT FOR PARTICIPATION IN THE HEARING SUPPORT PROGRAM

XYZ Rehabilitation Hospital and its staff are dedicated to positive patient outcomes. Toward this goal, we have established a Hearing Support Program for patients with hearing impairment. The program was established to facilitate patients' communication during their stay at our facility. Below are the various components of the program and their contribution to meeting the communication needs of our patients. The program is offered to you at no cost with the exception of the purchase of hearing aids. Please read each component and circle "yes" if you consent to participating in each component, "no" if you do not, and then sign and date this form in the spaces provided below.

- Yes No **Staff Notification:** Staff are notified of patients' hearing loss by signs placed over beds indicating types of assistance needed and by color codes used in patients' charts. Staff notification is critical to ensure that patient communication is optimized for rehabilitation.

- Yes No **Hearing Aid Monitoring:** Patients' hearing aids undergo a daily visual and listening check by our staff. It is important for patients' hearing aids to be functioning for maximum benefit from rehabilitation therapies.

- Yes No **Audiologic Services:** As part of patients' assessment, all patients are screened for hearing function. Those failing the screening are scheduled for complete audiologic evaluations. Aural rehabilitation is provided for patients with hearing loss, which includes hearing aid evaluations, hearing aid deliveries, hearing aid orientation, communication tips, and speechreading.

- Yes No **Assistive Listening Device Program:** Assistive listening devices that aid patients in communicating with staff, on the telephone, and in listening to television are available for patient use during their hospital stay.

_____   _____
Patient Signature   Date

_____   _____
Witness Signature   Date

APPENDIX VII-B

Notification of Patient Participation in Hearing Support Program

XYZ REHABILITATION HOSPITAL
On the road to your recovery...

HEARING SUPPORT PROGRAM

Hearing aids

Assistance needed:

- Securing of aid
- Insertion/removal
- Battery manipulation
- Hearing aid check

XYZ REHABILITATION HOSPITAL
On the road to your recovery...

HEARING SUPPORT PROGRAM

Assistive listening devices used during all waking hours

APPENDIX VII-C

Otoacoustic Emissions Fact Sheet[1]

XYZ REHABILITATION HOSPITAL

On the road to your recovery...

Otoacoustic Emissions Fact Sheet

➢ ***Otoacoustic emissions (OAEs) are cost-efficient, nonbehavioral, and noninvasive measures*** of inner ear, outer hair cell function, and are used for hearing screenings and numerous innovative audiologic applications for patients of all ages and cognitive abilities.

➢ ***OAEs are extremely valid and reliable screening measures*** for correctly identifying patients with hearing loss and dismissing those with normal hearing.

➢ ***There are two types of OAEs,*** distortion product otoacoustic emissions (DPOAE) and transient evoked otoacoustic emissions (TEOAE). Both types require computer equipment, either laptop or desktop models. Some hand-held screeners are even available. Costs for equipment range from $4,500 to $12,000, not including the cost of a suitable computer and printer. Equipment can be rented for as low as $200 a month.

➢ ***OAEs can be tested in both ears in less than five minutes.*** Even less time is needed for screening; that is a vast improvement over traditional pure-tone hearing screenings.

➢ ***Audiologic support personnel can be trained to test for OAEs,*** freeing the audiologists' valuable time to attend to other aspects of service delivery.

➢ ***OAEs increase patient referrals*** from hospitals, a wide variety of physicians, industry, attorneys, insurance companies, and "special program" schools.

➢ ***OAE tests are attractive measures to managed care*** because at a cost of $75, they may provide enough information to eliminate the need for more costly testing, such as a $150 auditory brainstem response (ABR) test or a $3,000 magnetic resonance imaging test (MRI).

➢ ***Reimbursement is often available,*** now that there are new OAE RVS codes for screening (92587) and in-depth diagnostics (92588).

---

[1]Adapted from "How Otoacoustic Emissions Testing Can Change Your Audiology Practice," by J. L. Danhauer, 1997, *The Hearing Journal, 50*(4), 62–69.

APPENDIX VII-D

Otoacoustic Emissions Test Equipment Manufacturers

BIO-LOGIC SYSTEMS CORPORATION
Mundelein, IL
(847) 949-5200

DANPLEX-HORTMANN, INCORPORATED
Dripping Springs, TX
(512) 858-1781

ELECTRO ACOUSTIC COMPANY,
INCORPORATED
San Jose, CA
(408) 445-3292

ETYMOTIC RESEARCH
Elk Grove Village, IL
(847) 228-0006

GRASON ASSOCIATES
Berlin, MA
(603) 672-0470

INTELLIGENT HEARING SYSTEMS
CORPORATION
Miami, FL
(305) 668-6102

MADSEN ELECTRONICS INCORPORATED
Minnetonka, MN
(612) 930-0804

OTODYNAMICS
Hatfied, England
(800) 659-7776

SONAMED CORPORATION
Waltham, MA
(781) 899-6499

STARKEY CALIFORNIA
Anaheim, CA
(714) 826-0824

WELCH ALLYN/GSI
Milford, NH
(603) 672-0470

APPENDIX VII-E

Inservice on Otoacoustic Emissions (OAEs) for Audiologic Support Personnel

Behavioral Objectives

Through participation in this inservice, attendees will be able to:
- Define otoacoustic emissions
- Describe the purpose of the screening program
- Understand the basic principles in testing
- Describe how OAE testing equipment works
- Describe anatomic regions involved in OAE measurement
- Describe preparation for OAE recording, protocols, troubleshooting procedures, and program documentation
- Demonstrate OAE measurement preparation, protocol, and troubleshooting of equipment

Suggested Time Allotment

About 3 hours
- Introduction (10 minutes)
- Basic principles and OAE testing equipment (30 minutes)
- Preparation for OAE recording, protocol, troubleshooting procedures, and program documentation (45 minutes)
- Break (5 minutes)
- Supervised practicum (1 hour, 10 minutes)
- Wrap-up: questions and answers (10 minutes)
- Quiz (10 minutes)

Format

Combination Informational and Skill-Based

Suggested Materials:

- Overhead projector
- OAE equipment and necessary accessories
- Otoscopes
- Appropriate handouts
- Appropriate overheads

Selected Participant Activities

- Complete otoscopy and OAE protocol on five peers.

HANDOUTS

BASICS OF OTOACOUSTIC EMISSIONS SCREENING PROGRAM
(Materials adapted from Hall & Mueller, 1997)

- **What are otoacoustic emissions (OAEs)?**

Otoacoustic emissions are little sounds that healthy hair cells in the inner ear produce either on their own or in response to sounds put into the ear. The ear's ability to make these little sounds is affected by mild amounts of hearing loss. OAE measurement is an ideal tool to use for hearing screening programs.

- **What is the purpose of the hearing screening program?**

The purpose of the hearing screening program is to identify patients with a hearing loss and to dismiss those with normal hearing.

- **What are the basic principles involved in OAE testing?**

In OAE testing, we present sounds of varying frequencies and intensities into the ear and measure the response from the inner ear hair cells that come back out. If there is an absence of such sounds, then the person probably has a hearing loss or other condition that precludes measurement of OAEs.

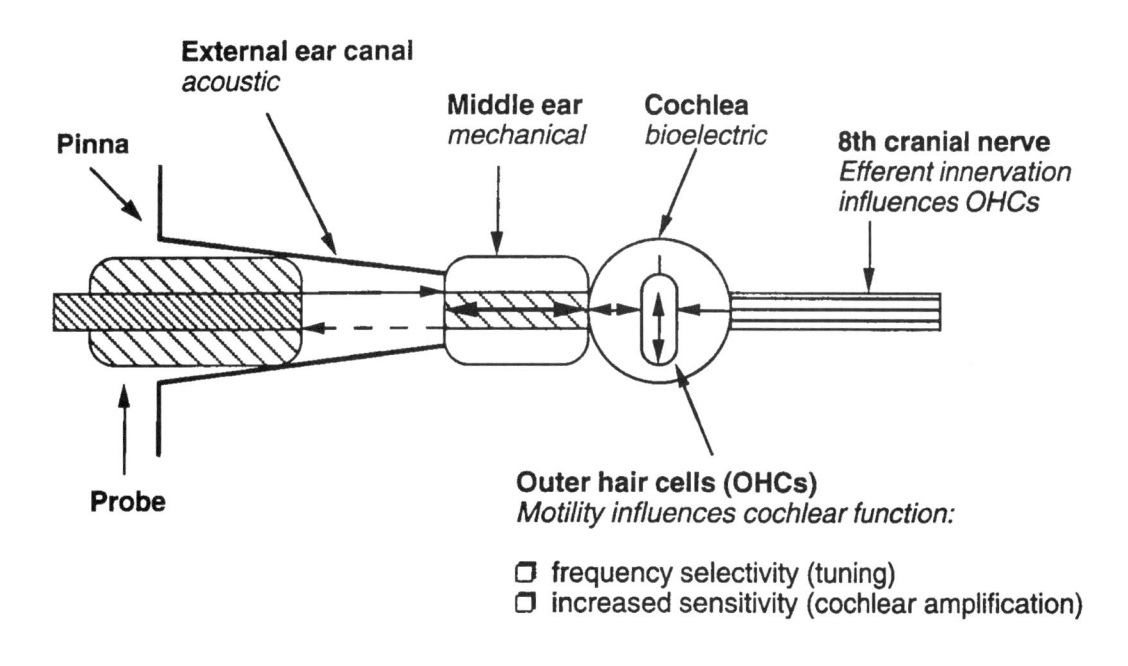

External ear canal
acoustic

Middle ear
mechanical

Cochlea
bioelectric

Pinna

8th cranial nerve
Efferent innervation influences OHCs

Probe

Outer hair cells (OHCs)
Motility influences cochlear function:

- frequency selectivity (tuning)
- increased sensitivity (cochlear amplification)

Inward propagation: acoustic - mechanical - bioelectric

Outward propagation: bioelectric - mechanical - acoustic

232 GUIDEBOOK FOR SUPPORT PROGRAMS IN AURAL REHABILITATION

■ How does the equipment work and what anatomical regions are involved?

A probe tip is placed snugly into the ear canal. The probe tip has a loudspeaker in it that will present two tones (DPOAEs) or a series of clicks (TEOAEs) to the ear that will go to the eardrum, travel through the middle ear, into the cochlea in the inner ear, and to the outer hair cells. If the outer hair cells are healthy, they will respond by emitting tiny sounds that will travel backward through the middle ear and into the ear canal so that a tiny microphone can pick them up and send them to the computer. The computer then analyzes those sounds to determine the functioning of the outer hair cells.

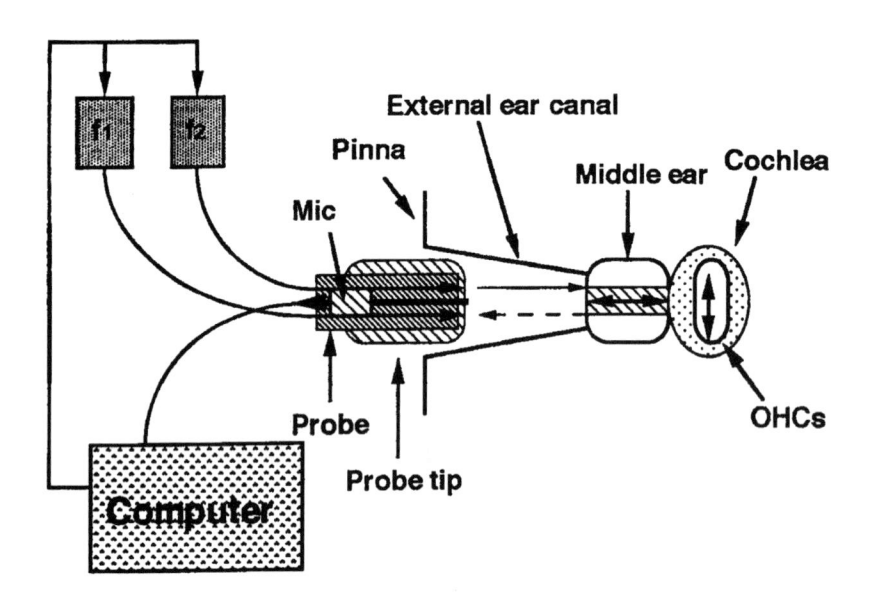

- **What preparations are involved for OAE recording?**

  ⇒ Turn on the computer.
  ⇒ Select the desired test protocol.
  ⇒ Select the appropriate OAE normative database for display on your screen. Norms have been established for patients based on age.
  ⇒ Instruct the patient to sit quietly.
  ⇒ Perform an otoscopic examination on each ear canal.
  ⇒ Locate the patient as far away from the OAE equipment and any other sources of noise as possible.
  ⇒ Select the proper tip size.
  ⇒ Fit the probe tip snugly and deeply into the external ear canal.
  ⇒ Verify that the OAE stimulus level, intensity, and spectrum are appropriate.
  ⇒ Perform a probe fit routine as recommended by the manufacturer.

- **What is a protocol and which will be used?**

  A protocol is a description of how something will be done. Our hospital has selected a protocol based on careful study of available research. The important parts of the protocol performed by audiologic support personnel are:

  ⇒ make the appropriate preparations described above,
  ⇒ screen both ears, and
  ⇒ save results on the computer and printout a hard copy for placement into the folder to be sent to the audiologist.

- **What happens if the equipment doesn't work?**

  ⇒ No sound?

  ➢ Check to make sure that the power for the external sound box is on.
  ➢ Check that all tubes and cords leading to and from the computer to the probe are appropriate and securely connected.

  ⇒ Very soft sound (as shown on the computer screen)?

  ➢ Check to make sure that you have the correct sound level by looking on the screen.
  ➢ Perform a listening check to determine if a sound is present at the level of the ear.
  ➢ Make sure that the probe is fit properly in the ear.
  ➢ Inspect probe ports and tubes for debris, such as earwax.
  ➢ Double check to see that the patient's ear canal is not full of earwax.

  ⇒ High noise levels?

  ➢ Is the patient quiet, not moving, not chewing, etc.?
  ➢ Is the door to the test room open?
  ➢ Is the room noisier than average?
  ➢ Is the test ear away from the OAE unit and other sources of sound in the test room?
  ➢ If you try all of these steps and it is still too noisy, contact the managing audiologist.

INTRUCTOR OVERHEADS

BASICS OF THE OTOACOUSTIC EMISSION SCREENING PROGRAM

- What are OTOACOUSTIC EMISSIONS (OAEs)?

- What is the PURPOSE of the hearing screening program?

- What are the BASIC PRINCIPLES involved in OAE testing?

- How does the EQUIPMENT WORK and what ANATOMICAL REGIONS are involved?

- What PREPARATIONS are involved for OAE recording?

- What is a test PROTOCOL and which one will be used?

- What happens when the equipment DOESN'T WORK?

    ⇒ No sound?
    ⇒ Very soft sound?
    ⇒ High noise levels?

BASIC PRINCIPLES OF OAEs

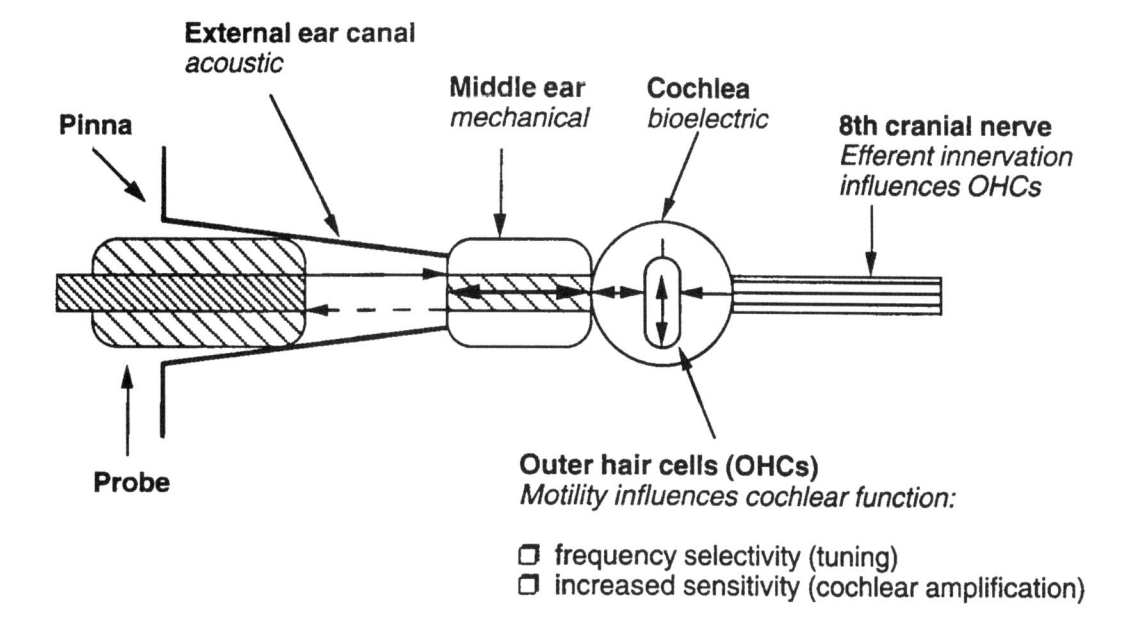

Pinna

External ear canal
acoustic

Middle ear
mechanical

Cochlea
bioelectric

8th cranial nerve
Efferent innervation influences OHCs

Probe

Outer hair cells (OHCs)
Motility influences cochlear function:

- frequency selectivity (tuning)
- increased sensitivity (cochlear amplification)

Inward propagation: acoustic - mechanical - bioelectric

Outward propagation: bioelectric - mechanical - acoustic

How does the EQUIPMENT WORK and what ANATOMICAL REGIONS are involved?

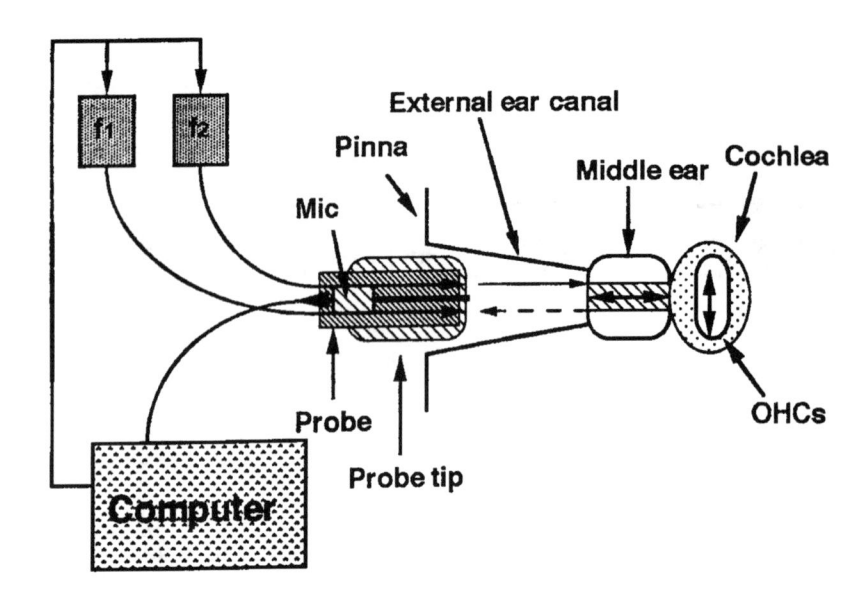

EQUIPMENT PREPARATIONS

⇒ **Turn on the computer.**

⇒ **Select the desired test protocol.**

⇒ **Select the appropriate OAE normative data base for display on your screen.**

⇒ **Instruct the patient.**

⇒ **Perform an otoscopic examination on each ear canal.**

⇒ **Locate the patient as far away from the OAE equipment and any other sources of noise as possible.**

⇒ **Select the proper tip size.**

⇒ **Fit the probe tip snugly and deeply into the external ear canal.**

⇒ **Make sure that the OAE stimulus level, intensity, and spectrum are appropriate.**

What happens if the equipment DOESN'T WORK?

⇒ **No sound?**

➢ Check to make sure that the power for the external sound box is on.
➢ Check that all tubes and cords leading to and from the computer and the probe are appropriate and securely connected.

⇒ **Very soft sound (as shown on the computer screen)?**

➢ Check to make sure that you have the correct sound level by looking on the screen.
➢ Perform a listening check to determine if a sound is present at the level of the ear.
➢ Make sure that the probe is fit properly in the ear.
➢ Inspect probe ports and tubes for debris, such as earwax.
➢ Double check to see that the patient's ear canal is not full of earwax.

⇒ **High noise levels?**

➢ Is the patient quiet, not moving, not chewing, etc.?
➢ Is the door to the test room open?
➢ Is the room noisier than average?
➢ Is the test ear away from the OAE unit and other sources of sound in the test room?
➢ If you try all of these steps and it is still too noisy, contact the managing audiologist.

APPENDIX VII-F

Hearing Screening Form

XYZ REHABILITATION HOSPITAL

On the road to your recovery...

HEARING SCREENING FORM

Name:_____ Date:_____

Chart No.:_____ Examiner:_____

Room No:_____

Circle one: Pass   Fail

Ear	250	500	1000	2000	4000	8000
Right						
Left						

APPENDIX VII-G

Hearing Handicap Inventory for the Elderly—Screening[1]

XYZ REHABILITATION HOSPITAL

On the road to your recovery...

Name:_____   Date:_____

Chart No.:_____   Score:_____

Room No:_____   Circle one: Pass   Fail

HEARING HANDICAP INVENTORY FOR THE ELDERLY—SCREENING

Please answer "yes," "no," or "sometimes" to each of the following items. Do not skip a question if you avoid a situation because of a hearing problem. If you wear a hearing aid, please answer the way you hear without the hearing aid.

Item	Yes (4)	No (0)	Sometimes (2)
E-1. Does a hearing problem cause you to feel embarrassed when you meet new people?	☐	☐	☐
E-2. Does a hearing problem cause you to feel frustrated when talking to members of your family?	☐	☐	☐
S-3. Do you have difficulty hearing when someone speaks in a whisper?	☐	☐	☐
E-4. Do you feel handicapped by a hearing problem?	☐	☐	☐
S-5. Does a hearing problem cause you difficulty when visiting friends, relatives, or neighbors?	☐	☐	☐
S-6. Does a hearing problem cause you to attend religious services less often than you would like?	☐	☐	☐
E-7. Does a hearing problem cause you to have arguments with family members?	☐	☐	☐
S-8. Does a hearing problem cause you difficulty when listening to a TV or radio?	☐	☐	☐
E-9. Do you feel that any difficulty with your hearing limits or hampers your personal or social life?	☐	☐	☐
S-10. Does a hearing problem cause you difficulty when in a restaurant with relatives or friends?	☐	☐	☐

[1]From "The Hearing Inventory for the Elderly: A New Tool," by I. Ventry and B. Weinstein, 1982, *Ear and Hearing, 3*, 128–134. Reprinted with permission.

APPENDIX VII-H

Hearing Handicap Inventory for Adults—Screening[1]

XYZ REHABILITATION HOSPITAL
On the road to your recovery...

Name:_____   Date:_____

Chart No.:_____   Score:_____

Room No:_____   Circle one: Pass   Fail

HEARING HANDICAP INVENTORY FOR ADULTS—SCREENING

Please answer "yes," "no," or "sometimes" to each of the following items. Do not skip a question if you avoid a situation because of a hearing problem. If you wear a hearing aid, please answer the way you hear without the hearing aid.

Item	Yes (4)	No (0)	Sometimes (2)
E-1. Does a hearing problem cause you to feel embarrassed when meeting new people?	☐	☐	☐
E-2. Does a hearing problem cause you to feel frustrated when talking to members of your family?	☐	☐	☐
S-3. Does a hearing problem cause you difficulty hearing/understanding coworkers, clients, or customers?	☐	☐	☐
E-4. Do you feel handicapped by a hearing problem?	☐	☐	☐
S-5. Does a hearing problem cause you difficulty when visiting friends, relatives, or neighbors?	☐	☐	☐
S-6. Does a hearing problem cause difficulty in the movies or theater?	☐	☐	☐
E-7. Does a hearing problem cause you to have arguments with family members?	☐	☐	☐
S-8. Does a hearing problem cause you difficulty when listening to a TV or radio?	☐	☐	☐
E-9. Do you feel that any difficulty with your hearing limits or hampers your personal or social life?	☐	☐	☐
S-10. Does a hearing problem cause you difficulty when in a meeting or conference?	☐	☐	☐

[1]From "Test-Retest Reliability of the Hearing Handicap Inventory for Adults," by C. W. Newman, B. E. Weinstein, G. P. Jacobson, and G. A. Hug, 1991, *Ear and Hearing, 12,* 355–357. Reprinted with permission.

APPENDIX VII-I

Letter to Patient and Family Regarding Hearing Screening Results

XYZ REHABILITATION HOSPITAL
On the road to your recovery...

June 28, 1999

Ima Patient & Family
Room 1111
XYZ Rehabilitation Hospital
Quality of Life City, CA 94545

Dear Ms. Patient & Family,

As part of its comprehensive approach to rehabilitation, XYZ Rehabilitation Hospital screens the hearing of all patients upon admission. The purpose of our hearing screening program is to identify patients who may have a hearing loss and need an audiologic evaluation. The results of your hearing screening indicate that a hearing loss may be present. We believe that hearing loss can negatively affect the rehabilitation process. I will be contacting you shortly to discuss the possibility of scheduling the evaluation. If you have any questions, please feel to call me at 555-1122.

Sincerely,

Starr Audiologist, Ph.D.
Certificate of Clinical Competence in Audiology
Fellow, American Academy of Audiology
Audiologist, XYZ Rehabilitation Hospital

APPENDIX VII-J

Hearing Aid Fitting Shopping List[1]

Speech in Noise (SIN) Test
Auditec of St. Louis
2515 S. Big Bend
St. Louis, MO 63143-2105

Hearing in Noise Test (HINT)
Starkey Laboratories, Inc.
Marketing Services
6700 Washington Ave. S
Eden Prairie, MN 55344

Dichotic Sentence Identification (DSI) Test
Auditec of St. Louis
2515 S. Big Bend
St. Louis, MO 63143-2105

3A Insert Earphones
Loretah Rowland
Cabot Safety Corporation
Auditory Systems Division
5407 West 79th St.
Indianapolis, IN 46268
(800) 624-5955
FAX (317) 692-3112

NAL Software
Denis Byrne
National Acoustics Laboratories
126 Greville St.
Chatswood, NSW 2067
Australia

FIG6 Software
Toni Gitles
Etymotic Research
61 Martin Lane
Elk Grove Village, IL 60007
(847) 228-0006

DSL 4.0 Software
Richard Seewald
Hearing Health Care Research
University of Western Ontario
Communication Disorders
London, Ontario N6G 1-H1 Canada
(519) 661-3901

Independent Hearing Aid Fitting Forum (IHAFF) Software
Dennis Van Vliet
Suite 130
17021 Yorba Linda Blvd.
Yorba Linda, CA 92686-3742
(714) 579-0717

Abbreviated Profile of Hearing Aid Benefit (APHAB) Software
Robyn Cox
University of Memphis
807 Jefferson Ave.
Memphis, TN 38105-5094

Hearing Handicap Inventory for the Elderly (HHIE)
Barbara Weinstein
Department of Speech and Theater
Bedford Park Blvd. West
Lehman College
Bronx, NY 10468-1589
(718) 960-8138

Hearing Aid Satisfaction Survey
Sergei Kochkin
1151 Maplewood Dr.
Itasca, IL 60143
(847) 250-5100

Count-The-Dot-Audiogram
The Hearing Journal
Volume 45, No. 9 (page 15)

---

[1]From "Hearing Aids and People: Strategies for a Successful Match," by H. G. Mueller, 1996, p. 28. *The Hearing Journal*, 49(4), 13–28. Reprinted with permission.

APPENDIX VII-K

Handouts for the Hearing Aid Delivery
XYZ REHABILITATION HOSPITAL
On the road to your recovery...

Do's and Don'ts for Maintaining Your Hearing Aid[1]

DO:

- Regularly remove earwax from the earmold or sound outlet of the hearing aids, using a wax removal brush or a wax loop remover.
- Routinely wipe the hearing aids with a clean, dry tissue.
- Open the battery case every night.
- Store hearing aids in your carrying case with a dry-pac and put in a safe place.
- Ensure your hands are clean and dry and free of creams before handling the hearing aids.
- Keep the hearing aids away from moisture.
- Carry a spare fresh battery with you when you are out.
- Check your batteries and replace when necessary.
- Turn off the hearing aid before taking it out of your ear to prevent feedback.
- Keep hearing aids away from dogs and cats.
- Remove your hearing aids when you are perspiring, such as on a very hot day or during strenuous exercise.
- Clean the earmolds and tubing on a weekly basis.

DON'T:

- Leave a dead battery in the battery drawer.
- Apply hair spray or face powder when wearing hearing aids.
- Bathe, shower, walk in the rain, or swim when wearing hearing aids.
- Take your hearing aids out while standing on a hard surface such as a tile floor; hearing aids are fragile and may break if dropped.
- Wear your hearing aids when using a hair dryer.
- Discard batteries in a place that is accessible to children or pets.
- Force the battery compartment closed. If it won't close, recheck the battery position or try another battery.

---

[1]Adapted from *Foundations of Aural Rehabilitation: Children, Adults, and Their Family Members*, by N. Tye-Murray, 1998. San Diego, CA: Singular Publishing Group.

XYZ REHABILITATION HOSPITAL
On the road to your recovery...

Appropriate Expectations for Hearing Aid Use[2]

➤ Many hearing aids may make speech somewhat clearer because they are adjusted to amplify the sounds with which you have the most difficulty.

➤ Hearing aids not only amplify speech but also noise in the background, so you will probably have difficulty understanding speech in noisy environments.

➤ Many hearing aids make soft sounds loud enough for you to hear but are designed to keep strong sounds from being uncomfortably loud.

➤ Even when wearing hearing aids, you may experience problems understanding people who are talking from a different room or locating where a sound is coming from.

➤ Hearing aids may not be helpful in reverberant listening conditions (e.g., rooms that have hard walls and floors and no draperies or carpet).

➤ Your voice and the voices of others may sound different. You might feel that your voice is emanating from inside of a barrel.

➤ Hearing aids will let you hear sounds that you have not heard for a while, such as your own breathing or clothes rustling.

➤ You may still have some difficulty understanding speech even though you are wearing hearing aids.

➤ Your hearing aids should be comfortable to wear. If not, then contact your audiologist.

---

[2]Adapted from *Foundations of Aural Rehabilitation: Children, Adults, and Their Family Members*, by N. Tye-Murray, 1998. San Diego, CA: Singular Publishing Group.

APPENDIX VII-L

Sequencing of Motor Skills for Hearing Aid Use and Manipulation

XYZ REHABILITATION HOSPITAL
On the road to your recovery...

MOTOR SKILLS AND SEQUENCING FOR HEARING AID USE AND MANIPULATION

One-Hand Functional Only

Battery Insertion:

- Position hearing aid and battery on a flat service.
- Pick-up hearing aid in hand.
- Manuever instrument so that hearing aid is held by all fingers except the index finger.
- Position the hearing aid so that index finger is able to "flick" open the battery door.
- Place the hearing aid down on the flat surface with door wide open.
- Pick up the battery with the "+" side up.
- Place it in the battery compartment.
- Close the battery compartment.

Insertion:

- Pick up hearing aid so that it is held by the middle finger, index finger, and thumb.
- Make sure that the hearing aid is oriented so it will sit in the ear:
  - ✔ top side up, bottom side down
  - ✔ inside (canal portion) toward the head, faceplate (controls, etc.) toward the outside
  - ✔ front of the hearing aid toward the anterior; back toward the posterior
- Raise arm so that the hearing aid is level with the ear.
- Insert the hearing aid into the ear by gently shoving it inward with the index finger.
- Once the hearing aid is secure in the ear, locate the on/off switch.
- "Flick" it with the index finger.
- Find the volume-control wheel with the index finger.
- Apply pressure to the wheel with the index finger.
- Roll the wheel back and forth through wrist and hand movement.
- Adjust the wheel so that sounds seem comfortable.

Note: If patient has behind-the-ear (BTE) hearing aids, the process is the same as above, but the earmold replaces the hearing aid, and an extra step of lifting the hearing aid and placing the BTE behind the pinna is added.

Removal:

- Raise arm so that the hand is at ear level.
- Find the volume wheel as described above.
- Turn the volume down or turn the hearing aid off as described above.
- Grip the hearing aid with middle finger, index finger, and thumb.
- Gently wiggle the hearing aid out of the ear.
- Place the hearing aid on a flat surface.
- Grip the hearing aid with the middle finger and the thumb so that the index finger can "flick" the battery compartment open.
- "Flick" the battery compartment open.
- Place the hearing aid in its box or container.

Note: For BTEs removal is similar, except after the hearing aid is turned off the BTE comes from behind the pinna. The earmold is removed just as if it were a hearing aid.

Both Hands Functional:

Battery Insertion

Dominant Hand	Other Hand
➢ Open battery compartment. ➢ Pick up battery with the "+" up. ➢ Place the battery in the battery compartment. ➢ Close the door.	➢ Holds hearing aid.

Insertion and removal are the same.

APPENDIX VII-M

Visualization and Imagery Task for CIC Insertion
XYZ REHABILITATION HOSPITAL
On the road to your recovery...

OUTLINE FOR VISUALIZATION AND IMAGERY TASK FOR CIC INSERTION FOR REHABILITATION-HOSPITAL PATIENTS[1]

JOINT REHABILITATION: Audiologist and Physical-Therapy Staff

➤ The audiologist and a member of the physical therapy (PT) staff will meet, review the patient's chart, and note any special circumstances that may interfere with success in using CICs. The PT staff member can be very helpful to the audiologist in understanding the patient's motoric limitations.

➤ The audiologist together with the PT staff member will educate the patient about the parts of the ear and the CICs prior to the initial insertion of the aids. The audiologist will have a model CIC for his/her own ear that can be used for demonstration with patients.

➤ The audiologist should have an intimate knowledge of the patient's ear canals through repeated otoscopic inspections.

➤ The audiologist should ensure that the patient's ear canal is free of cerumen and debris so that there is an unobstructed pathway.

➤ The audiologist should insert the CICs into the patient's ears to be sure that they fit properly and can be inserted without discomfort to the patient. If not, the audiologist should make the necessary modifications to the shells (e.g., buffing where too tight or building up where to loose) before proceeding.

➤ Have the patient close his or her eyes and create a visual image of a large, long tunnel with bends in it that are analogous to the first and second turns of the patient's ear canal (these correspond to the shape of the patient's CIC shell for each ear).

➤ Once the patient can visualize the tunnel, have him/her open the eyes and view the hearing aid, noting the turns that serve as the road map through the tunnel to complete the visualization association.

➤ Have the patient grasp the extraction string of the CIC with the thumb and forefinger of the hand corresponding to the hearing aid to be inserted.

➤ Remind the patient to be *patient* and *gentle.* The patient should insert the CIC into the ear canal while continuing to visualize the tunnel imaged previously. Note: It helps to lubricate the tunnel with mineral oil to ease the insertion.

➤ If successful, have the patient close his/her eyes and again visualize how the CIC went into the ear.

---

[1]Adapted from "Solving CIC Hearing Aid Insertion and Comfort Problems," by J. L. Danhauer and K. J. Danhauer, 1997. In M. Chasin (Ed.), *CIC Handbook* (pp. 169–191). San Diego, CA: Singular Publishing Group.

- Again, have the patient grasp extraction string and slowly and gently remove the CIC by pulling it straight out of the canal.

- Have the patient visualize the tunnel again and using the same procedure as above, reinsert the CIC into the ear canal. Use the same procedure and have the patient insert the other CIC into the other ear.

- Repeat this process several times to instill the image, ingrain it in his/her mind, and ensure success before ending the initial sessions and having the patient return to his/her room.

- At this point, the audiologist and the member of the physical therapy staff will contact the nursing station near the patient's room and schedule an appointment with the attending nurse(s) to go over these procedures.

- If the patient has extreme motoric difficulty with the CICs, hearing aid maintenance (e.g., insertion and removal) will be targeted as a behavioral objective for physical therapy.

- The nurses will assist the patient in inserting and removing the hearing aids as needed during the hospital stay. The nurses will report to the audiologist and the physical therapist as to how much difficulty the patient has had between appointments with the audiologist.

- At the next session with the patient, determine if the CICs are in the ears properly, how many hours per day they have been worn, and if there were any problems since the last appointment. If family members or the nurses are present, it is helpful to have them verify the patient's answers to these questions and to voice their impressions about how the CICs are performing for the patient.

- Ask if there are any sore spots in the ear canals. Ask the patient to remove the CICs. Inspect the canals thoroughly with an otoscope to ensure that there are no problems. If there are, note them in the patient's chart (with diagrams and comments) and make appropriate modifications before reinserting. Any necessary adjustments to the circuitry can also be made at this time and compared to the real-ear measures obtained during the first fitting session. Independent ear aided pure-tone and speech audiometry measures can also be completed at this time to help verify the fitting.

- If all is well, have the patient demonstrate that he/she can indeed insert the CICs without difficulty. This helps patients build confidence and feel good about themsleves, the CICs, their disability, and the entire process—especially if they had considerable difficulty inserting them previously.

- For the finale, have your patients insert each CIC while you time them with a stopwatch. We find that patients, who at first struggled and failed for several minutes attempting to insert their CICs, can usually insert them in under five seconds once they know how to insert them correctly. This serves as a real confidence builder and solidifies the process.

250 GUIDEBOOK FOR SUPPORT PROGRAMS IN AURAL REHABILITATION

➢ The picture below can assist in the process.

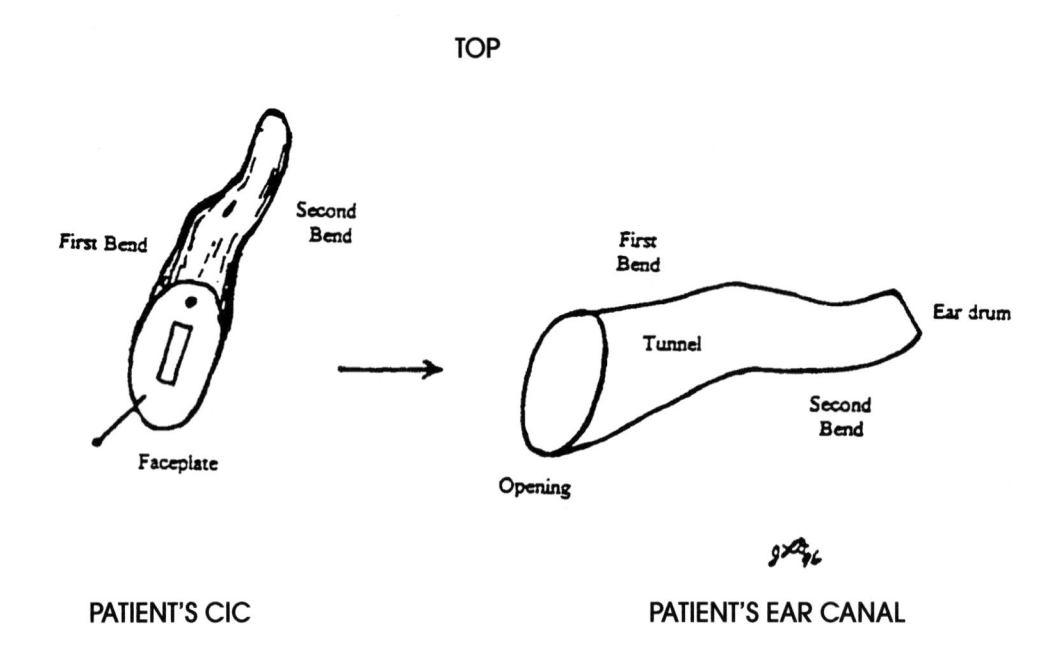

TOP

PATIENT'S CIC → **PATIENT'S EAR CANAL**

APPENDIX VII-N

Patients' Hearing Aid Status List

XYZ REHABILITATION HOSPITAL

On the road to your recovery...

PATIENTS' HEARING AID STATUS LIST

FLOOR: FIRST

Patient's Name: Chester A. Arthur
Room Number: 1001
Hearing Aid Make, Model, and Serial Number: Oticon E38-P (R#12345/L#67891)
Ears Fitted: Right and Left
Hearing Aid Battery Size: 675
Level of Assistance: Independent
Comments: Remind patient to check his aid at the Hearing Aid Check Station every morning.

Patient's Name: Betsy Ross
Room Number: 1007
Hearing Aid Make, Model, and Serial Number: Phonic Ear 805CD (R#00002)
Ears Fitted: Right
Hearing Aid Battery Size: 675
Level of Assistance: Partial Assistance
Comments: Attending nurse should work on physical therapy goals regarding hearing aid care with patient. See patient chart.

APPENDIX VII-O

Chart Note: Patient's Hearing Aid Status

XYZ REHABILITATION HOSPITAL

On the road to your recovery...

CHART NOTE

6/28/99

To: Nursing Staff on First Floor
From: Starr Audiologist, Ph.D., CCC-A, FAAA
      Certificate of Clinical Competence in Audiology
      Fellow of the American Academy of Audiology

Re: Status of Chester A. Arthur's Hearing Aid

The above patient has undergone a complete audiologic evaluation and hearing aid check. Below please note his hearing aid status. Please include him in the Hearing Aid Monitoring Program. He is at the Independent Level of Assistance, meaning that he can independently manage his amplification needs. Please show him the Hearing Aid Check Station, and demonstrate how to check his hearing aids and to fill out the daily Hearing Aid Check Sheet.

Please add this information to the Hearing Aid Status List posted at your station. The information will be permanently added to your list next week.

Patient's Name: Chester A. Arthur
Floor/Room: First/1001
Hearing Aid Make, Model, and Serial Number: Oticon E38-P (R#12345/L#67891)
Ears Fitted: Right and Left
Hearing Aid Battery Size: 675
Level of Assistance: Independent
Comments: Remind patient to check hearing aids at Hearing Aid Check Station every morning.
Method of Pay: Private Pay

APPENDIX VII-P

Hearing Aid Check Sheet

XYZ REHABILITATION HOSPITAL
On the road to your recovery...

HEARING AID CHECK SHEET

Name:_____

Room:_____

Hearing Aid Make/Model/Serial #:_____

Place the CHECK in the box if OK.

Item to Check	Date							
Visual								
■ Case clean & uncracked		☐	☐	☐	☐	☐	☐	☐
■ Sound bore clear of wax		☐	☐	☐	☐	☐	☐	☐
■ Tubing undamaged		☐	☐	☐	☐	☐	☐	☐
■ Battery contacts uncorroded		☐	☐	☐	☐	☐	☐	☐
■ Battery charged		☐	☐	☐	☐	☐	☐	☐
■ Free of moisture		☐	☐	☐	☐	☐	☐	☐
Listening								
■ Adequate volume		☐	☐	☐	☐	☐	☐	☐
■ Good sound quality		☐	☐	☐	☐	☐	☐	☐
■ Volume wheel moves smoothly		☐	☐	☐	☐	☐	☐	☐
■ No unusual sounds		☐	☐	☐	☐	☐	☐	☐

Comments:

APPENDIX VII-Q

Daily Log of Hearing Aid Use for Patients Requiring Assistance

XYZ REHABILITATION HOSPITAL

On the road to your recovery...

DAILY LOG OF HEARING AID USE FOR PATIENTS NEEDING ASSISTANCE WITH THEIR HEARING AIDS

Patient's Name:_____

Floor/Room Number:_____

Day of the Week	Time in	Sign	Time out	Sign
Sunday				
Monday				
Tuesday				
Wednesday				
Thursday				
Friday				
Saturday				

APPENDIX VII-R

Facility Communication Accessibility Checklist

XYZ REHABILITATION HOSPITAL
On the road to your recovery...

FACILITY COMMUNICATION ACCESSIBILITY CHECKLIST

FEATURE	YES	NO
Does your facility:		
■ Have an ADA committee or task force?	☐	☐
■ Have nondiscriminatory policies toward the disabled?	☐	☐
■ Provide auxiliary communication aids and services? (If yes to the last question, then answer these questions appearing between the lines of stars.)	☐	☐
***		
Regarding communication aids and services, does your facility:		
➢ Respond to auxiliary aids and services requests?	☐	☐
➢ Maintain the communication devices in good working condition?	☐	☐
➢ Provide TDD and accessible telephones or alternative services?	☐	☐
➢ Provide means for two-way communication in emergency situations?	☐	☐
➢ Provide closed-caption recorders?	☐	☐
***		
Does your facility:		
■ Inform the public of available accommodations using appropriate signs and symbols?	☐	☐
■ Make aurally (via hearing) delivered information available to persons with speech and hearing deficits?	☐	☐
■ Have staff display appropriate attitudes, behaviors, and communication strategies for interacting with patients with speech and hearing deficits?	☐	☐
■ Consider the effects of visually related, acoustically related, attitudinal, and prejudicial barriers on communication?	☐	☐
■ Seek to remove barriers to communication?	☐	☐
■ Obtain technical assistance and consult with rehabilitation professionals, disability organizations, consumers, and federal agencies as appropriate?	☐	☐

APPENDIX VII-S

Listening Questionnaire

XYZ REHABILITATION HOSPITAL

On the road to your recovery...

LISTENING QUESTIONNAIRE[1]

Patient's Name:_____ Date:_____

The information you provide by completing this questionnaire will assist us in providing you with the most comprehensive service. Please check the box for your response for each situation. If the situation does not apply to you, please check N/A (not applicable). Thank you.

Do you now wear hearing aid   YES   NO

If your answer is NO, skip Sections I and II and complete all of Sections III, IV, and V.

If your answer is YES, complete Sections I and II. Answer the questions for the times you ARE wearing your hearing aid(s). Then proceed to Sections III and IV and answer for the times you ARE NOT wearing your hearing aid(s) and then complete Section V.

SECTION I: WHILE WEARING MY HEARING AID(S), I HAVE DIFFICULTY UNDERSTANDING:

Situation	Yes	Sometimes	No	N/A
■ in an automobile	☐	☐	☐	☐
■ the television	☐	☐	☐	☐
■ the radio	☐	☐	☐	☐
■ over the telephone	☐	☐	☐	☐
■ in a restaurant or dining room	☐	☐	☐	☐
■ at a conference table	☐	☐	☐	☐
■ at a party	☐	☐	☐	☐
■ in a small family group	☐	☐	☐	☐
■ in the theater, movie, or play	☐	☐	☐	☐
■ in a house of worship	☐	☐	☐	☐
■ on the job	☐	☐	☐	☐
■ other	☐	☐	☐	☐

Describe:_____

[1]From "Beyond Hearing Aids: Use of Auxiliary Aids," by S. A. Sandridge, 1995, pp. 159–161. In P. B. Kricos and S. A. Lesner (Eds.), *Hearing Care for the Older Adult: Audiologic Rehabilitation* (pp. 127–166). Boston, MA: Butterworth-Heinemann. Reprinted with permission.

SECTION II: WHILE WEARING MY HEARING AID(S), I HAVE DIFFICULTY HEARING:

Situation	Yes	Sometimes	No	N/A
■ the telephone ring	☐	☐	☐	☐
when?_____	☐	☐	☐	☐
■ the doorbell when I'm in another room	☐	☐	☐	☐
■ someone knocking at the door	☐	☐	☐	☐
■ someone calling to me from another room	☐	☐	☐	☐
when?_____	☐	☐	☐	☐
■ the smoke detector at home or in hotels	☐	☐	☐	☐

SECTION III: WITHOUT HEARING AID(S), I HAVE DIFFICULTY UNDERSTANDING:

Situation	Yes	Sometimes	No	N/A
■ in an automobile	☐	☐	☐	☐
■ the television	☐	☐	☐	☐
■ the radio	☐	☐	☐	☐
■ over the telephone	☐	☐	☐	☐
■ in a restaurant or dining room	☐	☐	☐	☐
■ at a conference table	☐	☐	☐	☐
■ at a party	☐	☐	☐	☐
■ in a small family group	☐	☐	☐	☐
■ in the theater, movie, or play	☐	☐	☐	☐
■ in a house of worship	☐	☐	☐	☐
■ on the job	☐	☐	☐	☐
■ other	☐	☐	☐	☐

Describe:_____

SECTION IV: I HAVE DIFFICULTY HEARING:

Situation	Yes	Sometimes	No	N/A
▪ the telephone ring when?_____	☐	☐	☐	☐
▪ the doorbell when I'm in another room	☐	☐	☐	☐
▪ someone knocking at the door	☐	☐	☐	☐
▪ someone calling to me from another room when?_____	☐	☐	☐	☐
▪ the smoke detector at home or in hotels	☐	☐	☐	☐

SECTION V: I HAVE KNOWLEDGE ABOUT THE FOLLOWING ITEMS:

Item	Yes	No
▪ my rights under the Americans with Disabilities Act	☐	☐
▪ devices available for alerting me to the doorbell, telephone ringing, etc.	☐	☐
▪ devices available to help me understand the television or radio	☐	☐
▪ devices I can use on the phone to help me understand	☐	☐
▪ theaters are now required to provide devices that assist me in hearing the movie or play	☐	☐

That completes this questionnaire. By answering these questions you have provided a more complete picture of your listening abilities so we may be able to serve you better. Thank you again.

APPENDIX VII-T

Considerations for Purchasing Auxiliary Devices

XYZ REHABILITATION HOSPITAL
On the road to your recovery...

CONSIDERATIONS FOR PURCHASING AUXILIARY DEVICES[1]

➤ ***Look for simple solutions.*** Low-tech items are usually less expensive and often easier to use. They tend to be more popular, break down less often, and are easier to replace. It also makes people feel more comfortable (normal) if they do not need to use a lot of special equipment.

➤ ***Consider the learning and the work style of the user.*** Does he or she enjoy using aids and devices? Does he or she resist equipment that sets him or her apart? What is the best way to compensate for a hearing or vision impairment?

➤ ***Consider the long-range implications of the hearing or vision impairment(s).*** How can these devices be coupled to the individual's hearing aid? Will this product or method be something that will work long term? Will there be the need to repeat this procedure if the person loses more hearing or vision? Are there options that will work for this individual for a longer period of time?

➤ ***Look at each piece of equipment.*** Keep the following considerations in mind:
- ✔ How easy is the device to assemble or set up?
- ✔ How easy is the device to use? To maintain?
- ✔ Is the device durable?
- ✔ Will it be outdated shortly? Can it be updated easily?
- ✔ Will the individual continue to have the same needs over time?
- ✔ Is the device easily adaptable to a wide variety of situations and uses?
- ✔ If portability is a factor, how portable is it?
- ✔ Does this device have a history of dependability? Durability?
- ✔ If it breaks, how easy is it to get the device fixed? Is there a service contract?
- ✔ Is technical support easily available (e.g., by phone) if there is a problem?

➤ ***Investigate all options.*** Talk to other consumers at consumer organizations, support groups, or rehabilitation agencies. Many agencies have technology centers where hands-on trials and lending libraries are available. Go to the exhibits at the Annual Convention of the American Academy of Audiology. Equipment manufacturers will be there to demonstrate the latest innovations in adaptive and assistive technology. Ask a lot of questions! In addition, send away for catalogs from manufacturers. For more technical equipment, ask the local distributor to make a presentation to demonstrate the equipment. Ask for a trial period for expensive pieces of equipment.

➤ ***Compare similar equipment from different manufacturers.*** Ask the following questions:
- ✔ What features and options does each have? What is needed for the task?
- ✔ Is the manufacturer or brand dependable? Will the manufacturer stand behind the equipment even if that model is discontinued?
- ✔ What are the pros and cons for each device?

➤ ***Purchase devices only after consulting with a professional in the field.***

---

[1]Adapted from "Assistive Technology for Individuals With Sensory Impairments," by R. Rothstein and J. M. Everson, 1994. In F. F. Flippo, K. J. Inge, and J. M. Barcus (Eds.), *Assistive Technology: A Resource for School, Work, and Community* (pp. 105–132). Baltimore, MD: Paul H. Brookes.

APPENDIX VII-U

Handout on "Clear Speech"

XYZ REHABILITATION HOSPITAL
On the road to your recovery...

CLEAR SPEECH[1]

IS *NOT*...

Communicating in a monotone
Loud shouting
Exaggerated
Artificial
Real staccato

IS...

Speaking slowly
Pausing between phrases and sentences
Emphasizing key words
Enunciating accurately and precisely
Communicating with a full range of inflections
Heightening volume

^^*^*^*^*^*^*^*^*^*^*^*^

Benefits of Clear Speech

- Maximizes effective communication
- Actively includes family and friends
- Creates a happier environment

---

[1] Adapted from "Beyond Hearing Aids: Clear Speech Training as an Intervention Strategy," by D. J. Schum, 1997. *The Hearing Journal, 50*(10), 36–38, 40; and S. H. Abel, 1998, "Clear Speech Handout," Auburn, AL: Author.

APPENDIX VII-V

Speechreading Materials

XYZ REHABILITATION HOSPITAL

On the road to your recovery...

ORIENTATION TO SPEECHREADING[1]

Speechreading is a process of putting information together to form a message in order to help you understand what people are trying to say. Speechreading is not just watching others' lips to identify the words they are saying. It also consists of using your mind to collect all the information available and then make a "best guess." Speechreading includes the following:

- ➤ *Lipreading.* Watching the lip movements of the talker. It is impossible to identify every word, but we can identify some words and sounds that give us some information about what is being said.

- ➤ *Facial expression.* It is possible to identify people's moods or how they feel by the expression on their faces.

- ➤ *Gesture, posture, and movement.* What people are doing, how they are sitting, and the gestures they make give clues to what they are thinking about and what they might say.

- ➤ *Situational cues.* We might anticipate what a person is going to talk about by the situation or place they (sic) are in and the relationships of the people present.

- ➤ *Knowing the topic.* It is easier to follow conversation when you know what the talker is talking about. The easiest way to find out is to ask someone else who is listening.

- ➤ *Knowledge of the language.* We might be able to make educated guesses about a particular word missed on the basis of sentence structure.

- ➤ *Keeping informed.* Knowing what news items or subjects are of current interest to people may help us anticipate what will be talked about. Read newspapers and magazines and watch the news on television.

- ➤ *Emotional factors.* Keep motivated and develop self-confidence even though there will be times that you make errors.

- ➤ *Use your hearing.* Although you have a hearing loss, you do hear sounds and words that may help you identify the message or idea.

Until now, you have been taking advantage of these clues to some extent. The goal is to make you more conscious of them so you can use them maximally. Using these clues, much of the message can be predicted. Some parts of the message are less predictable (e.g., hearing a new name), making them more difficult. Therefore, you must use two kinds of information: (a) the part of the message you did understand and (b) any additional knowledge that can help you fill in the gaps in order to figure out the whole message.

---

[1]"Speechreading Instruction for Adults: Issues and Approaches," by R. Cherry and A. Rubenstein, 1988, p. 302. *The Volta Review 90*(5), 289–306. Reprinted with permission.

XYZ REHABILITATION HOSPITAL
On the road to your recovery...

GROUPS OF CONSONANTS THAT LOOK THE SAME ON THE MOUTH[1]

The following are groups of consonants that *look the same on a person's mouth* when they are made. Some consonants are voiced (v), while others are voiceless (vs). All vowels are voiced. We are interested in sounds, not letters (different letters can make the same sound, e.g., k, ck, c).

Consonant groups	Visible Characteristics	Examples
(vs) p, (v) b, (v) m	Lips closed	Pan Ban Man
(vs) f, (v) v	Upper teeth touch lower lip	Fan Van
(vs) th, (v) th	Tongue between teeth	THink THey
v wh, (v) r	Lips rounded	WHeel Reel
(vs) sh, (v) zh, (vs) tsh, (v) dzh	Teeth together; lips rounded	SHe aZure CHeck JUdge
(vs) s, (v) z	Teeth closed; lips in a smile	Say Zoo
(vs) t, (v) d, (v) n, (v) l	Tongue tip up	Ten Den Net Let
(vs) k, (v) g, (v) ng	Back of tongue tip	iKa iGa iNGa

---

[1] From "Speechreading Instruction for Adults: Issues and Approaches," by R. Cherry and A. Rubenstein, 1988, p. 305. *The Volta Review* 90(5), 289–306. Reprinted with permission.

CHAPTER 8

Establishing Support Programs in Long-Term Residential Care Facilities for the Elderly

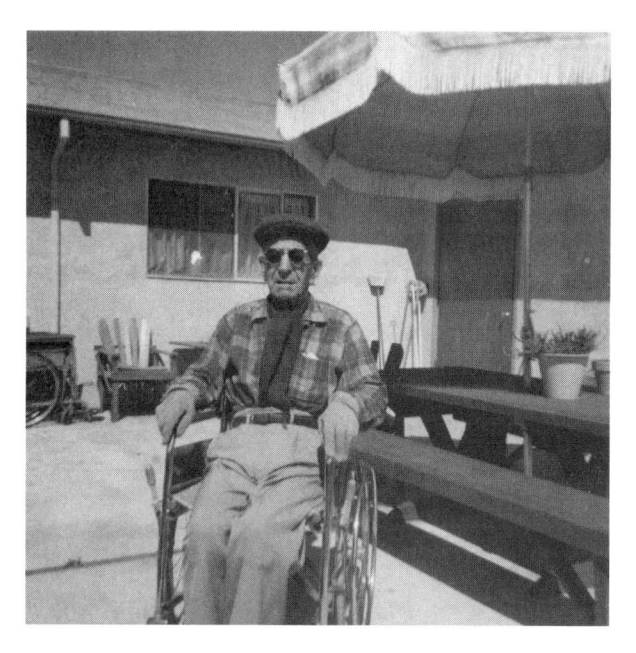

Figure 8-1. Elderly nursing-home resident with a hearing impairment.

INTRODUCTION

Approximately 23 to 28 million individuals in the United States have some form of hearing impairment (Kochkin, 1996). Half of these individuals are over the age of 65 (Bridges & Bentler, 1998). In addition, the number of patients over 65 years old with hearing impairment is expected to increase sharply in the next millenium due to the aging of the U.S. population (Bridges & Bentler, 1998). By the year 2020, 50 million persons in the United States are expected to be over 65 years of age (U.S. Bureau of the Census, 1996). The Baby Boomers, the generation that wanted to change the world, is expected to change the way we view the aging process. Who knows, maybe being "over fifty will be nifty." Marketing will be aimed at these individuals because they will have the most buying power. Some people even expect the faces on advertisements to change. Instead of using actors 30 years of age or younger in ads, "real people" of all ages will sell products. Having a hearing loss, traditionally associated with old age, may be just another acceptable part of life. Likewise, because the Baby Boomer generation is "high-tech," the hearing industry may focus on the technological aspects of hearing instruments' performance.

It is hoped that the aging Boomers will organize politically to ensure that their generation will have an adequate supply of housing. As has been the case with other generations, many aged Boomers may not be able to live in their own homes for a variety of reasons (e.g., deteriorating physical or mental health) and may need to reside in some sort of health-care facility. The term "health-care facility" is currently used to describe any facility that provides either short-term or long-term residential care for older adults who require medical or other health services beyond those provided by a hospital (Hull, 1995). In addition, Boomers may lobby to ensure that adequate health-care services, including audiologic care, are provided to all residents of these facilities at a reasonable cost. Establishment of support programs for elderly residents with hearing impairment would be one way to accomplish this goal. To do so successfully, audiologists need to understand the different aspects of aging, the reasons to provide audiologic services to the elderly, the continuum of housing available for the elderly, and components of a complete support program for elderly patients with hearing impairment residing in assisted-living/semidependent and dependent-care facilities. The purpose of this chapter is to discuss issues relating to the establishment of support programs in these facilities. Figure 8–2 shows one such facility.

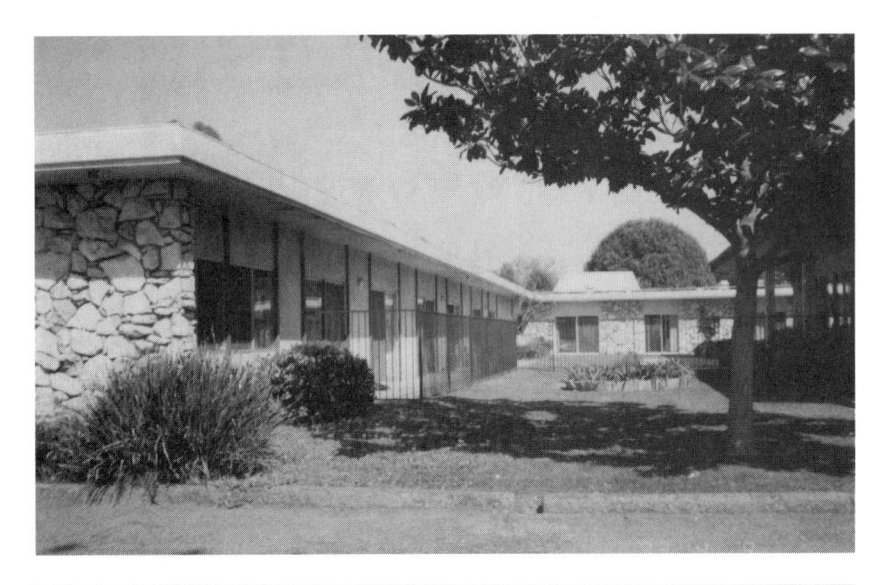

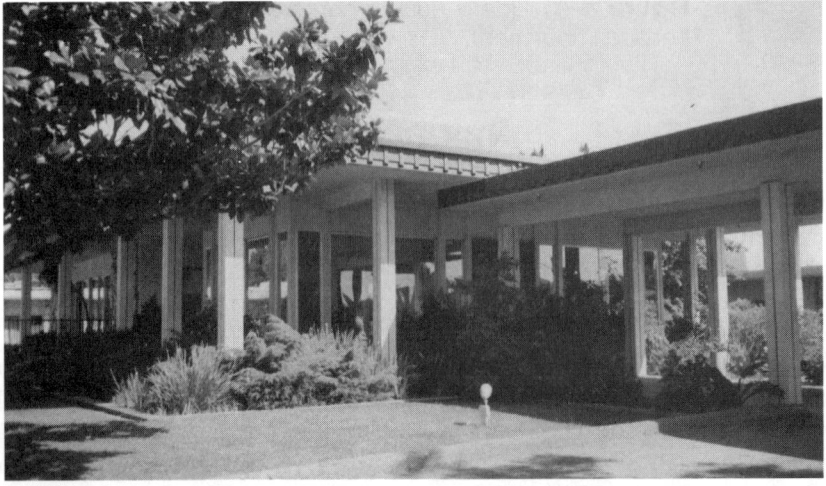

Figure 8–2. Pictures of a typical long-term residential care facility for the elderly.

> **LEARNING OBJECTIVES**
>
> **This chapter will enable the reader to:**
>
> - Understand the myths versus the realities of aging
> - Understand why audiologists should provide services to the elderly in long-term residential care facilities
> - Acknowledge the reasons for and effects of admitting the elderly to long-term residential care facilities
> - Discuss audiologic service delivery in long-term residential care facilities for the elderly
> - Understand the continuum of housing for the elderly
> - Understand the importance of preservice assessment of long-term residential care facilities for the elderly
> - Acknowledge nursing-home residents' bill of rights
> - List components of a full-service audiology support program in long-term residential care facilities for the elderly
> - Establish a complete support program at long-term care facilities for residents with hearing impairment

ASPECTS OF AGING: MYTHS VERSUS REALITY

Many of us dread the thought of growing old. Our fears are often driven by many of the myths concerning the elderly segment of the population. For example, Kricos (1995) reported several common myths of aging that are listed below, along with some of the realities (in parentheses):

- The elderly have difficulty walking (only about 20% actually do [Cox, 1988]).
- The elderly experience difficulties thinking clearly (only about 5 to 15% actually do [Cox (1988]).
- The elderly experience limitations in daily activities (only about 10 to 40% actually do [Cox, 1988]).
- The elderly are often alienated from their families.
- Most of the elderly are institutionalized (only about 5% actually are [Nussbaum, Thompson, & Robinson, 1989]).
- The elderly are senile (only about 5 to 15% actually are [Nussbaum et al., 1989]).

If we can believe the actual data cited above, then many of the myths associated with aging are, in fact, only myths. Many older individuals look, feel, and act much younger than their chronological age reflects, but the opposite can also be true (i.e., people who appear to be quite a bit older than their age). There is some truth in the old saying, "you are as young (or old) as you feel." In fact, elderly persons can be placed along a continuum of vitality (i.e., mental, emotional, and physical performance) ranging from the "super-old" to the "old-old" (Kricos, 1995; Piscopo, 1985). The "old-old" are frail with limited vitality while the "super-old" are those who lead very active lives. For example, at age 77, John Glenn represents an example of a "super-old" senior citizen. John Glenn, after serving as a state senator for several years, retrained diligently with astronauts nearly half his age to make an historic second trip into space. Conversely, a 77-year-old person who simply lies in bed all day and watches television is an example of someone at the "old-old" end of the continuum. Certainly, audiologists will see and serve members from both extremes, as well as those in between, but they should not rush to judge someone by age alone. Figure 8–3 contrasts uninvolved seniors to those who actively enjoy bingo with their peers.

Even though there are many healthy and active Americans over the age of 65, audiologists

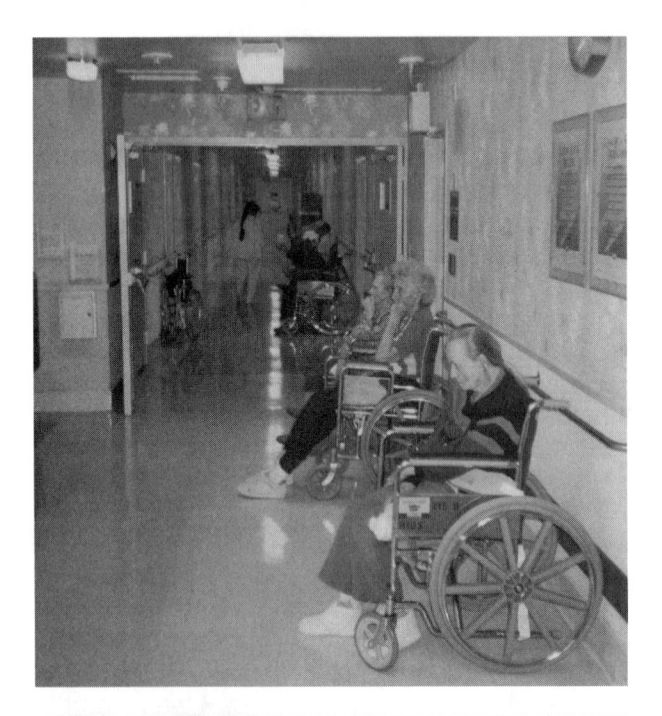

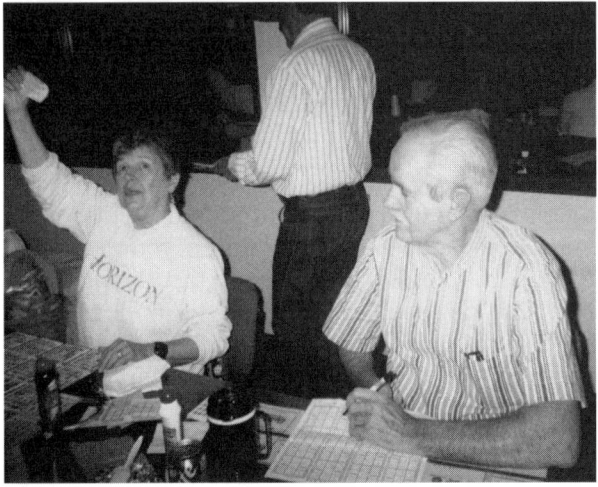

Figure 8-3. Several uninvolved seniors (top) who might benefit from stimulating activities and (bottom) who enjoy activities (e.g., Bingo) with their peers.

must acknowledge some of the grim realities of aging in order to serve this population adequately. Many of the elderly suffer from a variety of communication disorders such as dysarthria (i.e, interference with the control of speech resulting in slurring or difficult-to-understand speech caused by poor articulation, poor breath control, and uncoordinated movements of lips, tongue, palate, and larynx); aphasia (i.e., reduced ability to understand what others are saying, to express oneself, or be understood); voice problems (i.e., caused by laryngectomy or removal of the larynx due to cancer); hearing problems; and other disorders (ASHA, 1998). The major causes of dysarthria include diseases such as parkinsonism, multiple sclerosis, and bulbar palsy, as well as accidents (ASHA, 1998). Furthermore, the major cause of aphasia is cerebral vascular accidents (CVAs). Brain disorders, such as Alzheimer's disease, can also cause communication disorders in the elderly. Alzheimer's disease is not a benign loss of memory and it is not a normal part of aging, however (Goldberg, 1996). Until recently, little was known about this disease in which the body eventually forgets how to perform essential tasks such as eating and breathing, resulting in death (Goldberg, 1996). If individuals are fortunate enough to reach 85 years of age, they have a 50/50 chance of getting the disease (Goldberg, 1996). Thus, audiologists can assume that almost half of the patients seen in long-term residential care facilities for the elderly have Alzheimer's related symptoms. Diagnosis of Alzheimer's disease, however, is assumptive until it can be confirmed through an autopsy (Bayles & Tomoeda, 1995).

The elderly also have a variety of chronic health problems, deterioration of sensory systems, loss of memory, drug abuse, and malnutrition. Chronic health problems in the elderly include arthritis, cataracts, sinusitis, diabetes, heart disease, hypertension, and orthopedic problems (Lesner & Kricos, 1995; National Center on Health Statistics, 1987). In addition to hearing loss, the elderly experience a reduction in the sensory systems of vision (Atchley, 1993) and touch (Botwinick, 1984). For example, 30 to 40% of persons over the age of 70 years have some visual impairment (Castles, 1993; Tye-Murray, 1998; Vinding, 1989). Thus, audiologists could again assume that many elderly persons living in long-term residential care facilities have visual problems that could preclude their ability to use the visual aspects of speech for lipreading. These problems combined with hearing loss can result in communication difficulties and isolationism that often mimic or are misdiagnosed as dementia, senility, or withdrawal.

Chronic illnesses and other life problems may result in elderly persons who are unable to take care of themselves, yet do not need hospitalization. These individuals are often placed in nursing homes. Some interesting facts regarding nursing homes include (Careguide, 1998):

- 40 to 45% of individuals turning age 65 years in 1990 will stay in a nursing home at least once in their lifetime.

- About 50% of those admitted to nursing homes will stay less than 6 months.
- One in 5 will stay 1 or more years, and 1 in 10 will stay 3 or more years.

The major reason people are placed in nursing homes is their state of mental or physical health (Gatz, Bengstron, & Blum, 1990). Other reasons may include loss of residence or lack of nearby relatives, adequate finances, or support systems (Hull, 1995). Family members who live nearby are often able to take care of the elderly. Well-to-do elderly persons who desire to live independently can hire caretakers to assist them with tasks of daily living, whereas lower-income elderly persons who do not have this option may have to be institutionalized. In many cases, falls (which are prevalent among the elderly) cause broken hips, and because there are no other options, otherwise healthy individuals are placed in convalescent hospitals or nursing homes—frequently for the rest of their lives.

Placement in a nursing home can have negative effects on elderly persons, such as depression, loneliness, lack of desire to receive rehabilitation, shock/stress, poor self-image, dependency on strangers, loss of contact with the outside world, personality changes, loss of independence, loss of personal control, dehumanization, lack of stimulation, and a reduction of sensory capabilities (Hull, 1995). Lack of personal hygiene is unfortunately commonplace among those in long-term residential care facilities for the elderly. Presence of a hearing loss or visual problem can exacerbate these negative effects. The lack of ability to communicate, for example, results not only in additional social isolation, irritability, and depression, but an increased loss of independence as well (Anand & Court, 1989). In addition, Crandell (1998) stated that persons with sensorineural hearing loss have higher incidence of health-related problems, such as arhythmias, ischemic heart disease, hypertension, and osteoarthritis, than persons with normal hearing.

The incidence of communication disorders in the elderly is high, especially sensorineural hearing loss. In one study, 70% of elderly patients in institutions who are not demented and 83% of those who were demented were found to have hearing loss (Weinstein & Amsel, 1986). In a similar study, Garahan, Waller, Houghton, Tisdale, and Runge (1992) found that out of 121 residents, 77% had at least a mild hearing loss in the better ear and 51% had at least a moderate-to-severe loss. In addition, a relatively low proportion of these elderly persons uses any form of amplification. Schow (1982) reported that only 10% of nursing home residents who have hearing losses over 40 dB HL use hearing aids. Furthermore, Thibodeau and Schmitt (1988) found that only 4% of 493 residents in 17 nursing homes and only 5% of 451 residents of 3 retirement centers used amplification. Other studies and personal experience further reveal that of those who possess hearing aids, most of these devices are frequently found to be broken, suffering from a dead battery, full of cerumen, lost, locked in the nurses' station, at home with the family, or simply not worn. Clearly, the elderly in most residential healthcare facilities are part of the unserved or underserved population with hearing impairment (Tye-Murray, 1998).

WHY SHOULD AUDIOLOGISTS CARE?

Shultz and Mowry (1995) listed the common obstacles in audiologic service delivery in nursing homes including the following:

- visiting the facility and finding the patient,
- cerumen management,
- lost hearing aids,
- lack of physician and staff involvement,
- personnel turnover,
- limited family involvement, and
- reimbursement issues.

Audiologists often choose not to provide services in these types of facilities for a number of reasons. First, most residents in these facilities are too ill, nonambulatory, or generally immobile to be seen in a routine office setting. Because they cannot go to the audiologist, the audiologist must then go to them. Second, the fact that these patients must be seen out of the office means that audiologists must have an array of portable equipment and supplies (from diagnostic equipment to hearing aids and assistive listening devices) that can be taken to patients. Bringing the practice to patients means added expense for equipment and travel. The audiologist may have to rely on less-than-optimal equipment that must be used in less-than-optimal, sound-attenuating environments. Providing services "in the field" represents a dramatic change in the way that most audiologists practice (i.e., with clinical diagnostic audiometers, hearing aid analyzers, sound-treated booths, etc.).

Third, cooperation, assistance, and support from administrators, nursing staff, residents, and their families are often less than optimal in these facilities. Daily-living, medical-care, and life-and-death issues clearly take precedence over hearing health care. Consider, for example, a nurse's assistant who is busy cleaning up an 84-year-old, blind, amputee, with congestive heart failure and pneumonia who has just soiled her clothing and bed linens with a nasty bowel movement. It may be difficult for the nurse's assistant to understand why an audiologist, who happens to be present at the facility for the first time in a month, can be so upset over the fact that the battery in the patient's hearing aid is dead. Audiologists must remember that there may be more pressing priorities in these facilities than the functioning of patients' hearing aids.

Fourth, Medicare and other third-party payers do not reimburse audiologists for providing aural rehabilitation services in these facilities. Fifth, audiologists are often bombarded with unpleasant sights, sounds, and smells that can assault the senses in these facilities, creating difficult working environments. Audiologic service delivery is often time-consuming and difficult. In addition, some investigators have found that aural rehabilitation services are often not successful in these settings. Schow (1982) attempted to provide aural rehabilitation and hearing aid services to residents in a 55-bed nursing home. Although 25 residents (almost half of the total) were identified as potential hearing aid candidates, only four residents from the group would participate in a hearing aid trial, and only two of those became hearing aid users.

So, that brings us to the question: Why would any audiologists in their right minds want to expend valuable time and effort providing services to patients who may have questionable outcomes, in an environment that is often depressing and barring on sanitary conditions, with little promise of fiscal viability? In fact, Schow (1982) concluded that audiologists should expend their efforts in trying to assist the larger number of "noninstitutionalized" elderly persons with hearing impairment. Unfortunately, ignoring this segment of the elderly population represents the "easy way out" and leaves at least 70% of patients in these facilities without adequate hearing health care. Clearly, ignoring these patients is not an optimal solution. As audiologists (and as a society in general), we cannot put our heads in the sand and pretend that these individuals do not exist.

The clear answer to the question is that elderly individuals in long-term residential care facilities do need and deserve audiologic services. They are human beings. Before they are our patients, they are our mothers, fathers, sisters, brothers—someone's family. Many are living out their remaining days in far less than optimal conditions. Many are so ill, frail, and in constant pain that they pray to be taken as soon as possible. Regardless of past success and socioeconomic status, some have spent their life's fortunes on their last few years of medical care. They may eventually have to rely on state or federal funding for their daily existence. Many are literally "locked away in a place where nobody cares" because there is nowhere else to go. They either have no family or friends left, or their loved ones never seem able to visit anymore. Visitors stop coming for a variety of reasons, including financial hardships, distance, work schedules, or an emotional inability to see their loved ones in such conditions. Many family members who do visit want to communicate, but cannot do so because of the elderly person's hearing loss. Many elderly persons are simply lonely and have all but given up on life; some have. Unfortunately, many elderly people are labeled as demented, depressed, lonely, senile, and withdrawn when they really suffer from sensory deprivation caused by hearing and visual impairments. Figure 8–4 shows nursing-home residents who could benefit from a hearing support program.

Given the predictions of increased life expectancies for the Baby Boomers, members of this generation may find themselves or their loved ones in such circumstances one day. Many are currently facing these issues as they attempt to find appropriate housing and care for grandparents or parents. These tasks are never pleasant. As elderly individuals cannot always be taken into the home to live with the family, alternative living arrangements must be made.

In spite of how the media portray the aging process, unless one dies young or peacefully at a ripe old age, all of the face lifts, geritol, minoxidil, and Viagra in the world cannot stop the aging process. Unfortunately, old age means seeing friends, relatives, and acquaintances known for a lifetime die. It means coping with aches, pains, and illnesses not known in earlier years. Some see themselves as wasting away; as one of

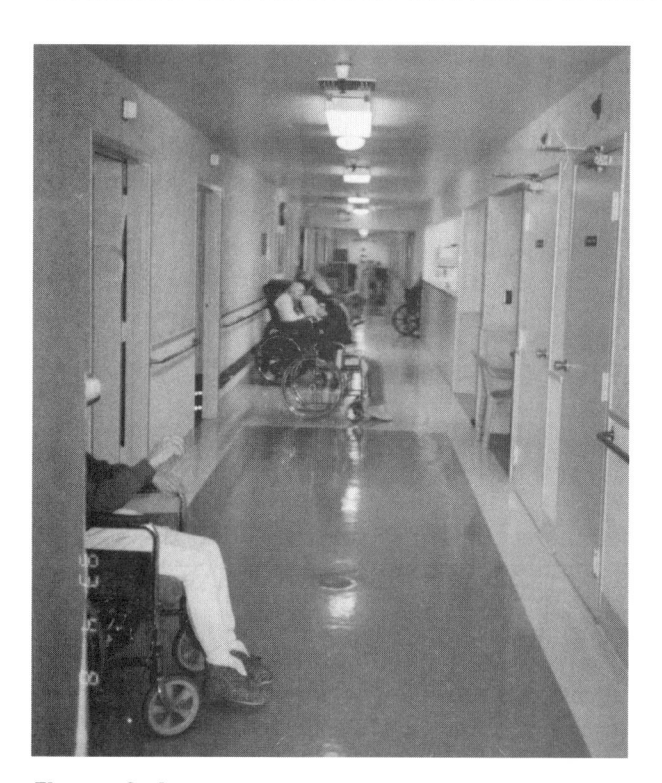

Figure 8–4. Patients who may benefit from a hearing support program.

our elderly patients recently put it, "getting old is not for the weak of heart."

After seeing literally thousands of patients in these facilities during our careers, one thing has become clear. All of these patients are human beings who have families and fascinating life experiences. Audiologists should take time to talk to these patients who, in their 8th, 9th, and 10th decades of life, often can vividly recall their pasts. How many of us take the time to interact with our own parents or grandparents, let alone patients in long-term residential care facilities for the elderly? Audiologists who do take the initiative to provide these services often may do so because they hope that someone else will do the same for their parents if they cannot be there to do it themselves. And yes, we all hope that someone will be there for us when we are in the same situation.

As a caring society, we can do better for our elderly. Indeed we owe it to them and to ourselves, because before too long, we may be among them. Audiologists need to find ways to provide hearing health care to these individuals because it is the right thing to do. We do not discriminate against our patients on the basis of race or creed. Likewise, we should not discriminate on the basis of age or living conditions. Indeed, not all audiologists are suited to work with patients in long-term residential care facilities for the elderly. Nevertheless, for those who can get past the difficult realities of these service-delivery sites and who truly enjoy and appreciate working with this population, these endeavors can be richly rewarding—both emotionally and for one's practice. Providing stellar services in these facilities can increase referrals through contact with administrators, nurses, nurse's assistants, nutritionists, physicians, psychologists, social workers, speech-language pathologists, and volunteers. The respect audiologists can gain in the community can carry over to other aspects of their practice as well. In addition, the smaller the community in which one practices, the more obvious one's contributions to elderly residents' quality of life becomes. Indeed, working with the elderly can enhance one's appreciation of life. Nonetheless, audiologists must understand the continuum of housing available to the elderly, use checklists for preservice assessment of the facility, and acknowledge the nursing-home residents' bill of rights.

CONTINUUM OF HOUSING FOR THE ELDERLY: IMPORTANT CONSIDERATIONS

Hull (1995) divided the health-care facilities available to elderly persons into three categories: (1) outpatient residential facilities (apartment or condominium living for ambulatory older persons), (2) short-term care (an intensive-care or skilled-nursing wing within a nursing home or skilled-nursing facility), and (3) intermediate- and long-term care facilities (nursing homes). The Careguide Web site (1998) uses a similar continuum: (1) independent living (senior apartments, retirement hotels, subsidized housing, small-group/supportive house, and matched housing); (2) semi-independent living or assisted-living facilities; and (3) dependent care (nursing homes, skilled-nursing facilities, extended-care homes, and continuing-care retirement communities). Appendix VIII-A lists these options with a description of the facility, requirements for residency, and some considerations for elderly persons and their significant others.

The focus of this chapter is the establishment of support programs for elderly persons with hearing impairment living in assisted-living/semiindependent and dependent-care facilities. When considering providing services to nursing homes, audiologists should assess the characteristics of the facility in much the same way as prospective residents and their significant others would in securing appropriate housing. Appendix VIII-B contains checklists for audiologists to assess assisted-living residences and nursing homes, adapted from the Careguide Web site (1998). The assisted-living residence checklist contains items pertaining to the physical environment, services, staff, activities, and other factors. The nursing-home checklist includes items to make general observations, as well as to assess the physical environment, medical services, payment issues, location, layout, maintenance, and other factors. Audiologists' preservice assessment of facilities can provide suggestions for improving residents' communication potential. Audiologists may suggest that community areas be carpeted to reduce the amount of reverberation, for example, or that the nursing home provide quiet areas without televisions or radios, or other noisy activities. In addition, preservice assessment of facilities allows audiologists to screen facilities prior to service provision. An audiologist may not wish to provide services to a facility that offers less-than-adequate care to its residents.

Facilities that offer less-than-adequate care may or may not be identifiable through a single visit. Obviously, inadequate facilities may be readily identifiable by unpleasant sights (e.g., ill-kept, half-clothed patients suffering from bedsores), heart-wrenching sounds (e.g., demented patients screaming obscenities or the wails of patients in pain), or by foul smells (e.g., urine and feces). Some inadequate facilities can disguise their shortcomings, however, by only allowing visitors into restricted areas that portray a clean, safe, stimulating, and wholesome environment. Facilities should allow visitors to see all public areas and have an opportunity to talk to residents. Audiologists should realize that even though most facilities conscientiously attempt to meet state and federal guidelines, many still fail to do so. Few are shining examples of where one would want loved ones to spend their remaining days, but many do provide an active, clean, and stimulating environment for residents by offering fun activities such as bingo, weekly visits by beauticians, pet therapy, piano recitals, and so on. Even the best long-term residential care facilities for the elderly periodically have unpleasant occurrences and must face difficult issues with some patients. Above all, all health-care providers and facility personnel should respect residents' rights.

Under federal regulations, all nursing homes must have written policies that describe residents' rights (Careguide, 1998). Nursing homes are required to make this policy available to any resident who requests to see it. A complete "Resident's Bill of Rights" should include patients' rights to:

- be informed of their rights and of the policies of the facility;
- be informed about the facility's services and charges;
- be informed about their medical condition;
- participate in their plan of care;
- choose their own physician;
- manage their own personal finances;
- maintain their privacy and dignity;
- be treated with respect;
- use their own clothing and possessions;
- be free from abuse and restraints;
- voice grievances without retaliation;
- be discharged or transferred only for medical reasons; and
- be accessible (accept or refuse visitors, as well as be guaranteed immediate access for family members, eight visiting hours per day, access for audiologists and other caregivers, confidentiality in communication, and access to legal services).

Audiologists must ensure that neither they nor any one else violate residents' rights. They should inform residents about charges for services, explain the results of audiologic evaluations, seek approval for aural rehabilitation plans, guarantee patients' confidentiality, allow for resident complaints about audiologic services, and understand residents' refusal of services. In addition, audiologists should report any suspected incidents of resident abuse to the appropriate authorities.

ESTABLISHING SUPPORT PROGRAMS IN RESIDENTIAL FACILITIES FOR THE ELDERLY

Clearly, not everyone is suited to provide services to patients in long-term residential care facilities for the elderly. Some cannot cope with the realities; some cannot tolerate the surroundings; others simply prefer to work with other populations. Those audiologists who do wish to practice in these facilities must acknowledge the types of service-delivery models available.

Contract-for-service and fee-for-service service-delivery models are the most common for audiologists practicing in assisted-living/semiindependent and dependent-care facilities. Contract-for-service audiologists in these settings face similar obstacles as those described earlier in this text for individuals practicing in educational settings. Nursing-home personnel may view audiologists as outsiders and refuse to follow directions when serving as audiologic support personnel. *Use of support personnel is critical in providing of optimal hearing health care to patients in long-term residential care facilities when the audiologist cannot be there on a daily basis.* Research has shown that the use of multiskilling and support personnel has been particularly effective in meeting the hearing healthcare needs of nursing-home residents with hearing impairment. Jordon, Worrall, Hickson, and Dodd (1993) investigated the efficacy of group-intervention programs using trained volunteers as agents of intervention with elderly nursing-home residents with hearing impairment. A six-week series of intervention programs was established in which residents could practice newly acquired skills. Results of the study indicated that some residents showed increases in communicative competence from pre- to postintervention. Unfortunately, not all assisted-living/semiindependent and dependent-care facilities attend to patients' hearing healthcare needs, resulting in a deterioration of physical and psychological well being. Consider Chester's experience:

> *Chester, an 84-year-old stroke survivor with a bilaterally severe sensorineural hearing loss was well cared for by his wife of 60 years, Ethyl. Ethyl enjoyed good health all of her life until she suddenly had a massive stroke and passed away. Chester was now all alone in the world except for his adult children John and Theodore, who both had moved to California years ago. Chester was heartbroken but pleased to see his children and their families who came to town to attend Ethyl's funeral. John and Theodore realized that their Dad could no longer live by himself. John's family and Theodore and his family returned to California immediately after the funeral. John stayed behind to help his father with his affairs. Although Chester had difficulty verbalizing and expressing his needs, he understood everything that was said to him when he wore his hearing aids. Chester had enjoyed visiting friends and going to church with his wife, but he was paralyzed on one side, making it difficult for him to insert and remove his hearing aids. Ethyl had done all that, and now she was gone.*
>
> *John put Chester's house up for sale and planned to move him into a nursing home. Chester did not like the idea, but there were few other alternatives. John visited the nursing home to discuss Chester's admission but failed to talk to staff or other residents. John was in a hurry to return to California. He told Chester that he and his family would visit at Christmas. Chester tearfully waved good-bye as he was taken to his room. In the evening, the nurse's assistant took off Chester's hearing aids and put them in his dresser drawer. The next morning, another nurse's assistant dressed Chester, placed him into a wheelchair, and took him to the cafeteria. He kept pointing to the dresser and his ears, but the nurse's assistant thought he was just senile. Chester ate, and then another assistant placed him in front of the television. Chester tried to gain the attention of nursing-home staff by vocalizing and pointing to his ears. They shook their heads and went about their tasks. Chester felt depressed. Soon it was time for lunch, more television, then dinner, and then bedtime. Day after day, Chester went through the same routine. He soon gave up.*
>
> *By Christmas time, Chester was withdrawn and noncommunicative. The staff physician grew increasingly concerned about Chester, who was losing weight and lying in bed all day. John and Theodore were shocked to see how much their Dad had deteriorated in just a few months. When they asked the staff about Chester's hearing aids, they said they didn't know he had any. John found his father's hearing aids pushed to the back of his dresser drawer.*

Unfortunately, this scenario is all too common in long-term care facilities without comprehensive, full-service audiology support programs for residents with hearing impairment. Shultz and Mowry (1995) provided the components of a full-service audiology program in three main areas: (1) patient services, (2) facility services, and (3) special services. Table 8–1 shows the individual components in each of the three areas.

Prior to program initiation, residents and their significant others should be informed of the hearing support program. Appendix VIII-C is an example of an audiologist's letter to patients and significant others, which includes the date and time of an informative meeting explaining all components of hearing support programs. Audiologists may find that residents and their families provide excellent suggestions on program logistics. In addition, these individuals should fill out an informed-consent form for participation in various aspects of the program. Audiologists may have difficulty dealing with residents whose families do not reside in the local community. In this case, audiologists should inquire if elderly residents have a geriatric case manager. Geriatric case managers are state licensed and/or certified professionals who have graduate degrees in the field of human services or the equivalent. They are trained in the assessment, coordination, monitoring, and direct delivery of services to the elderly and their families (Careguide, 1998). They can assist in communicating with residents' families about meeting the hearing health-care needs of their loved one.

Hearing support programs in a long-term residential care facility should ensure continuity of management of residents' hearing health-care needs from admission to discharge. Unlike rehabilitation hospitals, not all nursing-home residents are discharged from these facilities. Many will live the remainder of their lives in assisted-living/semiindependent or dependent-care facilities. Thus, it is imperative to include patients' hearing health-care status as part of

Table 8–1. Components for a full-service audiology program for long-term residential care facilities for the elderly.

Patient Services

- Audiometric and receptive-communication screening
- Individual patient screening report
- Diagnostic hearing evaluation
- Hearing aid fitting
- Hearing aid evaluation
- Hearing aid repair
- Hearing aid maintenance program
- Assistive listening devices: Selection, fitting, and orientation
- Cerumen management program
- Direct consultation with residents, physicians, families, social workers, nursing staff, and significant others
- Weekly in-house visits
- Emergency services

Facility Services

- Ombudsman Reconciliation Act: Receptive communication classification of all new admissions—Minimum Data Sheet (MDS)
- Patient-specific screening report for medical records
- Inservice training for nursing and administrative staff (continuing-education unit (CEU approved))
- Inservice training for ancillary personnel (CEU approved)
- Americans with Disabilities Act (ADA) review and recommendations for compliance
- Family lecture night series

Special Services

- Hospice patient care: Evaluations and loaner amplification devices
- Amplification devices acquired through charitable organizations
- Hearing aid safety cords for patients who cannot manage their own devices because of physical or mental conditions

Source: From "Older Adults in Long-term Care Facilities," by D. Schultz and R. B. Mowry, 1995, pp. 183–184. In P. B. Kricos and S. A. Lesner (Eds.), *Hearing Care for the Older Adult: Audiologic Rehabilitation* (pp. 167–184). Boston: Butterworth-Heinemann. Reprinted with permission.

the preadmission intake interview. Patients and their families should be asked about prior audiologic evaluations, the existence of confirmed or suspected hearing loss, additional communication problems, the history of hearing aid use, and the presence of any other communication disorders. Appendix VIII-D contains a brief case history intake form that can be used for this purpose. Likewise, audiologists and other professionals may find the "Communication/Environment Assessment and Planning Guide" by Lubinski (1995), which appears in Appendix VIII-E, helpful for environmental assessment and subsequent development of plans of action. From this information, audiologists can initiate delivery of patient services.

PATIENT SERVICES

Audiometric and Receptive Communication Screening

All residents, current and newly admitted, should be screened for hearing sensitivity and receptive communication to identify those in need of audiologic or medical services. Hearing screenings and necessary referrals should be made within the first 2 weeks of admission into a long-term care facility (ASHA, 1997a; OBRA, 1987). A variety of professionals can make the referral, including hospital-discharge planners, intake personnel, nurses, social workers, speech-language pathologists, physicians, or home health-care providers.

The Omnibus Budget Reconciliation Act (OBRA, 1987) determined the nature of care delivered to residents in nursing homes. Under this act, all nursing-home residents receiving federal support must be assessed using a standardized form known as the Minimum Data Set for Nursing Home Resident Assessment and Care Screening (MDS). The MDS is administered to all nursing-home residents to obtain a comprehensive approach to assessment, problem identification, and individualized care planning (ASHA, 1997a). Section C of the MDS, "Communication/Hearing Patterns," has two questions used to determine the adequacy of patients' hearing for everyday functioning with patients' hearing instruments. Appendix VIII-F contains these two questions and respective rating scales. If responses to the questions indicate problems, then more detailed assessments are indicated through the Resident Assessment Protocols (RAPs) (ASHA, 1997a).

Otoscopy and pure-tone screening should be completed whenever possible. An otoscopic examination should be completed to rule out the presence of impacted cerumen and collapsing ear canals, as well as to assess the integrity of the tympanic membrane (Shultz & Mowry, 1995). Referrals for cerumen management should be made if necessary. Residents passing the otoscopic inspection and those who have had cerumen management should undergo pure-tone air-conduction screening at 500 (if possible), 1000, 2000, and 4000 Hz at 30 dB hearing level (HL) in a quiet environment (Shultz & Mowry, 1995). If logistical and time constraints do not allow for pure-tone screening, audiologists should consider the following questions for residents (ASHA, 1997a):

- Does the person require repetition of verbal questions, instructions, or messages?
- Has a family member or caregiver voiced concern about the adequacy of the individual's hearing?
- Does the person complain of current or past history of difficulty hearing or understanding?
- Does the person complain of current or past history of head noise, ear pain, or ear discharge?

If a "yes" response is provided to one of these questions or if residents' cognitive condition limits judgments that can made regarding hearing status, a referral should be made for audiologic services, otolaryngologic services, or both (ASHA, 1997a). Other screening tools, such as the *Hearing Handicap Inventory for the Elderly-Screening Version* (HHIE-S) (Ventry & Weinstein, 1982) can be used as well. The use of this instrument is discussed in Chapter 7 and appears in Appendix VII-G. Patients failing hearing screenings should be referred for audiologic evaluation.

Cerumen Management

Cerumen management is within the scope of practice for audiologists (ASHA, 1992; Ballachanda, 1995) and is very useful within long-term residential care facilities (Shultz & Mowry, 1995). Each practitioner should take the following precautions before initiating this part of the hearing support program (ASHA, 1992):

- inform institutional and/or regulatory bodies about limited cerumen management as being within the scope of practice for audiologists;
- check with state and appropriate state licensure boards to determine any limitations or restrictions regarding cerumen management;
- check professional liability insurance for any limitations in coverage in practicing cerumen management;
- follow Universal Precautions;
- know who to contact in the event of an emergency; and
- obtain informed consent from residents.

Audiologists know that cerumen (along with dead batteries) is probably the biggest enemy to successful hearing aid use among elderly individuals in long-term residential care facilities. Therefore, even if audiologists choose not to provide cerumen management, they must be prepared to identify its presence and to make appropriate referrals to ensure that it is done. Otherwise, any attempt to establish support programs for these patients may fail because of simple problems with earwax. Figure 8–5 shows an audiologist performing cerumen management on an elderly patient.

Diagnostic Hearing Evaluation

Audiologic evaluations for nursing-home residents can be difficult for contract-for-service audiologists who may not have the necessary equipment or appropriate test environment available to them on-site. If possible, residents can be transported to facilities with the necessary equipment to carry out routine audiologic evaluations. In addition, portable audiometers equipped with insert earphones may suffice in quieter areas of long-term residential care facilities. Although we discuss and advocate proper guidelines and protocols for audiologic screening and evaluations in this service-delivery site, audiologists must be prepared to make acceptable and appropriate modifications as needed to these standard procedures for elderly patients. Unfortunately, audiologists must frequently provide hearing evaluations in less than optimal acoustic environments in which sound-treated booths are not available, and space for testing may be limited. They may find themselves conducting tests in rooms that are also used as beauty shops, dining halls, and recreational rooms, or in patients' rooms for those who are bedridden. Sometimes, as in testing infants and young children, getting any response from elderly patients is better than getting nothing at all. An appropriate audiologic evaluation should include the following (ASHA, 1997a):

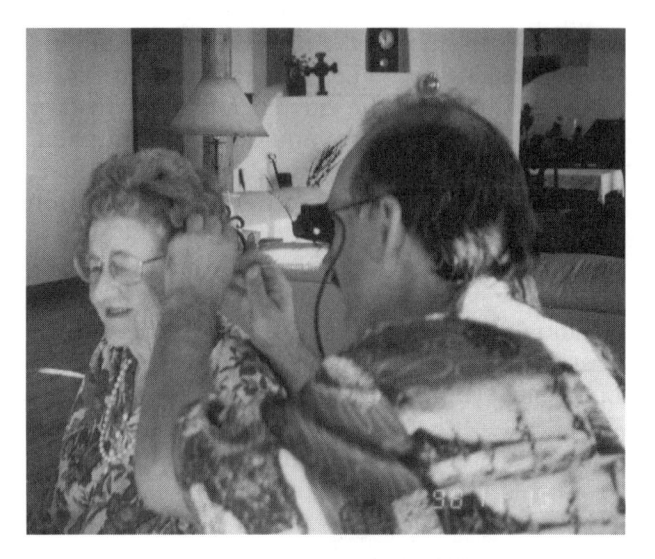

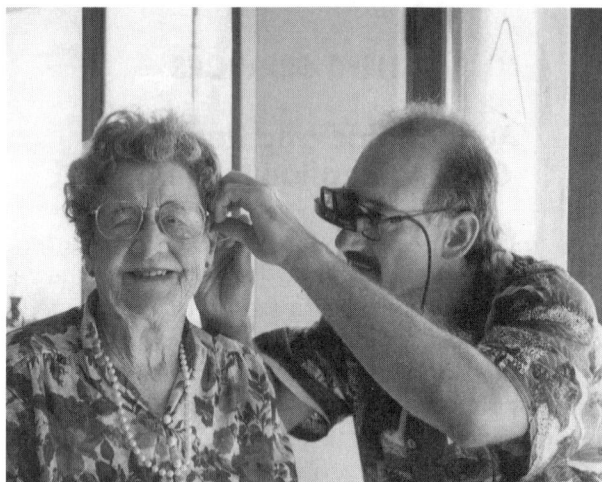

Figure 8–5. Audiologist performing cerumen management on an elderly patient.

- otoscopic examination;
- pure-tone air-conduction testing at 250, 500, 1000, 2000, 3000, 4000, and 8000 Hz, with the frequencies of 250 and 500 omitted if ambient noise levels exceed ANSI standards (ANSI, 1991) or if immittance testing is done;
- pure-tone bone-conduction testing at 250 to 4000 Hz or at those frequencies for which ambient-noise levels are within ANSI standards (ANSI, 1991);
- speech recognition or speech detection thresholds;
- suprathreshold word recognition testing;

- assessment of most comfortable listening levels (MCLs) and loudness discomfort levels (LDLs);
- immittance testing;
- reliable and valid functional communication assessment scale; and
- functional status on an annual basis to determine any significant changes.

Audiologists are reminded that it is often necessary to make modifications in testing procedures for elderly patients. Table 8–2 has some specific suggestions for modifying audiologic test procedures for these patients as provided by Weinstein (1995). When applicable, the audiologic evaluation should include the visual and listening check, electroacoustic analyses, and real-ear probe-tube microphone measurements of residents' hearing aids.

Whenever possible, audiologists should consider performing rehabilitation evaluations on residents. Although difficult, audiologists should strive to design individualized aural rehabilitation plans for each resident. Lesner and Kricos (1995) suggested a holistic approach to aural rehabilitation that includes considering strengths, capabilities, and needs in four global-assessment domains: (1) physical status (general health, visual status, dexterity, and fine motor skills), (2) psychologic status (mental status, motivation, attitude, and depression), (3) sociologic status (financial status, social environment, and physical environment), and (4) communication status (hearing handicap or disability, auditory speech reception, speechreading, audiovisual speech reception, and conversational fluency). Appendix VIII-G contains a quick check sheet of holistic factors to consider when designing individual aural rehabilitation programs for residents.

Residents and their families should be counseled regarding the results of audiologic evaluations. Audiologic counseling should not be taken lightly, as it is the cornerstone of rehabilitative audiology (Erdman, 1993). The effectiveness of counseling determines the success of other hearing-support-program components. Counseling in this situation has two purposes: (1) impart information and (2) discuss the need for hearing aids. Information counseling involves (Sanders, 1993):

Table 8–2. Suggestions for modifications in audiologic evaluation for elderly patients.

Behavior	*Test Modification*
Poor memory	- Simplify instructions - Use repetition - Check comprehension - Use frequent conditioning/reconditioning trials - Offer extensive opportunities for practice - Offer verbal reinforcement and reassurances
Movement deficits	- Evaluate different strategies before initiating testing - Select natural and easy responses - Select responses in patient's behavioral repetoire (e.g., hand raising, waving tissue) - Be consistent in choice of response behavior
Disorientation	- Allow patient to listen to spoken voice prior to initiation of test
Fading attention, Distractable	- Reduce length of test sessions - Limit sessions to a maximum of 20 to 30 minutes - Schedule 2 to 3 sessions, if necessary, to complete the test battery
Slower response time	- Slow down rate of tonal presentation - Allow patient's behavior to dictate the pace
Speech and language	- Evaluate speech reception and word recognition using relevant materials - Use simple commands and common questions - Consider eliminating speech perception testing for patients with severe word-finding difficulties, failing memory of recent events, or reduction of vocabulary

Source: Adapted from "Auditory Testing and Rehabilitation of the Hearing Impaired," by B. E. Weinstein, 1995. In R. Lubinski (Ed.), *Communication and Dementia* (pp. 223–227). San Diego, CA: Singular Publishing Group.

- clearly reporting what you know about the problem,
- using the audiogram to explain how residents' disability impacts communication,
- explaining how others react to communication breakdown,
- explaining side effects (e.g., inattention, memory problems, embarrassment, withdrawal), and
- explaining ways to cope with hearing loss.

Appendix VIII-H contains a protocol by Alpiner, Meline, and Holifield (1990) consisting of a series of questions for audiologists and elderly persons and their families to discuss in preparation for amplification.

Hearing Aid Evaluation and Fitting Program

As stated in Chapter 7, audiologists must be adequately prepared to fit their patients with hearing aids equipped with the latest high-performance hearing aid features. Recall that matching "high-tech" hearing aid features to elderly persons in assisted-living/semiindependent and dependent-care facilities can be a difficult or even an impossible task unless audiologists' hearing aid evaluation, selection, and fitting protocols are complete and up-to-date. Mueller's (1996) description of a complete protocol was discussed in Chapter 7.

There are little or no data suggesting that the elderly have any more difficulty with high-performance hearing aids than do younger patients. A large proportion of residents of assistive-living/semiindependent and dependent-care facilities may benefit from high-performance hearing aids. Keidser (1995) found that age had no effect on patients' benefit in using multimemory hearing aids. Similarly, Kuk (1996) found that age had no effect on patients' benefit from multimicrophone technology. Matching these devices to elderly hearing aid candidates can be problematic, however. Audiologists must consider multiple patient characteristics (e.g., chronic health problems, socioeconomic factors, and so on) that can affect the prognosis for aural rehabilitation and hearing aid use. The selection of appropriate high-performance hearing aid features for elderly patients should focus on: (1) high-performance hearing aid styles, (2) multichannel capabilities, (3) multimemory or programmable hearing aids, (4) multimicrophone technology, and (5) digital hearing aids. While these hearing aids may be quite appropriate for elderly persons in assistive-living/semiindependent situations, audiologists must carefully consider individual patient characteristics when preselecting hearing aids for patients of dependent-care facilities for the elderly.

High-Performance Hearing Aid Styles: Completely-in-the-Canals (CICs)

Completely-in-the-canal (CIC) hearing aids are high-performance technology with numerous advantages including: (1) increased gain, (2) increased output, (3) reduced distortion, (4) minimization of the occlusion effect, (5) reduction of feedback, (6) ease of insertion and removal from the ear, (7) comfort of fit, (8) security of fit, (9) natural telephone use, (10) capability of listening with headsets, (11) no volume-control wheel, (12) improved localization, (13) reduction of wind noise, (14) use during sleep, and (15) cosmetic appeal (Mueller & Ebinger, 1996).

Generally, audiologists should not rule out the use of CIC hearing aids for their elderly patients. In fact, Ebinger, Holland, Holland, and Mueller (1995) found no significant difference between the amount of benefit (as measured by the APHAB) experienced by CIC users who were under or over the age of 75. CIC hearing aids are especially appealing to "cosmetically sensitive" patients (Johnson & Danhauer, 1997a), and it is a mistake to believe that elderly patients are unconcerned about how their hearing aids look (Johnson & Danhauer, 1997b). We see many nursing-home patients who have little or no social life but are still very concerned about how their hearing aids look and want the least noticeable devices possible. CIC hearing aids can be a very appropriate fitting for elderly patients provided audiologists take a holistic approach to considering patient-selection criteria in the four assessment domains (Lesner & Kricos, 1995). Figure 8–6 depicts the decision chart for determining elderly patients' candidacy for CIC hearing aids.

Regarding the communication domain, patients' audiologic profiles are one of the most important considerations in determining the prognosis for CIC candidacy. Generally, CICs are best for patients with hearing loss up to about 60 dB HL in the low frequencies and up to about 80 dB HL in the mid-to-high frequencies (Mueller & Ebinger, 1996; Voll & Jones, 1998). Voll and Jones (1998) described three

COMMUNICATION	PHYSICAL	PSYCHOLOGICAL	SOCIAL
Audiometric Data	Ear	Fear of Stigma and Motivation	Financial/Family Support
Does the patient have ➤ thresholds better than 60 dB HL in the low frequencies and better than 80 dB HL in the highs? ➤ sloping high-fequency hearing loss? ↓ IF SO, THEN THE PATIENT IS A GOOD CIC CANDIDATE. If not, does the patient have a ➤ flat or reverse-slope loss? ➤ steeply sloping loss with normal thresholds up to 2000 Hz? ➤ severe to profound hearing loss? ↓ THEN THE PATIENT MAY BE MORE DIFFICULT TO FIT WITH CICs.	Does the patient's outer ear have ➤ round ear canals? ➤ a medium to firm texture? ➤ average length or long ear canals ➤ easily identifiable 1st and 2nd bends? ➤ minimal jaw movement in the cartilaginous portion? ↓ IF SO, THEN THE PATIENT IS A GOOD CIC CANDIDATE. If not, does the patient have ➤ collapsing ear canals? ➤ short canals? ➤ extremely sharp turns in the ear canals? ➤ straight canals? ➤ excessive jaw movement in the cartilaginous portion? ➤ excessive cerumen? ↓ IF SO, THE PATIENT MAY BE MORE DIFFICULT TO FIT WITH CICs. Does the patient have ➤ growths in the external canal (exostoses or osteomas)? ➤ chronic external otitis with drainage?	Is the patient ➤ cosmetically sensitive? ➤ highly motivated? ↓ IF SO, THEN THE PATIENT IS A GOOD CIC CANDIDATE. Is the patient ➤ depressed? ➤ cognitively impaired? ↓ IF SO, THEN THE PATIENT IS NOT A GOOD CIC CANDIDATE.	Does the patient have ➤ adequate financial resources for CIC purchase? ➤ a supportive family? ➤ supportive caregivers in the residential facility? ↓ IF SO, THEN THE PATIENT IS A GOOD CIC CANDIDATE. If not ↓ THEN THE PATIENT MAY NEED ASSISTANCE FOR FINANCING AND/OR MAY NOT BE A GOOD CIC CANDIDATE, OR MAY NEED ASSISTANCE IN CIC USE FROM A SIGNIFICANT OTHER. Environmental Does the patient have difficulty with the following with other styles of hearing aids: ➤ telephone use? ➤ wind noise? ➤ directionality? ↓ IF SO, PATIENT IS A GOOD CIC CANDIDATE.

Figure 8-6. Decision chart using for assessment domains for considering CICs for elderly patients.
(continued)

	↓ IF SO, THEN THE PATIENT IS A POOR CIC CANDIDATE. Vision Does the patient have good corrected vision? ↓ IF SO, THEN PATIENT IS A GOOD CIC CANDIDATE. If not ➢ is the patient legally blind, even when wearing glasses? ↓ IF SO, THEN THE PATIENT MAY NEED ADDITIONAL PRACTICE, VISUALIZATION AND IMAGERY TECHNIQUES, AND ASSISTANCE. Motor Ability Can the patient ➢ raise his/her arms so that his/her hands are at ear level (proximal-arm function)? ➢ use his/her hands and fingers proficiently to complete tasks requiring manual dexterity? ↓ IF SO, PATIENT IS A GOOD CIC CANDIDATE. If not, PATIENT MAY NEED EXTRA PRACTICE OR ASSISTANCE FROM A FAMILY MEMBER OR FROM FACILITY STAFF FOR CIC USE.		

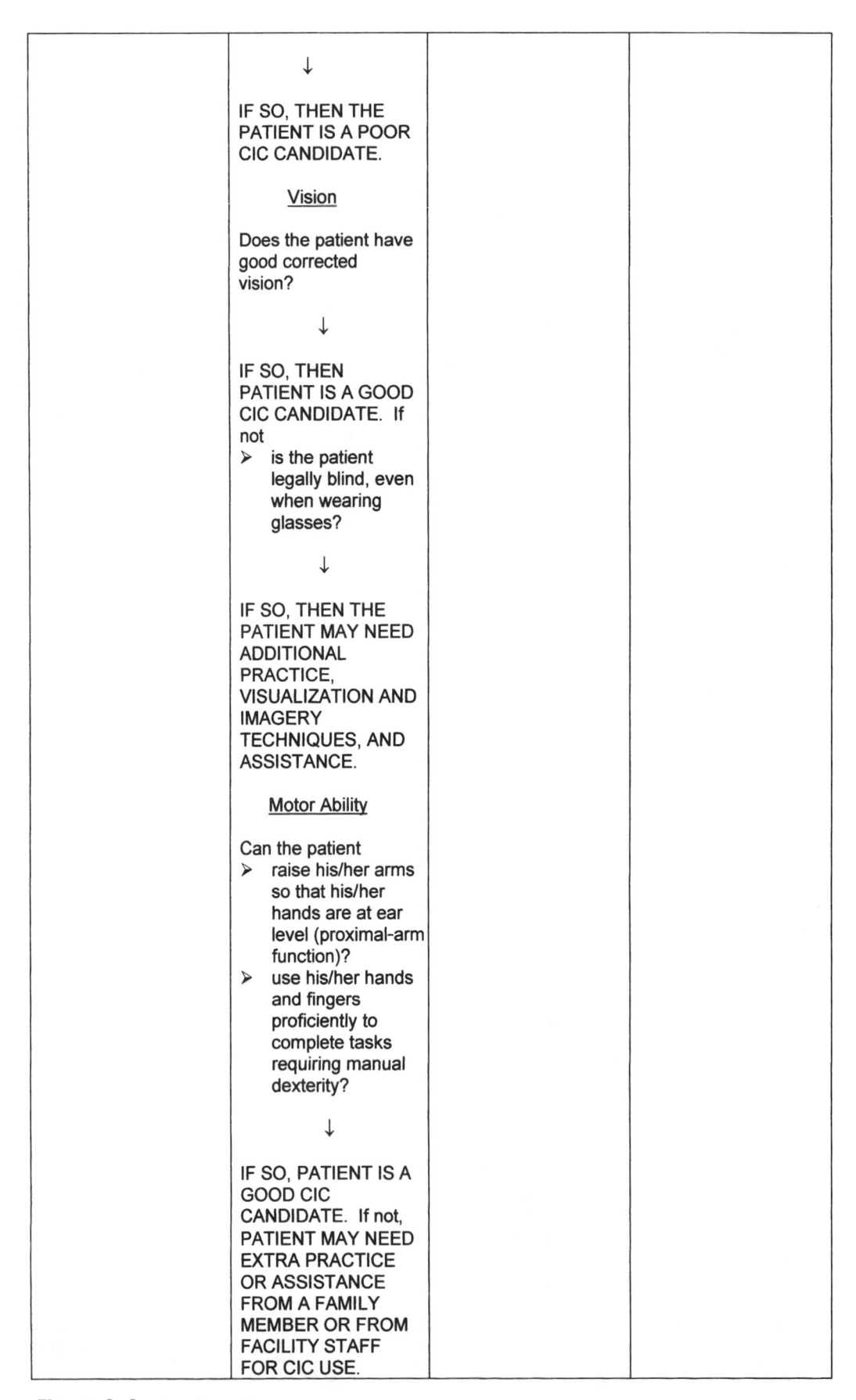

Figure 8-6. *(continued)*

types of hearing losses that are difficult to fit with CICs. First, flat or reverse-slope losses can be difficult to fit because the output from CICs may be unable to reach low-frequency targets. We have found, however, that two-channel and digital CICs with more advanced circuitry can offer the flexibility to reach such losses. Second, sharply sloping losses with normal thresholds out to about 2000 Hz are difficult to fit because patients may have negative reactions to the occlusion effect or circuit noise. In this case, we have found that "step microphones," which essentially eliminate gain below about 1500 Hz, in combination with two-channel and digital circuitry can help with this problem. Third, severe-to-profound hearing losses are difficult to fit because the size of the components needed limits the amount of gain available. Although this is true, we have found that real-ear gain from CICs (especially those with power circuits) often provides substantially more gain (sometimes as much as 10 to 20 dB) in the mid-to-high frequencies than would be expected from coupler measurements. Thus, one should not categorically rule out CICs for all severe losses. Being difficult to fit should not be the sole reason for failing to use CICs with elderly patients. The small size of the CIC may be an issue for patients in long-term residential care facilities for the elderly, however. In case of loss, audiologists should be sure that extended insurance coverage is part of any CIC fitting, as with any style of hearing aid. Hearing health-care professionals should consider important factors in the other assessment domains as well.

With regard to the physical domain, three key areas are important for the determination of CIC candidacy in elderly patients: (1) outer ear characteristics, (2) vision, and (3) proximal-and distal-arm function. First, CICs are best for elderly patients who have round outer ear canals, medium-to-firm outer ear texture, easily discernable first and second bends in the ear canal, and minimum jaw movement in the cartilaginous area (Voll & Jones, 1998). Possible contraindications for CIC candidacy include a collapsing, short, or sharply turning outer ear canal; excessive cerumen; tissue loss; or chronic external otitis (Jahn & Cook, 1997; Voll & Jones, 1998). Fortunately, dynamic impressions and future possibilities with soft-shell technology can assist with troublesome ear canals, but chronic external otitis can still complicate CIC use, especially if there is any type of drainage, which can severely shorten the life of a CIC (Perrie & Arndt, 1997). Elderly patients have a higher incidence of collapsing ear canals, overproduction of cerumen, and loss of tissue than do younger patients (Jahn & Cook, 1997). Use of CICs may push cerumen down the ear canal, and loss of tissue may cause the pinna to sag and misshape the ear canal (Jahn & Cook, 1997). Although not eliminating the possibility of CIC use, these issues must be identified, considered, and dealt with among patients of any age group, but especially among the elderly.

Adequate vision and proximal- and distal-arm function are also positive predictive factors for successful CIC use by elderly patients, especially for manipulating tiny 5A and 10A batteries. Poor vision does not preclude the use of CICs with this population, as it can be overcome with visualization and imagery techniques (Danhauer & Danhauer, 1997) (See Appendix VII-M) and a keen sense of touch (Lesner & Kricos, 1995). Another positive predictive factor for successful CIC use is adequate proximal- and distal-arm function. Proximal-arm function is the ability to raise the arms to an appropriate height in preparation for insertion or removal of CICs from patients' ears (Lesner & Kricos, 1995; Johnson & Danhauer, 1997b). Distal-arm function involves manual dexterity necessary for the insertion of the CIC into the ear and for manipulation of tiny batteries (Lesner & Kricos, 1995; Johnson & Danhauer, 1997b). Deterioration of the sensitivity of the ear canal and fingers may occur in the elderly due to changes in the skin and loss of nerve endings (Lesner & Kricos, 1995). Elderly patients who have poor distal-arm function, but adequate proximal-arm function may find CICs easier to manipulate than other styles of hearing aids. Although insertion may be tricky, removal is easier for elderly patients and their caregivers, who simply have to pull on CIC extraction strings. Moreover, a keen sense of touch is needed to manipulate the volume-control wheels in more conventional styles of hearing aids that are not a user-controlled option on most CICs. The use of nonlinear circuitry helps immensely in this case and makes this option useful for patients in long-term residential care facilities for the elderly who may not be able to manipulate volume-control wheels on their own. In addition, Upfold, May, and Battaglia (1990) found that when using the telephone, elderly patients had more difficulty with behind-the-ear (BTE) hearing aids than any other style. With CICs, elderly patients can use the phone naturally, a potential benefit for nursing-home residents who hope to maintain contact with family and friends. (Before advocating phone use for residents, audiologists should check facility policies.) In summary, elderly patients with manual-dexterity problems may become successful CIC users, provided that they have adequate counseling, practice, and assistance from significant others or caregivers as necessary.

The psychological and social assessment domains also contain important predictive factors for successful CIC use by elderly patients. Motivation and a sensitivity for hearing aid cosmetics are positive psychological patient characteristics for successful CIC use. Cosmetically sensitive elderly patients are excellent candidates for CICs because they are already motivated to be successful at the outset. Patient motivation is often necessary for a successful fit because about 75% of CICs need modification at the time of fitting and around 20% are returned to the manufacturer for modification, requiring several postfitting appointments with the audiologist (Voll & Lyons, 1995). Postfitting appointments may be difficult for some residents in dependent-care facilities if the audiologist is not able to make multiple visits to ensure the proper fit and use of CICs. Necessary postfitting appointments are less of a problem for those in semidependent-care facilities who are able to make visits to the audiologist's office.

Negative psychological patient characteristics for CIC use include depression and cognitive impairments, which make some elderly individuals poor candidates for most other aural rehabilitation efforts as well. Audiologists and other consulting professionals must determine if these diagnoses are accurate, however, and not simply reflections of hearing loss. Similarly, positive social patient characteristics for CIC use include a supportive family and adequate financial resources for their purchase. Unfortunately, many elderly patients on fixed incomes cannot afford CICs that are presently more expensive than more conventional hearing aids. The hearing aid industry must strive to make CIC and other high-performance technology more affordable to increase their availability to patients with modest resources. Other positive-social patient selection criteria for CICs include difficulty with telephone use, aversiveness to wind noise, and localization difficulties with other hearing aid styles (Kochkin, 1996). As mentioned above, elderly patients with poor manual dexterity can be successful CIC users with the daily support of a spouse, significant other, family member, friend, or caregiver who can help with CIC insertion and manipulation of the batteries. Figure 8–7 shows an audiologist instructing an elderly lady on CIC battery insertion.

In summary, the four assessment domains contain numerous positive and negative patient

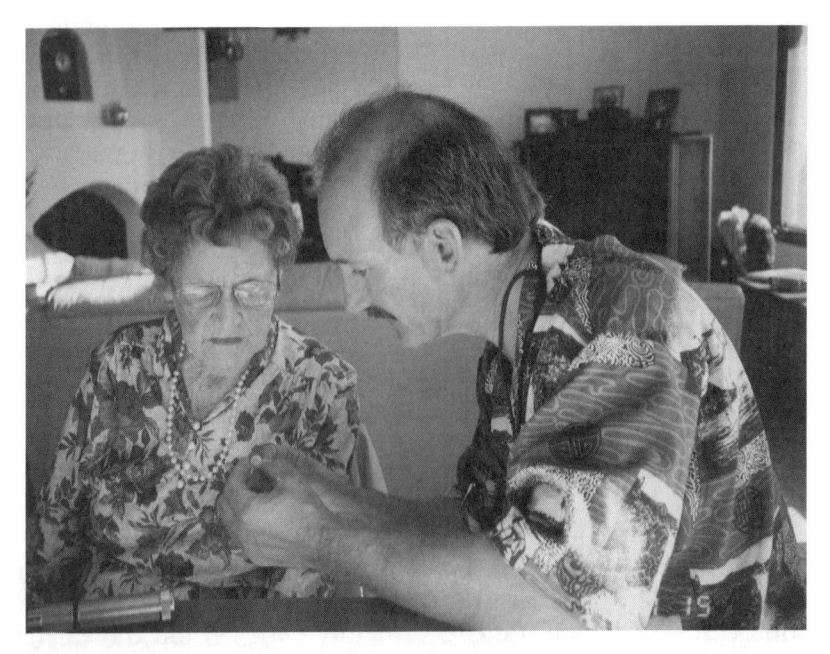

Figure 8-7. Audiologist showing elderly lady how to insert batteries into a CIC.

characteristics that need to be dealt with when considering CICs for elderly patients. Although it is impossible to create a universally applicable decision chart for this purpose, the one presented in Figure 8–6 can be used with the following considerations in mind. First, *each elderly patient is a unique individual and must be managed as such.* Hearing health-care professionals should not prejudge all elderly patients as being poor candidates for CICs just because they share similar characteristics with other elderly CIC users who were unsuccessful. Second, *existence of one negative factor should not preclude the use of CIC instruments for an elderly patient.* Audiologists who are skilled at making ear canal impressions may be successful in fitting CICs on patients with sharply turning or aberrant ear canals. Third, *strengths in one area can overcome weaknesses in others.* Highly motivated but difficult-to-fit patients may have the patience to try anything to make CICs work for them. The decision chart shown in Figure 8-6 can assist audiologists who are considering CICs for their elderly patients.

CICs have one very important benefit for elderly patients: the extraction string. Because CICs offer increased ease in inserting and removing the hearing aid with the extraction string, we now include strings on almost all nursing-home residents' hearing aids. The extraction strings work well on in-the-ear (ITE) and in-the-canal (ITC) hearing aids. Caregivers can use extraction strings rather than battery doors for insertion and removal (which are often broken in the process), which decreases needless repairs. Further, adding the patient's initials and jeweler's loops with bright-colored yarn attached to clothing by alligator clips can reduce hearing aid loss. We caution that they must be taken off before clothing is laundered, however.

Selection of High-Performance Compression Circuitry

Compression systems are nonlinear amplifiers (i.e., the relationship between input and output to the hearing aid is not one-to-one) that are useful for fitting individuals with reduced dynamic ranges (Walker & Dillon, 1982). Compression systems should be fitted to elderly patients for a variety of reasons including (Dillon, 1995): (1) limiting maximum output without distortion, (2) reducing intensity differences between speech syllables, (3) reducing the long-term intensity differences in speech, and (4) improving loudness normalization. Today a wide variety of high-performance compression circuitry exists for audiologists to use with their elderly patients who often require less gain and have greater recruitment than younger listeners with similar hearing losses (Holmes, 1995). Selection of high-performance compression circuitry can be difficult to master and match to particular patient characteristics considering the complex terminology (e.g., automatic gain control, automatic signal processing, single-channel, multichannel, etc.) and proprietary jargon used by manufacturers in attempt to distinguish their products from those of others. Hickson (1994) presented a complete description of much of the compression circuitry presently available. Although a holistic approach has been advocated here, selection of high-performance hearing aid circuitry for elderly patients is heavily based on audiometric information from the communication assessment domain. Figure 8–8 illustrates a simple decision chart for selecting high-performance compression circuitry for elderly patients.

As mentioned earlier, although patients' most comfortable listening levels (MCLs) and loudness discomfort levels (LDLs) traditionally have been obtained for speech stimuli, more descriptive patient loudness growth data should be considered for the selection of high-performance compression circuitry. VIOLA software, for example, provides input-output functions in two frequency regions (e.g., 500 and 3000 Hz) based on loudness ratings obtained from the Contour Test of the Independent Hearing Aid Fitting Forum protocol (IHAFF, 1994; Cox, 1995). These two input-output functions can be used to determine patients' needs for either single-channel or multichannel compression. Single-channel systems uniformly compress the input signal across the entire frequency response, while multichannel systems filter the input signal into a number of frequency bands for independent adjustment of gain and compression characteristics. Single-channel compression can be considered for patients with similar input-output functions for both low and high frequencies, while multichannel should be selected for patients whose functions differ across frequencies. Usually, measures like VIOLA and the Contour Test of the IHAFF protocol may be too complicated to perform in many nursing-home facilities with portable equipment. Thus, single-channel compression is used more often in these circumstances. Multichannel options should,

Does patient have a reduced dynamic range?
↓

| If not, then either select linear or nonlinear systems, depending on patients' profile and needs | ⇔ | If so, perform frequency-specific, input-output functions (e.g., VIOLA for 500 & 3000 Hz); proceed to decision chart below. |

| If dynamic range is the same across frequency range, then select: SINGLE-CHANNEL COMPRESSION. | If dynamic range is different across frequency range, then select: MULTICHANNEL COMPRESSION. |

⇓ ⇓ ⇓ ⇓

| If severely reduced dynamic range and poor word-recognition scores, select compression with lower input levels (e.g., AGC or syllabic compression). | If wide dynamic range and relatively good word-recognition scores, select compression for high input levels (e.g., compression limiting or K-AMP). | If hearing sensitivity in the low frequencies is normal or near-normal, select lower compression threshold for low-frequency regions to reduce upward spread of masking. | If dynamic range is severely reduced in high-frequency region, select higher compression levels for this region to improve intelligibility. |

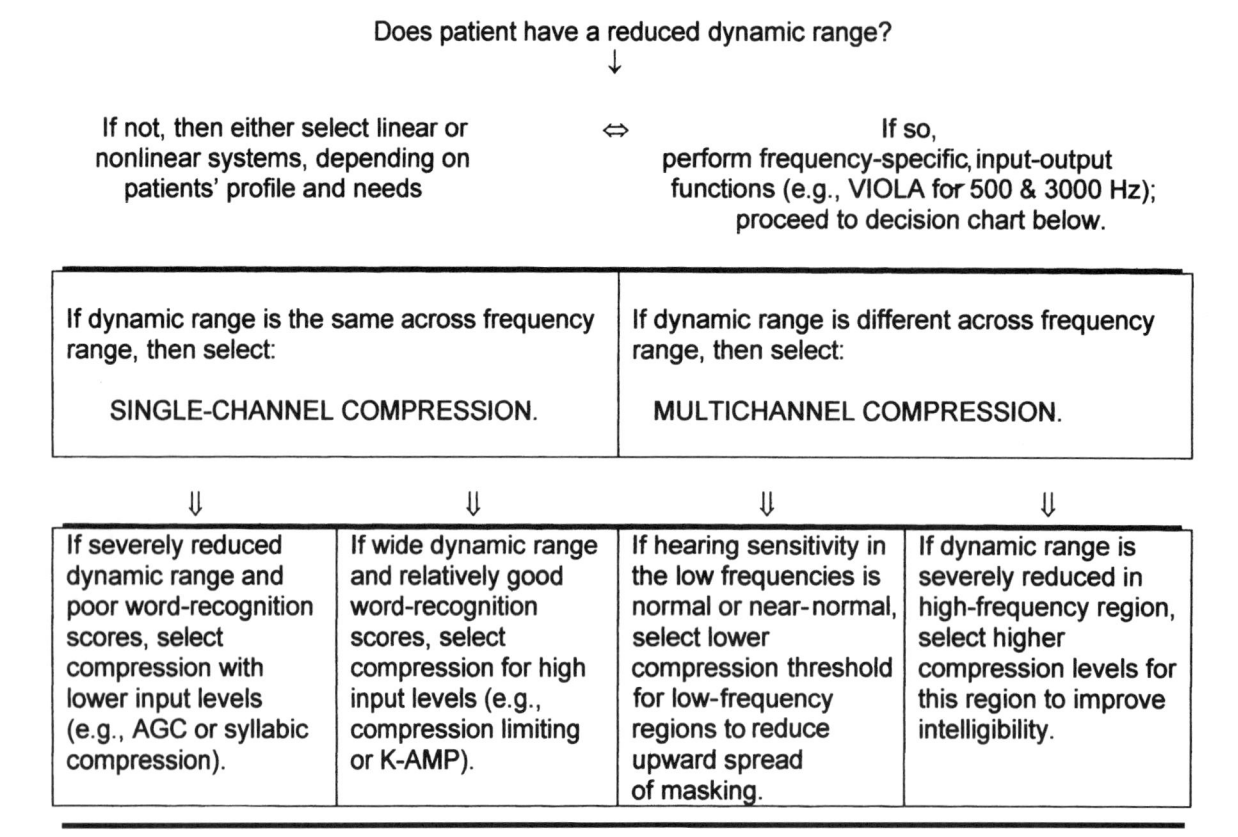

Figure 8–8. Decision chart for considering high-performance compression circuitry for elderly patients.

however, be available for high-functioning residents, particularly those who are able to leave the facility for appointments to the audiologist's office and home where such circuitry would be appropriate.

Single-Channel Systems. When single-channel compression is used, audiologists should select the type that would be most beneficial for each elderly patient's needs. Hickson (1994) stated that types of single-channel compression vary on the basis of both static (i.e., compression threshold and compression ratio) and dynamic (i.e., attack and release times) characteristics. The four main types of single-channel compression are:

- **Syllabic compression systems:** characterized by short attack times, short release times, low-compression thresholds, and low-compression ratios
- **Automatic gain control (AGC) systems:** characterized by low-compression thresholds and high-compression ratios
- **Compression limiting systems:** characterized by short attack times, high-compression thresholds, and high-compression ratios

- **K-AMP systems:** four-stage amplifiers with the greatest gain for low-level inputs, less gain for moderate levels, no gain for high levels, and compression limiting for the highest levels.

Referring to Figure 8–8, compression circuits that have low-compression thresholds provide wide dynamic range compression (WDRC). Kuk (1998) stated that patients with the following characteristics benefit most from wide dynamic range compression (WDRC): (1) mild-to-moderate hearing losses, (2) relatively good word recognition, (3) severe intolerance to moderately intense sounds, and (4) communication situations that are mostly quiet or mildly noisy. For patients who have a severely reduced dynamic range and poor word-recognition scores, however, AGC and syllabic compression systems may also be good choices. Dillon (1995) stated that the loudness differences between syllables might appear greater to patients with loudness recruitment than to individuals with normal hearing sensitivity. He explained that when the most intense syllables are heard at levels that are as loud as is comfortable, the less intense syllables may not be heard at all or at sensation levels below those required for correct identification, particularly in nursing-home environments where noise is loud and ever present. For many patients, both AGC and syllabic compression systems offer low-compression thresholds and optimal level differences between syllables that enhance speech intelligibility within a reduced dynamic range. Alternatively, for elderly patients with wider dynamic ranges and relatively good word recognition, compression limiting or K-AMP systems may provide enhanced listening at low levels, along with sufficient compression at higher input levels.

Multichannel compression systems can provide flexibility in the selection of compression characteristics for different frequency regions when needed (Keidser, Dillon, & Byrne, 1996). When hearing sensitivity in the low-frequency region is normal or near-normal, use of a lower compression for the low-frequency bands should assist in the reduction of the upward spread of masking and possibly improve speech intelligibility. If the dynamic range in the higher frequency region is severely reduced, then increased compression (higher compression ratios) may be needed for the higher frequency bands to enhance intelligibility within the restricted dynamic range.

The social domain should also be considered in the selection of multichannel compression features. For example, Keidser (1995) found that substantial high-frequency compression is preferred for ease in the understanding of multiple talkers whose voices differ in overall level by 10 dB in quiet environments. Similarly, Keidser found that low-frequency compression may improve speech understanding in environments with significant low-frequency background noise, such as multitalker babble. In summary, although selection of these features cannot be relegated to a simple decision chart as shown in Figure 8–8, it can provide a starting point for audiologists to use this circuitry for their elderly patients. Specific living arrangements and the health status of elderly patients will help dictate whether this technology is appropriate.

Selection of Other High-Performance Hearing Aid Features: Multimemory, Multimicrophones, and Digital Hearing Aids

Multimemory hearing aids have more than one set of electroacoustic characteristics that can be controlled by the hearing aid user (Fabry, 1996). Although multimemory hearing aids have received a high degree of patient satisfaction (Kochkin, 1996), they may not be for everyone. Sweetow and Shelton (1996) stated that patient satisfaction depends on audiologists' instrumentation skills and programming abilities, as well as their ability to convey realistic expectations and match these features appropriately to patients. Because patient selection criteria for multimemory hearing aids often encompasses much more than audiologic considerations, a holistic approach is useful when fitting elderly patients. Figure 8–9 shows a decision chart for considering multimemory hearing aids for elderly patients.

The social assessment domain is perhaps the most important area for considering the use of multimemory hearing aids for elderly patients. Multimemory hearing aids are probably not necessary for retired persons who live alone, rarely socialize, and simply wish to hear the television or radio a little bit better (Fabry, 1996). Likewise, they typically are not appropriate for patients in dependent-care facilities. Fabry stated that in many cases, however, hearing healthcare professionals should not preclude the use of multimemory hearing aids based on elderly patients' *present* lifestyle, but rather on their vision of what they would like their lives to be like in the future. Recall that many elderly persons become less social and are forced to stay at home because of their current hearing handicaps. Likewise, patients in dependent-care facilities, when left without amplification, tend to withdraw and have similar experiences to that of Chester, who was discussed in an earlier example. Multimemory hearing aids may help them in different situations. Similarly, elderly persons living in assisted-living/semiindependent-care facilities who have active lifestyles or who wish to expand their horizons to include more activities are good candidates for multimemory hearing aids.

Aside from lifestyle, elderly patients who have difficulty with speech recognition in reverberant and noisy environments (e.g., nursing homes) may be good candidates for multimemory hearing aids. In fact, the elderly are considered "special listeners" because they have a relatively more difficult time with speech recognition in reverberation and noise than do young adults (Nabelek & Nabelek, 1994). Long-term residential care facilities are noted for having excessive noise, and in some cases multimemory hearing aids may be quite appropriate for higher functioning residents in these environments. Use of the *Abbreviated Profile Hearing*

Determination of Candidacy for Multimemory Hearing Aids

SOCIAL	COMMUNICATION	PSYCHOLOGICAL
<u>Lifestyle</u> Does the patient ➤ have an active lifestyle requiring communication in difficult acoustic conditions? ➤ have a desire to expand his/her social life to include activities requiring communication in difficult acoustic conditions? ➤ not mind carrying a programmer (in purse or pocket)? ➤ have a facility staff who can assist him/her with programmer? ↓ IF SO, PATIENT IS A GOOD MULTIMEMORY HEARING AID CANDIDATE. If not, does the patient live a solitary life in a quiet environment? ↓ IF SO, THEN PATIENT MAY NOT BE A GOOD MULTIMEMORY HEARING AID CANDIDATE. <u>Physical Environment</u> Does the patient frequently communicate in difficult acoustic conditions involving ➤ noise? ➤ reverberation? ↓ IF SO, THEN PATIENT IS A GOOD MULTIMEMORY HEARING AID CANDIDATE. If not,	<u>Audiometric Data</u> Does the patient have ➤ an average high-frequency hearing loss (mean @ 2000, 3000, & 4000 Hz) of greater than or equal to 55 dB HL? ➤ a possibility of adjusting low-frequency gain by 5 dB? ↓ IF SO, PATIENT IS A GOOD MULTIMEMORY HEARING AID CANDIDATE.	Does the patient ➤ like to control his/her environment? ➤ seem flexible? ➤ seem motivated? ↓ IF SO, THEN THE PATIENT IS A GOOD MULTIMEMORY HEARING AID CANDIDATE.

Figure 8–9. Decision chart for considering multimemory hearing aids for elderly patients. *(continued)*

↓		
PATIENT MAY NOT BE A GOOD MULTIMEMORY HEARING AID CANDIDATE.		

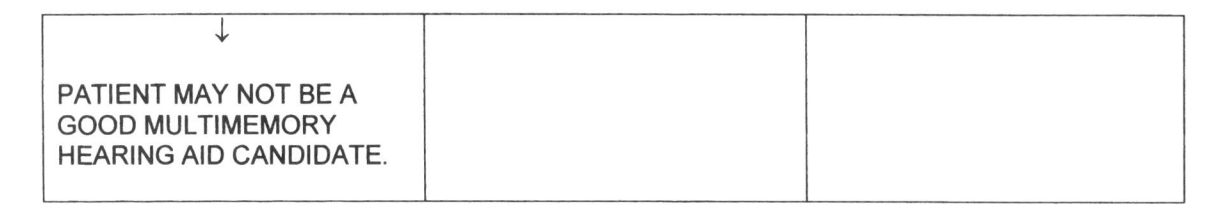

Selection of Multimemory Features

Number of Memories	Types of Processing	Remote Control or Button on Hearing Aid
Does patient have, need, or want a volume-control wheel? ↓ IF SO, THEN TWO TO THREE PROGRAMS SHOULD BE ENOUGH. If not ↓ SEVEN OR EIGHT MAY BE NEEDED PROVIDING TWO TO THREE VOLUME SETTINGS FOR EACH RESPONSE.	If patient communicates ➢ in quiet meetings with two or more talkers whose levels differ by at least 10 dB ↓ THEN USE HIGH-FREQUENCY COMPRESSION. ➢ in low-frequency background noise ↓ THEN REDUCE GAIN AND OUTPUT IN LOW FREQUENCIES. ➢ on the phone with significant feedback ↓ THEN USE RESPONSES THAT ATTENUATE ABOVE 3000 Hz.	Does patient have manual-dexterity problem? ↓ IF SO, THEN USE REMOTE CONTROL. Is patient absent-minded? ↓ IF SO, THEN USE BUTTON ON HEARING AID. Does patient mind using remote control? ↓ IF NOT, USE REMOTE CONTROL. IF SO, USE BUTTON ON HEARING AID OR SOME OTHER STYLE CIRCUIT.

Figure 8–9. *(continued)*

Aid Benefit (APHAB) (Cox & Alexander, 1995) and the *Client Oriented Scale of Improvement* (COSI) (Dillon, James, & Ginis, 1997) with elderly patients may assist the audiologist in this regard. Time and residents' limitations may preclude use of formal versions of these tests, but modified versions of these scales can be adapted for patients as appropriate.

Elderly patients' limited incomes are also obstacles to their use of multimemory hearing aids. Unfortunately, the cost of these hearing aids is too high for many who live on a limited or fixed income. Fabry (1996) believed that the industry must find ways of efficiently and economically marketing these devices to this population.

The psychological assessment domain also has important considerations for the possible use of multimemory hearing aids with elderly patients. Those who are flexible and desire to have some control over their environment may be good candidates for multimemory hearing aids (Fabry, 1996). Many elderly patients' need for psychological control over communication in social settings may hasten their decision to seek high-performance hearing solutions, including those provided by multimemory hearing aids (Garstecki & Erler, 1998). Certainly, we all have patients well into their 80s who are still very active socially, and may entertain, hold positions on boards, interact frequently with their families, and even date. For many of them, the benefits of high-performance hearing aid features outweigh their increased costs. Whether this is the case for all elderly persons in long-term residential care facilities must be determined on an individual basis, but it may be applicable for those in assisted-living/semidependent levels of care.

Audiometric data from the communication assessment domain is also important when considering multimemory hearing aids for elderly patients. Specifically, Keidser, Dillion, and Byrne (1995) and Keidser et al. (1996) found that multimemory hearing aids work well for patients who have an average high-frequency hearing loss of 55 dB HL (at 2000, 3000, and 4000 Hz) and for whom low-frequency gain can be varied by at least 5 dB. Once an elderly patient has been deemed to be a good candidate for multimemory hearing aids, then other decisions must be made regarding the number of memories, how parameters are varied in different listening conditions, and whether a remote control or button on the hearing aid itself should be used. Fabry (1996) stated that if elderly patients' hearing aids have a volume-control wheel (VCW), then two to three memories should suffice; if not, then seven to eight memories may be needed with two or three volume settings for each response. Audiologists who routinely work with elderly patients know that two to three memories are challenging enough to master and that seven or eight would be problematic even for younger patients. If patients have difficulty with background noise, then one program could reduce the gain and output in the low frequencies relative to the standard response (Fabry, 1996; Keidser, 1995; Keidser et al., 1996). Again, high-frequency compression should be considered for situations involving multiple talkers whose voices differ in overall level by at least 10 dB in quiet environments such as meetings (Keidser, 1995; Keidser et al., 1996). In addition, a second program that attenuates the frequencies above 3000 Hz would help patients who have difficulty with feedback during telephone use (Fabry, 1996). Audiologists will need to consider whether to use remote controls or buttons on the hearing aids for elderly patients on an individual basis. Fabry (1996) suggested that absent-minded patients should not use remote controls that can be lost easily; this would probably be the case for many patients in long-term residential care facilities for the elderly. If patients often misplace their keys, they are not good candidates for remote controls. Alternatively, remote controls could be helpful for elderly patients with limited distal-arm function or manual-dexterity problems (Fabry, 1996; Lesner & Kricos, 1995).

Multimicrophone technology (e.g., Phonak's Audio-Zoom) is another high-performance programmable hearing aid feature that may be beneficial for elderly patients. The Audio-Zoom is a three-memory programmable hearing instrument that employs multiple-microphone technology (MMT) to achieve the switchable directional effect by having two omnidirectional microphones in the hearing aid case (Kuk, 1996). Etymotic Research has recently designed and marketed a directional microphone circuit that can be used with traditional ITE hearing aids. These directional microphones may be an important option for elderly patients in noisy listening environments because it can be accessed through a switch on the faceplate rather than through a special programmer. As mentioned earlier, Kuk (1996) found that age had no effect on listeners' satisfaction or ability to benefit from this technology. Elderly patients who need to communicate face-to-face with individuals in environments such as noisy restaurants, bingo parlors, bridge tournaments, and so on should benefit from multimicrophone technology.

Digital hearing aids are rapidly becoming favorites of patients, audiologists, and the industry. Although until recently only two manufacturers provided digital instruments, their popularity, flexibility, ease of fitting, and availability in all hearing aid styles (including CICs) is a strong indication that more and more manufacturers will add digital devices to the market in the near future. Presently the increased cost is the main impediment to market penetration of digital hearing aids, especially to elderly consumers on limited or fixed incomes. It is hoped that prices will be reduced in the future. So far, everything we have said about other high-performance hearing aid features is also true for digital circuitry. Digital technology takes some time and effort from audiologists to learn about the nuances of each device so that they can make them available to their patients. Many elderly patients can afford and do desire digital technology. For them, the benefits outweigh the costs, but it is important to ensure that extended insurance coverage is in effect. We should not rule out digital devices for elderly patients.

In summary, a holistic approach is needed to match high-performance hearing aid features to the many characteristics of elderly patients. Experienced audiologists know that there are no "easy answers" for achieving high-performance hearing solutions for elderly patients, especially in long-term residential care facilities. It is hoped that this discussion has provided a starting point for clinicians who must determine elderly patients' candidacy for high-performance hearing aid features.

One may ask why we spent so much time discussing high-performance hearing aid features for elderly patients in long-term residential care facilities. Recall that we have covered a continuum of living options in which elderly persons may find themselves, ranging from independent-living environments to acute-care settings. Because support programs for residents who have hearing impairments should be adapted to the specific population being served, and because amplification systems available today cover a broad spectrum, we felt that it was important to present high-performance hearing solutions for higher functioning elderly patients. Later on in the chapter, less technical amplification devices are discussed (i.e., pocket talkers) for lower-functioning patients. As there is a range of living experiences that elderly patients encounter, there is also a continuum of amplification options available. It is up to the audiologist to match appropriate amplification systems to each patient.

Hearing Aid Delivery

New hearing aid users should be given instructions describing the care, maintenance, use, and appropriate expectations of hearing aids. Recall that Appendix VII-K contains handouts for the hearing aid delivery. Modifications to those materials may be needed for elderly residents. Audiologists may find, for example, that enlarging the font on the handouts may be helpful to those residents with visual problems. In addition, significant others should attend residents' hearing aid deliveries, if possible. Spouses, close friends, or family members who live nearby or in the same long-term residential care facility should attend the residents' hearing aid delivery. These individuals can assist residents with the hearing aid adjustment process. Residents should also be required to demonstrate basic hearing aid skills to promote their independence. If possible, residents should be required to insert and remove their hearing aids, manipulate the batteries, and even perform basic visual and listening checks on their hearing instruments. During the hearing aid delivery, audiologists can determine residents' level of assistance required for hearing aid care, maintenance, and use.

Audiologists must realize that hearing aid deliveries to elderly patients in these long-term residential care facilities can be quite time-consuming. Audiologists cannot simply drop them off at the nurse's station and hope that they will make it to the patient. Some elderly persons need additional time and practice to master the most simple of tasks. Sometimes providing instructions in the simplest way can cue these individuals into succeeding at certain aspects of hearing aid care. Elderly persons often forget which way to turn the volume-control wheel to make the sound louder or softer, for example. One effective strategy has been to use a picture showing that turning the wheel forward (i.e., toward the eyes) makes the sound louder (i.e., demonstrated with a large font) and turning the wheel backward (i.e., away from the eyes) makes the sound softer (i.e., depicted with a small font). In addition, elderly residents with memory problems may forget the sequence of steps necessary to use their hearing aids on the telephone. Behind-the-ear hearing aids with telecoils can be especially problematic for elderly hearing aid users.

Sometimes providing residents with a simple list of steps, printed in a large font, that can be placed near the phone can help tremendously. We cannot stress enough the importance of supervised practice in learning these skills, particularly the use of hearing aids on the telephone. Elderly persons must be quick in accessing the telecoils on their hearing aids, for example, because the person calling them may hang up after only a few rings. Also when initiating calls, elderly persons must be able to hear the dial tone and dial the appropriate numbers in the allotted time before the call is disconnected.

Hearing aid use and maintenance skills can be included in OT and PT rehabilitation plans for residents who have a particularly difficult time with these tasks. Via multiskilling, members of these departments must have knowledge of the sequence of motor skills involved in the insertion and removal and care of hearing aids. Appendix VII-L contains an informational sheet for OT and PT staff that presents the sequence of steps for each of these tasks. Furthermore, residents who are current CIC wearers or who are fit with this style of hearing aid at the facility may have difficulty inserting these aids into their ears. (Refer to Appendix VII-M.)

Hearing Aid Monitoring and Maintenance

All residents who own or who are fit with hearing aids should participate in a hearing aid monitoring and maintenance program upon consent. The hearing aid monitoring and maintenance program is exactly the same as that described in Chapter 7, "Establishing Support Programs in Rehabilitation Hospitals" and has four levels of assistance for care of residents' hearing aids: (1) independent, (2) partial assistance, (3) full assistance, and (4) supervised use (ASHA, 1997a). All of the necessary forms can be found in the appendices of Chapter 7, including signs placed over residents' beds indicating that special assistance with hearing aids may be needed. Some patients who cannot manage their own devices due to physical or mental conditions may require the use of hearing aid safety cords. As described earlier, many patients may need the nursing staff to insert their hearing aids in the morning and remove them at bedtime. The hearing aids of some residents who need full assistance and those who need supervised use should be locked in the nurse's cart at night for safekeeping. Because the cart may contain several hearing aids that look alike, the chance of loss or misplacement is high. The use of the patients' initials on the shells of their hearing aids avoids confusion. The initials can either be placed in the shell by the manufacturer during fabrication or engraved by the audiologist. The hearing aid monitoring and maintenance program ensures that residents' hearing aids are worn, safe, and functioning properly, which is critical for improving their quality of life (Bridges & Bentler, 1998). Ideally, residents' hearing aids should undergo a complete visual and listening check each day. Recall that the visual and listening check procedures vary according to the level of assistance needed for hearing aid care.

The success of hearing aid monitoring and maintenance programs depends on the communication infrastructure among audiologists, physicians, ancillary personnel, social workers, residents, and their families. Figure 8–10 shows a model communication network that works between and among these professionals, residents, and significant others.

Again, communication is the key. Residents must have direct and efficient ways to notify staff members about problems with their hearing aids; the staff may then request immediate assistance with malfunctioning hearing aids from audiologists. Therefore, audiologists must identify which staff members will serve as audiologic support personnel through selection of an appropriate multiskilling model. Most often, members of the nursing staff serve in this capacity. In this case, both collateral (i.e., registered nurses) and collateral-subordinate (i.e., licensed-practical nurses and nurse's assistants) models are used. In addition, audiologists must be diplomatic in their requests for staff to participate as audiologic support personnel and use the appropriate lines of communication. Audiologists should talk to both the director of the nursing department and administrators when requesting the participation of the staff as audiologic support personnel, for example.

Audiologists and audiologic support personnel must maintain a high profile in the facility so that everyone will know who has the training to assist residents with their hearing aids. Ideally, audiologists should make weekly visits to these facilities to maintain personal contact with residents and maintain the necessary professional visibility for support-program viability. In reality, this will rarely happen. Therefore, audiologists should have their office phone number and e-mail address posted throughout the facility so that residents and staff members can consult directly with audiologists at most any time. E-mail can be a far more efficient method of communication than phone calls. Unlike phone messages, e-mail does not get jumbled by receptionists or lost on someone's desk. Audiologists must be diligent in reading and responding to their e-mail, however. Although it is rarely necessary, audiologists must be willing to make emergency visits to the facility as needed. Unfortunately, many of these calls are the result of problems that have simple so-

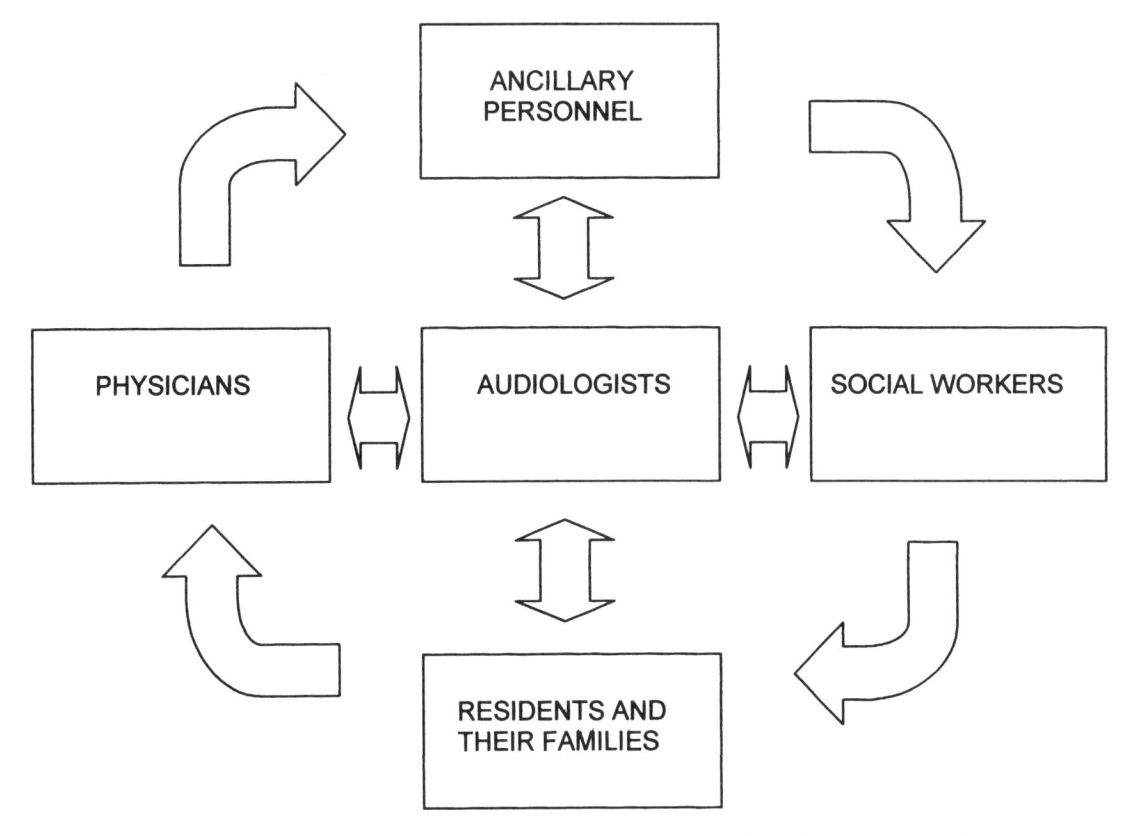

Figure 8-10. Communication network for support programs in long-term residential care facilities for the elderly.

lutions. In the future, audiologists will be able to consult with facility personnel through videoconferencing via the Internet. This may resolve many potential problems without having to leave the office.

Group and Individual Aural Rehabilitation Services

Group Aural Rehabilitation Programs

Group aural rehabilitation in long-term residential care facilities has been found to be beneficial for residents with hearing impairment, their significant others, and audiologists (Hull, 1995; Kricos & Lesner, 1997; Krutt & Shea, 1998; Lesner, 1995). Several different levels of group therapy may be needed for long-term residential care facilities that provide several levels of care. Audiologists may want to group residents by the level of assistance needed with daily tasks such as managing their hearing aids. Group aural rehabilitation sessions are particularly beneficial for residents who are new hearing aid wearers. In addition, establishment of ongoing "Hearing Clubs" can be instrumental in optimizing and maintaining residents' communication skills. Unfortunately, there are few prepackaged group aural rehabilitation programs for elderly residents in long-term residential care facilities (Krutt & Shea, 1998), and audiologists may have to construct their own programs to meet their groups' special needs.

Group aural rehabilitation sessions should be an ongoing aspect of support programs for residents of long-term care facilities. Audiologists should schedule group sessions as needed for those residents who are new hearing aid wearers. Residents who are alumni or experienced hearing aid users may wish to receive refresher courses periodically as well. The added stimulation provided can be helpful for them even if they have already learned to manage their hearing aids. In turn, they serve as role models and mentors for the new hearing aid wearers in the group. Group aural rehabilitation sessions should be advertised throughout the facility for all interested residents to see. Ideally, the group should have between 6 and 10 members, which is small enough to allow residents to get involved if they want to, yet large enough to reduce any pressure they may feel to participate (Lesner, 1995).

Preparations for group aural rehabilitation sessions involve scheduling meeting times, selecting topics, orientating members, selecting the environment, and creating an atmosphere of trust. Generally, group aural rehabilitation sessions should be scheduled for 1 to 1½ hours for 4 to 5 consecutive weeks, meeting on the same day, and at the same time if possible (Lesner, 1995). Some audiologists, however, prefer scheduling five sessions during a 2-week period (Krutt & Shea, 1998). The scheduling of sessions for group aural rehabilitation can have a significant impact on the success of the program (Krutt & Shea, 1998) and involves the consideration of several factors. First, audiologists should schedule adult group aural rehabilitation sessions on the same day of weekly visits to the facility for cost effectiveness. It is not uncommon for members of the group to have particular problems with their hearing aids that can be dealt with directly before the session. Second, audiologists should select a time of day that is conducive for all potential members of the group. Group sessions should be scheduled in the mid-to-late morning or about 1 or 2 hours after lunch when residents are up, bathed, dressed, and have had a meal so they are more alert (Hull, 1995; Krutt & Shea, 1998). Recall that many elderly individuals take quite a bit longer than younger people to awaken and get ready for the day, especially if they need assistance with dressing, medications, or wheelchairs. Third, sessions should be scheduled such that they do not conflict with residents' favorite activities, such as organized facility events. Also, residents may not attend if sessions are scheduled during their favorite television shows. Audiologists should be sensitive to these issues. Fourth, scheduling of sessions depends of the availability of the room selected for group aural rehabilitation sessions. In busy nursing homes where space is limited, it is not uncommon for the same room to be used for numerous activities. Although it may not always be possible, audiologists should try to use the same room for all session to avoid confusion.

Some scheduling problems can be eliminated if administrators designate a room in the facility for all aural rehabilitation support-program activities including, but not limited to, hearing screening, cerumen management, ALD center, resource library, and group aural rehabilitation sessions. Audiologists should be selective if given several rooms to choose from, which is not very likely to be the case. If at all possible, these factors should be considered when selecting a site (Lesner, 1995):

- Sufficient space
- Accessibility for people with handicaps
- Low ambient noise (low S/N and use of assistive listening devices)
- Nonskid carpeting, as opposed to scatter rugs
- Comfortable temperature
- Adequate ventilation
- Sufficient lighting with minimal glare
- No distractions
- Appropriate acoustic environment
- Large easy-to-read signs posted at eye level
- Comfortable seating, that provides support, and is easy for residents to lower themselves onto and rise up from

In addition, seating arrangements should allow participants to be close to each other and at optimal angular orientations for speechreading (Lesner, 1995). The optimal angle for speechreading is 0 to 45 degrees (Tye-Murray, 1998). In addition, audiologists should try not to use tables, but simply arrange participants' chairs or wheelchairs into a semicircle to increase the intimacy and reduce the distance among participants (Lesner, 1995). Audiologists should use audiologic support personnel to help manage the group. These individuals can sit beside participants with visual problems or provide needed assistance during group activities. Figure 8–11 shows an optimal room arrangement for group aural rehabilitation sessions. It is also a good idea to have an adequate supply of tissues, paper towels, and drinking water available because many patients will have coughing spells, drooling, and so forth that could otherwise interrupt the group if you had to go search for such items when they are needed. In addition, sessions should be situated as close to a wheelchair accessible restroom as possible.

Creating a supportive environment for group aural rehabilitation sessions begins with the administrators' commitment to support audiologists' efforts in managing residents' hearing health-care needs. Administrators generally do not support programs that they believe do not improve residents' level of independence, quality of life, and self-esteem (Kemp, 1990). Facility personnel generally know administrators' attitudes toward hearing support programs. Unfortunately, aural rehabilitation efforts will often

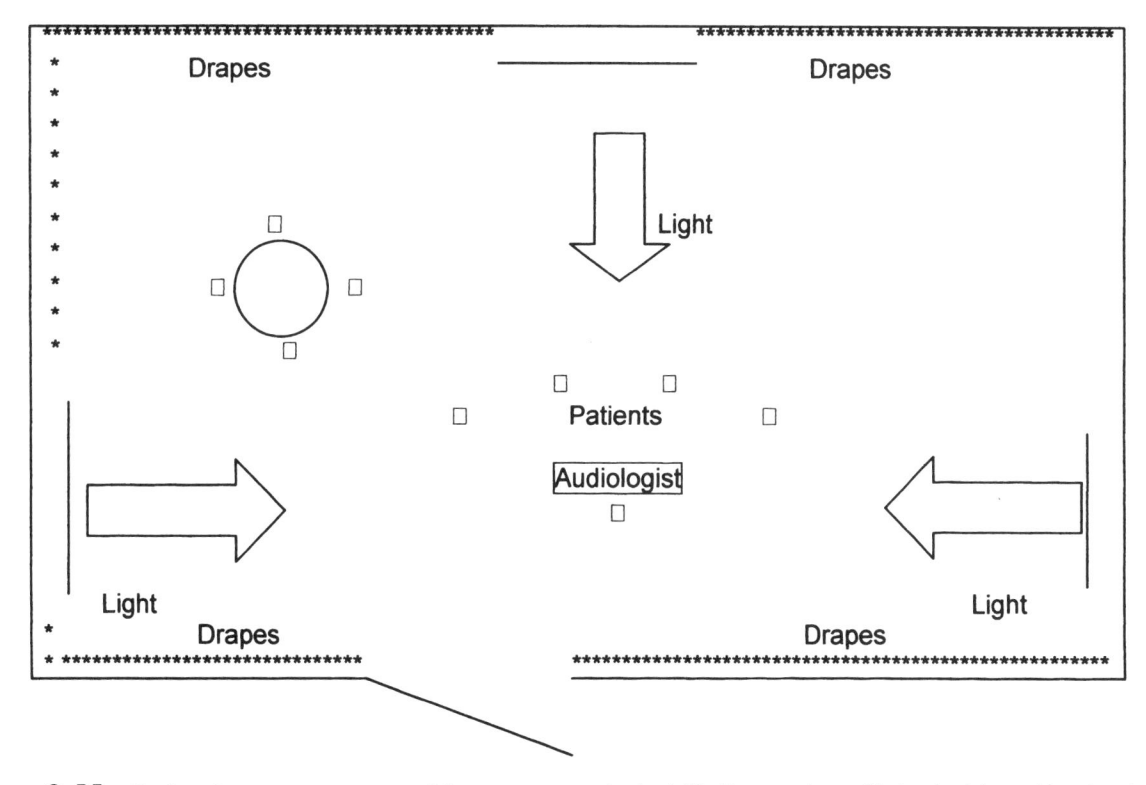

Figure 8–11. Optimal room arrangement for group aural rehabilitation sessions. (Adapted from *Hearing in Aging*, by R. H. Hull, 1995. San Diego, CA: Singular Publishing Group.)

fail unless the staff members involved believe they can succeed. In addition, residents can sense whether personnel are excited about and believe in the potential success of the program.

Content of group aural rehabilitation programs can vary based on the needs of the individual patients. Appendix VIII-I contains a highly detailed, specific-content protocol designed by Lesner (1995). Her protocol consists of five sessions on the topics of: (1) hearing aids and their function, (2) hearing and hearing loss, (3) assistive technology, (4) the auditory and visual nature of speech, and (5) communication strategies. Similarly, Krutt and Shea (1998) have developed a more simplified specific-content protocol, which also covers five sessions, that is presented in Appendix VIII-J. Audiologists must be able to adapt these protocols to the needs of residents who have varying competency levels. It is difficult to gauge the appropriate level for each group, but it is best to gear the presentation to the lowest level of expected competence within the group. In addition, written material should be printed using a large font and at about a sixth-grade reading level. Audiologists should not be afraid of insulting participants' intelligence, as all should derive some benefit from the group.

There are two types of group aural rehabilitation sessions: (1) instructional groups and (2) interactive groups (Kricos & Lesner, 1997). The general goal of instructional groups is for participants to learn information presented to them by audiologists or other professionals in a clear, concise, and motivating manner. Interactive groups are those in which participants learn from each other about coping strategies, behaviors, or factors that influence communication with audiologists talking no more than 30% of the time. Successful instructional groups are those that document improvement in participants' knowledge or skill level from baseline to post-treatment. Thus, audiologists must devise both formal and informal methods of assessing participants' immediate understanding, as well as their short-term (i.e., weekly) and long-term retention of knowledge or skills to determine efficacy of instruction and interaction. Assessment of participants' immediate understanding of material can be informally assessed at the end of each weekly session through fun group activities. Participants might enjoy games that promote friendly competition such as, "Name that ALD!" or "Speechreading Bingo."

Participants' improvement in knowledge or skills from baseline to posttreatment can be assessed through written quizzes or skill-based competency tests. In addition, participants can be given a skill-based competency test in which they must successfully troubleshoot a hearing aid on their own. Observational assessment tools can also be used as measures of group aural rehabilitation sessions. Audiologists can observe residents' skill level with their new aids to determine if further individual instruction is needed, for example. Appendix VIII-K contains a checklist for this purpose (Kricos & Lesner, 1997). In addition, Appendix VIII-L contains an additional checklist (Kricos & Lesner, 1997) that assesses participants' use of important communication strategies emphasized in group therapy. Audiologists and other audiologic support personnel can use this checklist to assess participants' interaction with each other and family members attending the group sessions. Audiologists and audiologic support personnel may wish to stage some problem interactions during the group's snack time to assess specific residents' spontaneous use of communication strategies.

Audiologists must realize that not all participants will benefit from group aural rehabilitation sessions. Kricos and Lesner (1997) defined characteristics of successful patients as those who show a willingness to:

- Learn and attend
- Participate
- Do homework
- Consider their longstanding communication habits
- Try new things
- Share insights and experiences with others
- Learn from peers
- Involve family and friends
- Inform others of communication problems or needs
- Be assertive
- Wear hearing aids and use ALDs when necessary
- Develop new skills and acquire new knowledge
- Be an advocate for self and others with hearing impairment

All residents completing the group aural rehabilitation program should receive a diploma easily made with various software programs. Some participants may enjoy the interaction with their peers with hearing impairment and want to continue with similar activities. Establishment of an ongoing peer support group or "Hearing Club" can have benefits for both participants and audiologists. In addition to ongoing peer support, members of the Hearing Club can assist audiologists with the support program. Depending on the facility and the competency levels of the residents, participants might manage the aural rehabilitation room, resource center, and ALD center. Often these participants can identify other residents with hearing difficulties who could benefit from audiologic services, thus, becoming in-house referral sources. Similarly, they can serve as an advocacy group for all residents with hearing impairment in the long-term care facility. They can work with administrators regarding facility compliance with the ADA. Members of the Hearing Club may want to establish their own Self-Help for the Hard-of-Hearing People (SHHH) chapter. Highly successful hearing aid users can serve as audiologic support personnel in assisting in the group aural rehabilitation program. Eventually, they may wish to conduct some of the sessions!

Individual Aural Rehabilitation Support Programs

The foregoing discussion was obviously based on residents with a fairly high level of functioning and represents the best-case scenario (i.e., those who are alert, motivated, and able to manage major aspects of their lives). Unfortunately, far more residents of dependent-care facilities, such as nursing homes and convalescent hospitals, may not possess that level of competence. They may be seriously ill, heavily sedated for pain, or less mentally alert than those described above. These individuals need aural rehabilitation services but probably would not benefit from group aural rehabilitation sessions. Thus, these residents may function better in limited individual aural rehabilitation sessions. In addition, even higher-functioning residents may continue to have difficulty with their hearing aids, need speechreading therapy, or additional counseling that can be handled best in individual therapy. Staffings may be required for some residents who have problems that need a multidisciplinary management plan. Audiologists may need to meet the nursing staff and physicians on duty to discuss establishment of an ongoing cerumen management program, for example. Similarly, audiologists may need to consult psychologists or social workers concerning residents who are having a particularly difficult time adjusting to hearing loss and other problems.

FACILITY SERVICES

Inservice Training for Nurses, Administrative Staff, and Ancillary Personnel

The success of support programs for elderly patients with hearing impairment residing in assisted-living/semiindependent, and dependent-care facilities depends on audiologists' inservice training of nursing staff. Hull (1995) stated that audiologists should provide regular and periodic inservice training for these individuals to participate in the support program by providing carry-over of therapeutic aspects into their daily lives. Recall that Chapter 5 provided specific suggestions and protocols for developing effective inservice programs. Generally, the inservice programs should include (ASHA, 1997a):

- Cause and functional effects of presbycusis
- Psychosocial effects of hearing loss
- Realistic expectations of hearing aids
- Hearing aid care, use, and troubleshooting procedures
- Methods to facilitate communication
- Procedures to report lost hearing aids

As with other service-delivery sites, all facility personnel should attend informational inservices about the Americans with Disabilities Act (ADA) (1990) (Appendix V-D), "Hearing Loss and its Effect on Communication" (Appendix V-E), and "How Do You Communicate with Someone with a Hearing Loss?" (Appendix V-F). In a sense, all staff members are audiologic support personnel by being sensitive to and facilitating the communication needs of elderly residents with hearing impairment. Audiologic support personnel need to understand the characteristics of elderly residents with dementia. Koury and Lubinski (1995) reported that dementia:

- Is a "brain disorder" that progressively gets worse
- Involves impairment of:
  ⇒ recent, short-term memory, and remote long-term memory
  ⇒ understanding (comprehension)
  ⇒ expression (linguistic and pragmatic skills)

Audiologic support personnel may find the following guidelines effective in interacting with elderly persons with dementia (Clark & Witte, 1995):

- Using calm and inviting facial expressions
- Assuming calm and nonthreatening body postures
- Approaching residents within their visual field
- Using touch to reassure
- Listening for resident's perspective and the feelings being expressed
- Facilitating with nondirective comments (e.g., "Let's do this together.")
- Using praise and compliments that are fitting for an adult
- Sharing information one point at a time
- Using the same spoken phrases to signal routine daily activities
- Making sure the situational, contextual, and verbal cues are harmonious so they contribute to the redundancy of information within the situation
- Speaking slowly

Caregivers may need practice to implement these guidelines. Interacting with elderly persons, particularly those with Alzheimer's disease, can be frustrating for new caregivers who have had little or no experience with this population. Inservices must quickly and efficiently provide instruction on effective communication with these patients. Role-play provides an action-oriented technique for personnel who benefit more from visualization and active participation in contrived scenarios than from listening to a lecture (Koury & Lubinski, 1995; Shadden, Raiford, & Shadden, 1983). Role-play encourages participants to "think on their feet," and engages them in scenarios that reinforce effective on-the-job behavior without any penalties within an informal, protected environment (Koury & Lubinski, 1995).

Koury and Lubinski (1995) stated that the role-play technique should be as "open-ended" as possible, allowing freedom for creativity for participants. Audiologists should ask for volunteers to assume roles of audiologic support personnel and residents engaged in contrived situations involving communication or some aspect of hearing health care. Koury and Lubinski (1995) provided the following guidelines:

- Stop the interaction if participants become anxious or "get stuck."
- Ask the audience to offer suggestions to participants.
- Provide hints to participants if they have difficulty coming up with appropriate ideas.

- Restart the role-play to give participants a second chance for a positive experience.
- Use videotape equipment to provide participants with visual feedback.
- Emphasize actions and attitudes by requiring participants to cope with emotionally charged statements and situations (e.g., "You're angry . . . . The patient just hit you.").
- Summarize communication-repair strategies frequently for participants each time the interaction stops.
- Derive a list with the audience of common strategies that were useful in the role-play scenarios.

Caregivers should also understand the role of the audiologist, functions of the hearing support program, and specific skills for serving as audiologic support personnel. Audiologic support personnel for the hearing aid monitoring and maintenance program should attend the combination informational and skill-based inservices on "Understanding Hearing Aids, Their Care and Their Use" (Appendix V-G). In addition, OT and PT staff members who work with residents in managing their hearing aids should also attend these inservices. Again, this may represent the "ideal" inservice situation. Many times the nursing staff is too busy to devote extended amounts of time to inservices. In some cases, audiologists must provide short segments of the formal inservice "on the fly" as a particular nurse is moving from one patient's room to another or in other impromptu situations. Although not as comprehensive or effective as a formal inservice, limited information conveyed in this matter is better than none at all. Audiologists may be able to demonstrate how to clean cerumen from the receiver of a hearing aid, for example, or how to change a battery without breaking the battery door during a short, informal session. In other words, audiologists have to be innovative and creative by taking advantage of these opportunities to educate other professionals. Such informal interactions might even convince nurses to attend future formal inservices. Figure 8-12 shows an audiologist providing one-on-one instruction to a nurse who was absent during a hearing aid inservice.

Other Facility Services

Audiologists should provide additional services to the facility. As discussed previously, audiologists should perform the receptive communication classification of all new admissions using the two questions in Appendix VIII-E concerning communication and hearing patterns. In addition, audiologists should prepare screening reports for patients' medical records. Again, audiologists must understand how and where in each patient's chart the facility wants to enter audiologic findings, reports, and progress notes. Different facilities have different ways of charting this information and enforce their procedures.

Audiologists can also review and make recommendations for facilities' compliance with the Americans with Disabilities Act (ADA) (1990). Appendix VII-R contains a checklist for facility compliance with the ADA that can be used for rehabilitation hospitals and long-term residential care facilities for the elderly. Audiologists can also help establish ALD centers and resource libraries for residents with hearing impairment and their families. Chapter 4 and Chapter 7 have suggestions for funding and procedures respectively for establishing ALD centers. Resource libraries can be established simply by designating an appropriate area and acquiring materials over time. Appendix VIII-M lists organizations that provide information that would be of interest to elderly residents with hearing impairment and their families.

We cautioned that our earlier discussion of high-performance hearing solutions for elderly persons must be taken into careful considera-

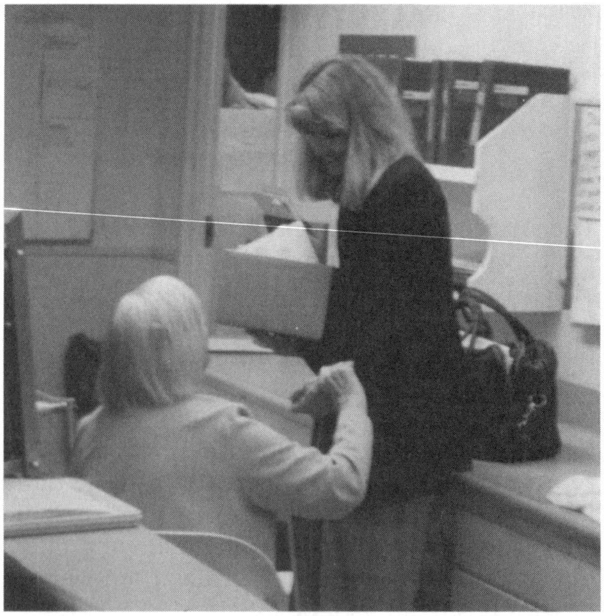

Figure 8-12. Audiologist providing one-on-one instruction to a nurse who missed a hearing aid inservice.

tion before fitting hearing aids with high-tech features to residents of long-term residential care facilities. Their use with these individuals should be implemented on a case-by-case basis, in consultation and with the support of the family and the facility, and only when extended warranties are in effect. Hearing aids in general tend to have short lives in long-term residential care facilities for the elderly. Due to high staff turnover and increased numbers of patients housed within the same facility, audiologists may find it difficult to keep track of any hearing aids, let alone those with high-performance features costing $5,000 or more. As stated earlier, hearing aids in these facilities are often lost or damaged. Sometimes they reappear, but in denture cups, trash cans, or the laundry. Of course, some patients are in transition to long-term residential care facilities from other living arrangements where high-performance hearing aids were fit previously. In these cases, audiologists must educate support personnel about the use, care, and cost of the devices. Together they can work to prevent loss of the hearing aids and ensure that patients continue to wear and benefit from the devices.

For many patients in long-term residential care facilities for the elderly, simpler ALDs like pocket talkers or others provided by electronics stores such as Radio Shack may be more appropriate. Radio Shack offers a wide variety of ALDs including phone-alerting devices (e.g., amplified ringers, outdoor bells, and phone flashers), special option phones and accessories (e.g., adjustable-volume handset, amplified ringers, amplifying handset, big buttons, extra-loud ringers, flash button, LED hold indicator, snap-on amplifiers, and three-way calling), text-viewing phones with special options (e.g., caller ID, printers, and real-time viewing), basic devices for one-on-one communication, and infrared television-listening systems. All of these devices can be purchased by a facility in development of an ALD center for less than $750. Furthermore, cheap does not necessarily mean inferior. An inexpensive Radio Shack ALD worn by a terminally ill patient who uses it to communicate with family members certainly provides a worthwhile benefit.

Although these ALDs will not provide the same sound quality as more expensive products, they can make sound audible for residents of facilities that must operate on a "shoe-string" budget. For those facilities without resources to stock a complete ALD center, some type of amplification device that assists in face-to-face communication should be kept at the nurse's station for use by families and physicians who need to communicate with residents who have hearing impairment. Universal health precautions (e.g., prevention of bodily injury and transmission of infectious disease) should be taken when using the same ALD for several patients (ASHA, 1997b). Decontamination, cleaning, disinfection, and sterilization before reuse of multiple-use ALDs should be carried out according to facility-specific infection control policies and procedures and according to manufacturers' instructions (ASHA, 1997b). Similarly, these devices may be ideal for patients who have limited funds or for less well-to-do families who wish to purchase ALDs for their parents or grandparents. When residents' personal ALDs are no longer needed (after death), they can be used immediately by someone else in the facility. Because ALDs are basically one-size-fits-all, audiologists need not worry about matching a specific style or circuitry to a resident. In fact, this is one aspect of the support program that audiologic support personnel can manage without the audiologist.

The American Speech-Language-Hearing Association has developed a preferred-practice pattern for ALD selection (ASHA, 1997b). The expected outcome for this procedure is for use of an ALD to reduce the impact of hearing loss on patients' lives and facilitate their listening in various acoustic environments. The clinical process includes (ASHA, 1997b):

- Demonstration of pre-established basis for provision of a product
- Consideration of the use of the device in both clinical and natural environments
- Addressing system/device compatibility, as many ALDs are used with hearing aids
- Careful control of output to minimize adverse affects, as there are no standards that specify sound level and other characteristics
- Informing the patient about safety concerns
- Obtaining outcomes information through the use of communication inventories

Documentation for ALD selection includes (ASHA, 1997b):

- rationale for the system/device,
- counseling provided,
- procedures involved in the assessment of the device/system,
- the patient's response to use,
- prognosis for benefit,

- plan for monitoring and orientation, and
- final disposition/reassessment plans.

Appendix VIII-N contains a form for documenting the selection of ALDs for patients in long-term residential care facilities for the elderly.

Compton, Lewis, Palmer, and Thelen (1994) developed a list of objectives for ALD fittings and orientations in which patients must:

- demonstrate the ability to install the device, turn the device on and off, change the batteries, use an AC power source, and clean and care for the device;
- determine with the audiologist the optimal method for coupling the device to their ears and to select the best coupling method for a variety of situations;
- demonstrate understanding the principle of sound/source-microphone proximity for proper operation of the device;
- demonstrate the ability to explain the presence of the device, what it is, what purpose it serves, and what the speaker needs to do to use it;
- develop with the audiologist an inventory of situations where the device may be useful;
- indicate in which situations they are willing to try using the device; and
- demonstrate the ability to troubleshoot potential problems with device installation, coupling, and operation.

Appendix VIII-D contains a checklist of these directives.

SPECIAL SERVICES

Audiologists may offer a variety of special services ranging from audiologic service provision to Hospice patient care and assisting residents in securing funding for hearing aids to supplying hearing aid safety cords.

The term hospice can be traced back to early Western civilization when it was used to describe a place of shelter and rest for weary or sick travelers who were on long journeys (National Hospice Organization, 1998). Today, the term hospice refers to an increasingly popular concept of humane and compassionate care of persons in the final phase of terminal illnesses in a variety of settings: patients' homes, hospitals, nursing homes, or freestanding inpatient facilities coordinated by local hospice centers affiliated with the National Hospice Organization (National Hospice Organization, 1998). Hospice services are available to persons who can no longer benefit from curative medical treatments and who have a life expectancy of six months or less. Services are provided by a team of trained professionals including physicians, nurses, counselors, therapists, social workers, aides, and volunteers who provide medical care to patients, their families, and their caregivers (National Hospice Organization, 1998). Hospice differs from other types of health care in the following ways by (National Hospice Organization, 1998):

- Offering palliative rather than curative treatment
- Treating the person, not the disease
- Emphasizing the quality, rather than length of life
- Considering the entire family, not just the patient as the "unit of care"
- Offering help and support to the patient on a 24-hours-a-day, 7-days-a-week basis.

Audiologists can serve as valuable members of the Hospice team by facilitating communication between hospice patients with hearing impairment and their families through the use of ALDs and effective communication strategies. In addition, audiologists should offer to provide in-services to Hospice team members regarding the importance of hearing to patients' quality of life, as well as on hearing aid care.

Audiologists can also offer the special service of practicing "strategic philanthropy" (Chartrand, 1998) in assisting residents with hearing impairment and their families to secure funding for the purchase of hearing instruments. Social workers can assist audiologists with this process. Chapter 4 discussed numerous ideas for assisting residents in this regard. Long-term residential care facilities may instead wish to establish their own bank of donated hearing aids form residents who either get new ones or who pass away. Audiologists can then match hearing aids to needy hearing aid candidates.

SUMMARY

This chapter was not an easy one to write because it deals with the highly emotional topic of providing support programs to elderly persons in a range of living situations. We began this chapter with demographic data and a continuum of vitality of elderly persons. The importance of adequately serving the elderly population was emphasized in anticipation of the glut of Baby Boomers who will be age 65 years and older by the year 2020. Although the myths about aging were discussed, the realities of the process were described graphically, but accurately. The continua of housing available for the elderly, ranging from independent living to dependent-care situations, was discussed. We also discussed the establishment of a complete support program (i.e., patient, facility, and special services) for elderly persons with hearing impairment who live in long-term residential care facilities. We tried to include program development for both assisted-living/semiindependent and dependent levels of care, as well as for Hospice care. We advocated a holistic approach (Lesner & Kricos, 1995) in matching high-performance hearing aid features to active elderly residents in assisted-living/semiindependent-care facilities. Alternatively, suggestions for hearing aid use (e.g., using colored yarn and alligator clips to prevent hearing aid loss, security procedures at nurses' stations) and the use of less technical amplification devices were discussed for patients needing more dependent care. We discussed the need for audiologists to present all options to patients, their families, and caregivers to select the most appropriate options for amplification. In addition, the use of multiskilling and audiologic support personnel is critical to monitoring and maintaining all amplification devices. Although the names, titles, and specific support personnel have changed from service-delivery site to another, their roles across support programs have remained similar. We depend on them in establishing stellar support programs for patients with hearing impairment in long-term residential care facilities for the elderly. Whether identifying patients with communication difficulties; assisting in group or individual aural rehabilitation sessions; monitoring, maintaining, or troubleshooting hearing aids; or securing administrative support for our programs, support personnel are vital to our success.

LEARNING ACTIVITIES

- Volunteer to visit with residents of a local nursing home one afternoon a week.
- Volunteer to provide an inservice on hearing aid care and maintenance to the nursing staff at a local nursing home.
- Visit a semi-independent care facility and a nursing home in the community and complete a preservice checklist for each.
- Develop a resource guide for elderly persons in the community with regard to hearing care.

REFERENCES

Abrahamson, J. (1995). Effective and relevant programming. In P. B. Kricos & S. A. Lesner (Eds.), *Hearing care for the older adult: Audiologic rehabilitation* (pp. 75–112). Boston, MA: Butterworth-Heinemann.

Alpiner, J. G. (1994). Counseling geriatric patients and their families. In J. G. Clark & F. N. Martin (Eds.), *Effective counseling in audiology: Perspectives and practice* (pp. 278–309). Englewood Cliffs, NJ: Prentice-Hall.

Alpiner, J. G., Meline, N. C., & Holifield, M. (1990). *Getting ready for hearing aids*. Birmingham, AL: Department of Veteran Affairs Medical Center.

American National Standards Institute. (1991). *Criteria for permissible ambient noise during audiometric testing*. New York: Author.

American Speech-Language-Hearing Association. (1992, March). External auditory canal examination and cerumen management. *Asha, 34*(Suppl. 7), 22–24.

American Speech-Language-Hearing Association. (1997a, Spring). Guidelines for service delivery in nursing homes. *Asha, 39*(Suppl. 17), 15–29.

American Speech-Language-Hearing Association. (1997b, November). *Preferred practice patterns for the profession of audiology*. Rockville, MD: Author.

American Speech-Language-Hearing Association. (1998). Available Internet: *www.asha.org*.

Americans with Disabilities Act of 1990, Public Law 101–336, 42, U.S.C. 12101 *et seq.*: *U.S. Statutes at Large, 104*, 327–378 (1991).

Anand, J. K., & Court, I. (1989). Hearing loss leading to impaired ability to communicate in residents of homes for the elderly. *British Medical Journal, 298*, 1429–1430.

Atchley, R. C. (1993). *The social forces and aging: An introduction to social gerontology*. Belmont, CA: Wadsworth.

Ballachanda, B. P. (1995). *The human ear canal.* San Diego, CA: Singular Publishing Group.

Bayles, K., & Tomoeda, C. (1995). *The ABCs of dementia.* Phoenix, AZ: Canyonlands Publishing.

Botwinick, J. (1984). *Aging and behavior.* New York: Springer Publishing.

Bridges, J. A., & Bentler, R. A. (1998). Relating hearing aid use to well-being among older adults. *The Hearing Journal 51*(7), 39, 42–44.

Careguide. (1998). Available Internet: *www.careguide.net.*

Castles, D. (1988). The oral interpreter. *Volta Review, 90,* 307–313.

Chartrand, M. S. (1998). Growing your practice/business with strategic philanthropy. *The Hearing Review, 5*(7), 35–36.

Clark, L. W., & Witte, K. (1995). Nature and efficacy of communication management in Alzheimer's disease. In R. Lubinski (Ed.), *Dementia and Communication* (pp. 238–256). San Diego, CA: Singular Publishing Group.

Compton, C., Lewis, D., Palmer, C., & Thelen, M. (1994). *Assistive technology: Too legit to quit.* Pittsburgh, PA: Support Syndicate for Audiology.

Cox, H. G. (1988). *Later life: The realities of aging.* Englewood Cliffs, NJ: Prentice Hall.

Cox, R. M. (1995). Page ten: Using loudness data for hearing aid selection: The IHAFF approach. *The Hearing Journal, 48*(2), 10, 39–41, 43–44.

Cox, R. M., & Alexander, G. C. (1995). The abbreviated profile of hearing aid benefit. *Ear and Hearing, 16,* 176–183.

Crandell, C. C. (1998). Hearing aids and functional health status. *Audiology Today, 10*(4), 20–21, 23.

Danhauer, J. L., & Danhauer, K. J. (1997). Solving CIC hearing aid insertion and comfort problems. In M. Chasin (Ed.), *CIC handbook* (pp. 169–191). San Diego, CA: Singular Publishing Group.

Dillon, H. (1995). Compression in hearing aids. In R. E. Sandlin (Ed.), *Handbook of hearing aid amplification, Vol. I: Theoretical and technical considerations* (pp. 121–145). San Diego, CA: Singular Publishing Group.

Dillon, H., James, A., & Ginis, J. (1997). Client oriented scale of improvement (COSI) and its relationship to several other measures of benefit and satisfaction provided by hearing aids. *Journal of the American Academy of Audiology, 8,* 27–43.

Ebinger, K. A., Holland, S. A., Holland, J., & Mueller, H. G. (1995, March). *Using the APHAB to assess benefit from CIC hearing aids.* Paper presented at the Annual Convention of the American Academy of Audiology, Dallas, TX.

Erdman, S. A. (1993). Counseling hearing impaired adults. In J. Alpiner & P. McCarthy (Eds.), *Rehabilitative audiology: Children and adults* (pp. 374–413). Baltimore, MD: Williams & Wilkins Co.

Fabry, D. A. (1996). Page ten: Clinical applications of multimemory hearing aids. *The Hearing Journal, 49*(8), 10, 53.

Garahan, M. B., Waller, J. A., Houghton, M., Tisdale, W.A., & Runge, C.F. (1992). Hearing loss prevalence and management in nursing home residents. *Journal of the American Geriatrics Society, 40*(2), 130–134.

Garstecki, D. C., & Erler, S. F. (1998). Hearing loss, control, and demographic factors influencing hearing aid use among older adults. *Journal of Speech, Language, and Hearing Research, 41,* 527–537.

Gatz, M., Bengstron, V. L., & Blum, M. J. (1990). Caregiving families. In J. E. Birren & K. W. Schaie (Eds.), *Handbook of the psychology of aging.* San Diego, CA: Academic Press.

Goldberg, B. (1996). A very long goodbye: The ravages of Alzheimer's disease. *Asha, 38*(4), 25–29, 31.

Hickson, L. M. H. (1994). Compression amplification in hearing aids. *American Journal of Audiology, A Journal of Clinical Practice, 3,* 51–65.

Holmes, A. E. (1995). Hearing aids and the older adult. In P.B . Kricos & S. A. Lesner (Eds.), *Hearing care for the older adult: Audiologic rehabilitation* (pp. 59–74). Boston: Butterworth-Heinemann.

Hull, R. H. (1995). *Hearing in aging.* San Diego, CA: Singular Publishing Group.

Independent Hearing Aid Fitting Forum (IHAFF). (1994). The unveiling of a comprehensive hearing aid fitting protocol for the 21st century. Presented at the Jackson Hole Rendezvous, Jackson Hole, WY.

Jahn, A. F., & Cook, E. W. (1997). Medical issues related to CIC fitting. In M. Chasin (Ed.), *CIC handbook,* (pp. 53–68). San Diego, CA: Singular Publishing Group.

Johnson, C. E., & Danhauer, J. L. (1997a). The "hearing aid effect" revisited: Can we achieve hearing solutions for cosmetically sensitive patients? *High Performance Hearing Solutions, 1,* 37–44.

Johnson, C. E., & Danhauer, J. L. (1997b). CIC instruments: Cosmetic issues. In M. Chasin (Ed.), *CIC Handbook* (pp. 151–167). San Diego, CA: Singular Publishing Group.

Jordon, F., Worrall, L. E., Hickson, L.M.H., & Dodd, B.J. (1993). The evaluation of intervention programs for communicatively impaired elderly people. *European Journal of Disorders of Communication, 28,* 63–85.

Keidser, G. (1995). The relationship between listening conditions and alternative amplification schemes for multiple memory hearing aids. *Ear and Hearing,16,* 575–586.

Keidser, G., Dillon, H., & Byrne, D. (1995). Candidates for multiple frequency response characteristics. *Ear and Hearing, 16,* 562–574.

Keidser, G., Dillon, H., & Byrne, D. (1996). Guidelines for fitting multiple memory hearing aids. *Journal of the American Academy of Audiology, 7,* 404–418.

Kemp, B. (1990). The psychosocial context of geriatric rehabilitation. In B. Kemp, K. Brummel-Smith, & J.W. Ramsdell (Eds.), *Geriatric rehabilitation* (pp. 41–57). Boston: Little, Brown.

Kochkin, S. (1996). Customer satisfaction and subjective benefit with high performance hearing aids. *The Hearing Review, 3*(12), 16–26.

Koury, L. N., & Lubinski, R. (1995). Effective in-service training for staff working with communication-impaired patients. In R. Lubinski (Ed.) *Dementia and communication* (pp. 279–291). San Diego, CA: Singular Publishing Group.

Kricos, P. B. (1995). Characteristics of the aged population. In P. B. Kricos & S. A. Lesner (Eds.), *Hearing care for the older adult: Audiologic rehabilitation* (pp. 1–20). Boston: Butterworth-Heinemann.

Kricos, P. B., & Lesner, S. A. (1997, April). *Evaluating the success of hearing aid orientation programs.* Instructional course presented at the Ninth Annual Convention of the American Academy of Audiology, Ft. Lauderdale, FL.

Krutt, S. S., & Shea, J. (1998, April). *Facilitation of aural rehabilitation programs in geriatric communities.* Instructional course presented at the Tenth Annual Convention of the American Academy of Audiology, Los Angeles, CA.

Kuk, F. K. (1996). Subjective performance for microphone types in daily listening environments. *The Hearing Journal, 49*(4), 29–30, 32–35.

Kuk, F. K. (1998). Using the I/O curve to help solve subjective complaints with WDRC hearing instruments. *The Hearing Review, 5*(1), 8, 10, 14, 16, & 59.

Lesner, S. A. (1995). Group hearing care for older adults. In P. B. Kricos & S. A. Lesner (Eds.), *Hearing care for the older adult: Audiologic rehabilitation* (pp. 203–226). Boston: Butterworth-Heinemann.

Lesner, S. A., & Kricos, P. B. (1995). Audiologic rehabilitation assessment: A holistic approach. In P. B. Kricos & S. A. Lesner (Eds.), *Hearing care for the older adult: Audiologic rehabilitation* (pp. 21–58). Boston: Butterworth-Heinemann.

Lubinski, R. (1995). Environmental considerations for elderly patients. In R. Lubinski (Ed.), *Dementia and Communication* (pp. 257–278). San Diego, CA: Singular Publishing Group.

Mueller, H. G. (1996). Hearing aids and people: Strategies for a successful match. *The Hearing Journal, 49*(4), 13–15, 19, 22–23, 26–28.

Mueller, H. G., & Ebinger, K. A. (1996) CIC hearing aids: Potential benefits and fitting strategies. *Seminars in Hearing, 17*(1), 61–80.

Mueller, H. G., Holland, S. A., & Ebinger, K. A. (1995). The CIC: More than just another pretty hearing aid. *Audiology Today, 7*(5), 19–20.

Nabelek, A. K., & Nabelek, I. V. (1994). Room acoustics and speech perception, In J. Katz (Ed.), *Handbook of clinical audiology* (4th ed., pp. 624–637). Baltimore, MD: Williams & Wilkins Co.

National Center for Health Statistics. (1987). Current estimates from the National Health Interview Survey: United States (*Vital and Health Statistics. Series 10*). Washington, DC: United States Government Printing Office.

National Hospice Organization. (1998). *The basics of hospice.* Available Internet: *www.nho.org/basics.html.*

Nussbaum, J. F., Thompson, T., & Robinson, J. D. (1989). *Communication and aging.* New York: Harper & Row.

Omnibus Budget Reconciliation Act (OBRA). (*1987; Suppl. 1989*). Public Law 100–203, 101 Stat. 1330 (Codified at 42 U.S.C.A. Sec. 1396).

Perrie, A., & Arndt, H. (1997). Engineering issues with CIC hearing aids: One manufacturer's view. In M. Chasin (Ed.), *CIC handbook* (pp. 137–149). San Diego, CA: Singular Publishing Group.

Piscopo, J. (1985). Physical health and wellness of older adults. In T. Tedrick (Ed.), *Aging: Issues and policies for the 1980s* (pp. 50–61). New York: Praeger.

Sanders, D. A. (1993). *Management of hearing handicap: Infants to elderly* (3rd ed.). Englewood Cliffs, NJ: Prentice Hall.

Sandridge, S. A. (1995). Beyond hearing aids: Use of auxiliary aids. In P. B. Kricos & S. A. Lesner (Eds.), *Hearing care for the older adult: Audiologic rehabilitation* (pp. 127–166). Boston: Butterworth-Heinemann.

Schow, R. L. (1982). Success of hearing aid fittings in nursing homes. *Ear and Hearing, 3*, 173–177.

Schultz, D., & Mowry, R. B. (1995). Older adults in long-term care facilities. In P. B. Kricos & S. A. Lesner (Eds.), *Hearing care for the older adult: Audiologic rehabilitation* (pp. 167–184). Boston: Butterworth-Heinemann.

Shadden, B. B., Raiford, C. A., & Shadden, H. S. (1983). *Coping with communication disorders in aging.* Tigard, OR: C.C. Publications.

Sweetow, R. W., & Shelton, C. W. (1996). Programmable vs. conventional instruments: Time/cost and satisfaction factors. *The Hearing Journal, 49*(4), 51–52, 54, 56–57.

Thibodeau, L. M., & Schmitt, L. (1988). A report on condition of hearing aids in nursing homes and retirement centers. *Journal of the American Academy of Rehabilitative Audiology, 21*, 113–119.

Tye-Murray, N. (1998). *Foundations of aural rehabilitation: Children, adults, and their family members.* San Diego, CA: Singular Publishing Group.

United States Bureau of the Census. (1996). *Current population reports, special studies, P-23 190, 65+ in the United States.* Washington, DC: U.S. Government Printing Office.

Upfold, L. J., May, A. E., & Battaglia, J. A. (1990). Hearing aid manipulation skills in the elderly population: A comparison of ITE, BTE, and ITC aids. *British Journal of Audiology, 24*, 311–318.

Ventry, I. M., & Weinstein, B. E. (1982). The hearing inventory for the elderly: A new tool. *Ear and Hearing, 3*, 128–134.

Vinding, T. (1989). Age-related macular degeneration: Macular changes, prevalence, and sex ratio. *Acta Ophthalmology, 67*, 609–616.

Voll, L. M., & Jones, C. H. (1998). CICs: Five years later, what have we learned? *The Hearing Review, 5*(4), 8, 10, 12.

Voll, L. M., & Lyons, P. (1995). Frequency and effectiveness of in-office modifications with CIC hearing instrument fittings. *The Hearing Review, 2*(7), 38–40, 50.

Walker, G., & Dillon, H. (1982). *Compression in hearing aids: An analysis, a review, and some recommendations (NAL report 90)*. Australian Government Printing Service.

Weinstein, B. E. (1995). Auditory testing and rehabilitation of the hearing impaired. In R. Lubinski (Ed.), *Communication and dementia* (pp. 223–237). San Diego, CA: Singular Publishing Group.

Weinstein, B., & Amsel, L. (1986). Hearing loss and dementia in the institutionalized elderly. *Clinical Gerontologist, 4*, 3–15.

APPENDIX VIII-A

Continuum of Housing for Elderly Persons[1]

INDEPENDENT LIVING

Senior Apartments

- ➢ Description
    - Apartment for individual or couple
    - No entrance fee
    - Meals, housekeeping, and a variety of social, recreational, and cultural programs provided
    - Dispense medications (case-by-case basis)
    - No hospital or 24-hour-care facilities on premises

- ➢ Reqirements
    - Must be mobile and capable of caring for self
    - Monthly fee covers rent only—extra charge for meals and other services
    - Inquire about age requirement

- ➢ Considerations
    - Prolonged illness or inability to care for self requires moving
    - Quality of facility and types of services vary widely—thorough research of options important

Retirement Hotels

- ➢ Description
    - Room with private or shared bath
    - May or may not be furnished
    - Maid and linen service available
    - Meals available
    - Dispensing medications and other medical services vary by facility

- ➢ Requirements
    - Must be mobile and capable of caring for self
    - Monthly fee covers rent—extra charge for meals and other services
    - Inquire about age requirement with facility

- ➢ Considerations
    - Few, if any, social programs
    - Prolonged illness or inability to care for self requires moving

Subsidized Housing

- ➢ Description
    - Apartment for individual or couple
    - State or federally subsidized low-income housing
    - Provide one to three meals a day, housekeeping and some social, recreational, and cultural programs
    - No hospital or 24-hour-care facilities on premises

---

[1] From Careguide, 1998. Available Internet: www.careguide.net

➢ Requirements
- Must be age 62 or older
- Specified income guidelines
- Must be able to care for self
- Monthly rental fee covers rent, meals, and programs

➢ Considerations
- Long waiting lists
- No medical care

Small Group/Supportive Housing

➢ Description
- Shared home for 5 to 20 residents
- Residents do all cooking and housekeeping chores
- May have full-time, live-in housekeeping managers
- Sponsored by churches, synagogues, or advocacy groups

➢ Requirements
- Monthly rent, plus shared expenses
- Must be mobile and capable of handling some household chores

➢ Considerations
- Home-like environment
- Living with strangers may be challenging for some people
- Residents take care of each other once they get to know one another
- Prolonged illness or inability to care for self requires moving
- Quality of facility varies widely

Matched Housing

➢ Description
- Parents (patients) stay in own home
- Rent room to someone in need of housing in exchange for household help

➢ Requirements
- Private arrangement

➢ Considerations
- Locating and trusting an individual to share your parents' (patients') home may be difficult

SEMI-INDEPENDENT LIVING

Assisted-Living Facilities

➢ Description
- Licensed facilities that range from a large private home to converted hotels with apartments, a shared dining room, and nurses
- Room with private or shared bath
- Provide all meals, housekeeping, and social programs
- Services include bathing, dressing, and other routine functions
- Medical services vary by facility

➢ Requirements
- Monthly fee
- Resident does not require skilled nursing or 24-hour care

- Considerations
  - If need for personal assistance increases, help is available on site
  - Prolonged illness requires moving to nursing home
  - Medicare does not cover this type of care
  - Medicaid may be available for a few facilities in some states
  - Cost and quality of care can vary

DEPENDENT CARE

Nursing Homes/Skilled Facilities/Extended-Care Homes

- Description
  - Licensed facilities
  - Private or semiprivate room with bath
  - Skilled nursing care 24 hours a day
  - Provides all meals, and social and cultural programs
  - Help with eating, bathing, and grooming
  - Dispenses medications

- Requirements
  - Daily fee (billed monthly)
  - Resident must need 24-hour skilled nursing care and/or rehabilitative services

- Considerations
  - Expensive
  - Medicaid generally takes over payment once the individual qualifies financially
  - Quality of care can vary by facility

Continuing-Care Retirement Communities

- Description
  - Rental or condominium apartment for individual or couple
  - Residents remain in community for the rest of their lives
  - Hospital and nursing-home facilities on premises (in most cases)
  - 24-hour care (as needed)

- Requirements
  - Good health when entering
  - High entrance fee as well as monthly maintenance
  - Age requirements vary by facility

- Considerations
  - Very expensive
  - Most flexible alternative
  - Over time, as parents' (patients') needs change, all levels of care are available
  - If one parent becomes ill, the other can remain in their nearby apartment
  - Facilities available in most parts of the country
  - Features, services, and quality of care can vary widely

APPENDIX VIII-B

Assisted-Living Residence (ALD) Checklist

All-PRO HEARING SERVICES
"So all may hear..."

ASSISTED LIVING RESIDENCE (ALR) CHECKLIST
PHYSICAL ENVIRONMENT

QUESTIONS	YES	NO
Do residents live in their own units?	☐	☐
Are there pleasant common areas in which residents enjoy spending time?	☐	☐
If so, are these rooms:		
➤ Away from high-noise areas?	☐	☐
➤ Free of glare?	☐	☐
➤ Without competing noise from television?	☐	☐
➤ Equipped with surfaces treated with absorptive material?	☐	☐
➤ Well lighted?	☐	☐

SERVICES

QUESTIONS	YES	NO
Are residents' personal care services included in the basic monthly rate (e.g., assistance with amplification)?	☐	☐
If such assistance is needed, is there an extra charge for patients?	☐	☐
Can residents select their own audiologist for services?	☐	☐

STAFF

QUESTIONS	YES	NO
Is the staff-to-resident ratio adequate?	☐	☐
Will the same staff tend to residents' needs (re: assistance with amplification)?	☐	☐
Is staff responsive to "hearing needs" of patients?	☐	☐
Does the ALR employ a sufficient number of staff who are capable of caring for residents with dementia?	☐	☐

ACTIVITIES

QUESTIONS	YES	NO
Are residents active in planning activities?	☐	☐
Is there a resident's council?	☐	☐
Are there activities that promote communication?	☐	☐
Can residents go to religious services?	☐	☐
Is there a support group for residents with hearing impairment?	☐	☐
Are ALDs available?	☐	☐

OTHER

QUESTIONS	YES	NO
Is the facility interested in including the cost of audiologic services in resident's fees?	☐	☐
Is the facility interested in offering hearing plans to residents?	☐	☐

COMMENTS:

Nursing-Home Checklist

All-PRO HEARING SERVICES
"So all may hear..."

NURSING-HOME CHECKLIST
GENERAL OBSERVATIONS

QUESTIONS	YES	NO
Do residents seem to enjoy being with staff?	☐	☐
Does staff know residents by name?	☐	☐
Does staff use adequate communication techniques?	☐	☐
Are residents involved in a variety of activities?	☐	☐
Does the nursing home have a resident's council?	☐	☐
Does the nursing home have a family council?	☐	☐
Does the nursing home have contact with community groups?	☐	☐

PHYSICAL ENVIRONMENT

QUESTIONS	YES	NO
Do residents live in their own units?	☐	☐
Are there pleasant common areas in which residents enjoy spending time?	☐	☐
If so, are these rooms:		
➢ Away from high-noise areas?	☐	☐
➢ Free of glare?	☐	☐
➢ Without competing noise from television?	☐	☐
➢ Equipped with surfaces treated with absorptive material?	☐	☐
➢ Well lighted?	☐	☐

MEDICAL SERVICES

QUESTIONS	YES	NO
Do the physician and nursing staffs meet with residents and their families to develop plans for treatment?	☐	☐
What is the extent of possible participation of medical staff in an aural rehabilitation support program?	☐	☐
Are there nurses or assistants at the facility?	☐	☐
Are licensed nurses on duty around the clock?	☐	☐
Is the confidentiality of medical records assured?	☐	☐
Does the home offer programs to restore lost physical functioning (e.g., physical therapy, occupational therapy, speech and language therapy)?	☐	☐
Does the home promote aural rehabilitation services?	☐	☐
Does the home have special services to meet the needs of residents?	☐	☐
Does the nursing home have a program to restrict the use of physical restraints?	☐	☐
Does the nursing home have an arrangement with a nearby hospital?	☐	☐

PAYMENT ISSUES

QUESTIONS	YES	NO
Is the facility certified for Medicare?	☐	☐
Is the facility certified for Medicaid?	☐	☐
Is the resident or the resident's family informed when charges are increased?	☐	☐

LOCATION, LAYOUT, AND MAINTENANCE

QUESTIONS	YES	NO
Is the outside of the nursing home clean and in good repair?	☐	☐
Is the same true for the inside?	☐	☐
Is the nursing home free from unpleasant odors?	☐	☐
Do noise levels fit the activities that are going on?	☐	☐

ADDITIONAL FACTORS

QUESTIONS	YES	NO
Does the nursing home have a good reputation in the community?	☐	☐
Does the nursing home have a list of references?	☐	☐

COMMENTS:

APPENDIX VIII-C

Sample Letter to Nursing-Home Residents and Their Families

SHADY PINES NURSING HOME
"For their golden years..."

June 28, 1999

Chester A. Brown and Family
Room 123
Shady Pines Nursing Home
123 Golden Sunset Lane
Quality of Life City, CA 94545

Dear Chester and Family,

My name is Starr Audiologist, Ph.D., CCC-A, FAAA. I am managing audiologist for Shady Pines Nursing Home in Quality of Life City. Shady Pines Nursing Home and its staff are dedicated to positive patient outcomes. Toward this goal, we are establishing a Hearing Support Program for residents with hearing impairment. The program was established to facilitate resident communication at Shady Pines utilizing several components:

- Hearing screening and evaluation
- Hearing aid fitting, evaluation, and repair
- Hearing aid maintenance program
- Assistive listening device program
- Cerumen-management program (earwax)
- Consultations with residents, medical personnel, and other personnel
- Weekly in-house audiologist visits
- Emergency services

I will be at Shady Pines on October 10th to discuss all aspects of the program and to answer any questions you may have. If you cannot attend this meeting or if I can be of any assistance to you, please feel free to call me at 555-1122. I will be sending an Informed Consent Form giving you the opportunity to participate in one or all aspects of the Hearing Support Program.

Sincerely,

Starr Audiologist, Ph.D., CCC-A, FAAA
Certificate of Clinical Competence in Audiology (CCC-A)
Fellow, American Academy of Audiology (FAAA)

APPENDIX VIII-D

Sample Case-History Intake Form

SHADY PINES NURSING HOME
"For their golden years..."

AUDIOLOGIC CASE-HISTORY INTAKE FORM

Name:_____ Date of Birth:_____

Birth:_____ Date:_____

Form filled out by: Self   Other

QUESTIONS	Yes	No	I don't know.
1. Have you had your hearing tested? If yes, when?_____	☐	☐	☐
2. Do you have a hearing loss? If yes, when did you first notice it? _____	☐	☐	☐
3. Any history of: Hearing loss in the family? Exposure to noise? Ear pain? Ear drainage? Dizziness?	☐ ☐ ☐ ☐ ☐	☐ ☐ ☐ ☐ ☐	☐ ☐ ☐ ☐ ☐
4. Do you have difficulty understanding speech: Talking on the phone? With one-on-one conversations in quiet? With one-on-one conservations in noise? In group meetings? At church? In restaurants?	☐ ☐ ☐ ☐ ☐ ☐	☐ ☐ ☐ ☐ ☐ ☐	☐ ☐ ☐ ☐ ☐ ☐
5. Do you wear hearing aids? 　If so, one ____ or two ____ 　If so, for how long?_____ 　Under warranty? 　Do you have your own audiologist? 　If so, who?_____ 　If not, have you in the past?	☐ ☐ ☐ ☐	☐ ☐ ☐ ☐	☐ ☐ ☐ ☐
6. Any other communication disorder?	☐	☐	☐

APPENDIX VIII-E

Communication/Environment Assessment and Planning Guide[1]

SHADY PINES NURSING HOME
"For their golden years..."

COMMUNICATION/ ENVIRONMENT ASSESSMENT AND PLANNING GUIDE

PHYSICAL ENVIRONMENT

General Visual Environment

Questions	Yes	No	Plan of Action
➢ Is there sufficient, diffuse lighting to see communication partners clearly?	☐	☐	
➢ Can lighting from lamps and windows be controlled?	☐	☐	
➢ Is indirect lighting available?	☐	☐	
➢ Do areas contain glare-resistant furniture, floors, and surfaces?	☐	☐	
➢ Is printed information presented clearly on contrasting background?	☐	☐	
➢ Are areas color or pattern coded by function (e.g., bedroom, toilet)?	☐	☐	
➢ Is the setting visually interesting in color, design, and topic?	☐	☐	
➢ Is visually stimulating material placed at eye level for most patients?	☐	☐	

Personal Visual Environment Needs (Consider for individual patients.)

Questions	Yes	No	Plan of Action
➢ Has the patient's vision been tested within the past 2 years?	☐	☐	
➢ Does the patient wear corrective lenses or use an assistive correction device?	☐	☐	

[1]From "Environmental Considerations for Elderly Patients," by R. Lubinski, 1995, pp. 274–278. In R. Lubinski (Ed.), *Dementia and Communication* (pp. 257–278). San Diego: Singular Publishing Group. Reprinted with permission.

Questions	Yes	No	Plan of Action
➢ Is the patient given daily assistance and encouragement to use glasses or visual assistance devices?	☐	☐	
➢ Do caregivers communicate at eye level with the individual?	☐	☐	
➢ Does the patient have access to large-print reading material or talking books?	☐	☐	

General Auditory Environment

Questions	Yes	No	Plan of Action
➢ Does the area contain sound-absorbent materials?	☐	☐	
➢ Can background noise be controlled during conversations?	☐	☐	
➢ Do caregivers control background noise during conversations and care?	☐	☐	
➢ Is information presented via intercoms or loudspeakers intelligible to patients?	☐	☐	
➢ Are there noise-reduced areas available for conversations with caregivers, friends?	☐	☐	
➢ Do caregivers come close enough to patients to facilitate hearing and visual cues?	☐	☐	

Personal Auditory Environment (Consider for individual patients.)

Questions	Yes	No	Plan of Action
➢ Has the patient's hearing been tested within the past 2 years?	☐	☐	
➢ Does the patient have a hearing aid for one or both ears?	☐	☐	
➢ Does the patient have an assistive listening device?	☐	☐	

Questions	Yes	No	Plan of Action
➢ Does the person wear hearing aids or an assistive listening device during conversations and activities?	☐	☐	
➢ Do caregivers know how to insert, control, and maintain hearing aids or assistive listening devices?	☐	☐	
➢ Are assistive listening devices easily available for use with caregivers?	☐	☐	
➢ Have caregivers been instructed in techniques for facilitating auditory reception/comprehension?	☐	☐	
➢ Do caregivers speak clearly and with moderate volume while facing the individual?	☐	☐	

General Tactile and Olfactory Environment

Questions	Yes	No	Plan of Action
➢ Does the setting contain a variety of textures?	☐	☐	
➢ Does the setting contain a variety of appropriate odors?	☐	☐	
➢ Does the setting appear to maximize multisensory cueing to facilitate orientation and thinking?	☐	☐	
➢ Do caregivers frequently and appropriately touch persons during conversations and care?	☐	☐	
➢ Does the person appear to benefit from touching people and objects?	☐	☐	

General Spatial Environment

Questions	Yes	No	Plan of Action
➢ Do patients have access to a variety of sites to pursue activities and conversations?	☐	☐	

Questions	Yes	No	Plan of Action
➤ Is physical accessibility to activities easily available to all patients?	☐	☐	
➤ Are most of activities held on the patient's own floor?	☐	☐	
➤ Is there a bathroom easily accessible at activity sites?	☐	☐	
➤ Can furniture be grouped to facilitate communication?	☐	☐	
➤ Are there private places for conversations?	☐	☐	
➤ Are patients' territorial needs respected by caregivers?	☐	☐	
➤ Do caregivers respect patients' private possessions?	☐	☐	

Personal Spatial Environment (Consider for individual patients.)

Questions	Yes	No	Plan of Action
➤ Does the patient have clearly defined personal space?	☐	☐	
➤ Do patients personalize their own space?	☐	☐	
➤ Does the patient's room reflect a personal identity?	☐	☐	
➤ Is ample seating available for the patient's visitors?	☐	☐	
➤ Is the patient's room conducive to privacy?	☐	☐	

PSYCHOSOCIAL ENVIRONMENT

General Psychological Environment

Questions	Yes	No	Plan of Action
➤ Do caregivers respect the dignity of the patient in care and conversations?	☐	☐	

Questions	Yes	No	Plan of Action
➤ Are patients encouraged to be decision-makers in their activities of daily living?	☐	☐	
➤ Are all forms of communication including complaining responded to appropriately?	☐	☐	
➤ Is communication an integral part of all interactions and activities?	☐	☐	
➤ Do caregivers monitor nonverbal cues they send during care and conversations?	☐	☐	
➤ Does the setting reflect seasonal changes, holidays, and special events?	☐	☐	
➤ Are staff members made aware of patients' former interests, vocations, and lifestyles?	☐	☐	
➤ Are patients given responsibilities that reflect a contribution to their environment?	☐	☐	
➤ Are patients encouraged to be both participants and observers of activities?	☐	☐	
➤ Are families encouraged to include patients in outside social activities?	☐	☐	
➤ Do caregivers have opportunities to discuss their perceptions, frustrations, and strategies for communication?	☐	☐	

Personal Psychosocial Environment Needs (Consider for individual patients.)

Questions	Yes	No	Plan of Action
➤ Do activities meet the patient's present and changing cognitive abilities?	☐	☐	
➤ Are daily activities reflective of patient's personal interests and abilities?	☐	☐	

Questions	Yes	No	Plan of Action
➢ Do caregivers inform and individually invite patients to activities?	☐	☐	
➢ Does the patient have at least one person of choice who is a primary communication partner?	☐	☐	
➢ Do caregivers use special techniques to facilitate comprehension and expression?	☐	☐	
➢ Do caregivers take special time to converse with the patient on a daily basis?	☐	☐	
➢ Do caregivers understand the nature of the patient's communication abilities and disabilities?	☐	☐	

NOTES:

APPENDIX VIII-F

Sample Items for the Resident Assessment Instrument: Communication/Hearing Patterns

1. Hearing: Resident's ability to hear (with hearing appliance, if used) during the LAST SEVEN DAYS.

   0. Hears adequately—normal talk, TV, phone
   1. Minimal difficulty—when not in quiet setting
   2. Hears in special situations only; speaker has to adjust tonal quality and speak distinctly
   3. Highly impaired or absence of useful hearing

2. Communication Devices/Techniques. (Check all that apply to the resident during the LAST SEVEN DAYS.)

   a. Hearing aid, present and used
   b. Hearing aid, present and not used
   c. Other receptive communication techniques used (i.e., lipreading)
   d. None of the above

APPENDIX VIII-G

Checklist of Holistic Factors in Planning Aural Rehabilitation[1]

SHADY PINES NURSING HOME
"For their golden years..."

Name:_____ Room:_____ Date:_____

CHECKLIST OF HOLISTIC FACTORS IN PLANNING AURAL REHABILITATION[1]

AREAS	ANSWERS		
PHYSICAL STATUS	Good	Average	Poor
➢ General health	☐	☐	☐
➢ Visual status (with glasses)	☐	☐	☐
➢ Manual dexterity	☐	☐	☐
➢ Fine motor skills	☐	☐	☐
PSYCHOLOGICAL STATUS	Good	Average	Poor
➢ Mental status	☐	☐	☐
➢ Motivation	☐	☐	☐
➢ Outlook	☐	☐	☐
SOCIAL STATUS	Good	Average	Poor
➢ Participates in community activities	☐	☐	☐
➢ Enjoys interacting with other residents	☐	☐	☐
➢ Communicates in noisy environments	☐	☐	☐
➢ Goes to church	☐	☐	☐
➢ Has spouse in same facility	☐	☐	☐
➢ Has supportive extended family	☐	☐	☐
COMMUNICATION STATUS	Good	Average	Poor
➢ Has overall communication skills	☐	☐	☐
FINANCIAL STATUS	Yes		No
➢ Needs assistance in purchasing hearing aids	☐		☐

[1] Adapted from "Audiologic Rehabilitation Assessment: A Holistic Approach," by S. A. Lesner and P. B. Kricos, 1995. In P. B. Kricos and S. A. Lesner (Eds.), *Hearing Care for the Older Adult: Audiologic Rehabilitation* (pp. 21–58). Boston: Butterworth-Heinemann.

APPENDIX VIII-H

Getting Elderly Patients Ready for Hearing Aids[1]

➤ DISCUSSION ASPECTS

✔ Why do you need hearing aids?

✔ Individuals have communication difficulties in various environments. What about you? Consider communication with family and friends, at work, in social gatherings, at recreational events, and in other situations.

✔ Do you have difficulties related to loudness, clarity, and frustration?

✔ Do any of the following apply to you?

- You may think people mumble.
- You may think people avoid you.
- You don't understand the words.
- It may seem easier to stay home and avoid people.

✔ Where do you have problems because of your hearing? Let's think for a moment. Let's name some of the problems.

✔ Why do you have these problems?

➤ INFORMATIONAL ASPECTS ABOUT DIFFERENT TYPES OF HEARING LOSS

✔ Conductive hearing loss.

✔ Sensorineural hearing loss.

✔ Mixed hearing loss.

➤ AMPLIFICATION

✔ What do you know about hearing aids and how do you think they can help?

✔ What are the different kinds of hearing aids?

✔ Do you know about other assistive devices that can help?

✔ What kind of hearing aid(s) are you going to get? Why are you getting this type?

✔ Are you getting one or two hearing aids? What make and model are you getting?

---

[1] From "Counseling Geriatric Patients and Their Families," by J. G. Alpiner, 1994, pp. 278–309. In J. G. Clark and F. N. Martin (Eds.), *Effective Counseling in Audiology: Perspective and Practice*. Englewood Cliffs, NJ: Prentice Hall; and *Getting Ready for Hearing Aids* by J. G. Alpiner, N. C. Meline, and M. Holifield. Birmingham, AL: Department of Veteran Affairs Medical Center.

APPENDIX VIII-I

Specific Content Protocol for Adult Group Aural Rehabilitation Sessions[1]

SESSION 1: HEARING AIDS AND THEIR FUNCTION

➢ Group Topics
- ✔ Professional staff
  - Name
  - Position
  - Background experience
  - Professional interests

- ✔ Participants
  - Name
  - Where they are from
  - Type of hearing problems
  - Interesting facts about self

- ✔ General review of program goals, procedures, and activities

- ✔ General introduction to hearing aids
  - Basic operation
  - Benefits
  - Limitations
  - Hearing aid fitting procedures

- ✔ Controls, parts, and functions of hearing aids
  - M-T-O switch
  - Volume control
  - Battery compartment
  - Microphone opening
  - Receiver opening
  - Earmold
  - Vents
  - Tubing

- ✔ Batteries
  - Types and sizes
  - Battery life
  - Storage of batteries
  - Costs and suggestions about where to purchase batteries
  - Battery testers
  - Accidental swallowing of batteries

- ✔ Care of hearing aids
  - How to clean the hearing aid and earmold
  - Wax removal tools and their use
  - Dehumidifiers, dry aid kits, and forced-air blowers
  - How to store the hearing aid when it is not being used
  - Situations to avoid: extremes of heat, humidity
  - Pets and hearing aids

---

[1] From "Group Hearing Care for Older Adults," by S. A. Lesner, 1995, pp. 220–226. In P. B. Kricos and S. A. Lesner (Eds.), *Hearing Health Care for the Older Adult: Audiologic Rehabilitation* (pp. 203–226). Boston: Butterworth-Heinemann. Reprinted with permission.

- ✔ Hearing aid warranties

- ✔ Hearing aid insurance

- ✔ General troubleshooting information
  - Causes and prevention of feedback
  - Problems related to batteries
  - Problems related to cerumen and moisture

➢ Group Counseling Topics

- ✔ Group conversation to introduce members

- ✔ Conversation about the following question: Have you been disappointed with your hearing aid?

➢ Individual Counseling or Testing

- ✔ Discuss and assess difficulties that patient identifies as most important

- ✔ Determine that patient can handle the hearing aids, including insertion of the hearing aid and battery and that patient can successfully manipulate the controls.

SESSION 2: HEARING AND HEARING LOSS

➢ Group Topics

- ✔ Anatomy of the ear

- ✔ Physiology of the ear

- ✔ Common disorders of the ear (emphasize problems encountered by participants)
  - Impacted cerumen
  - External otitis
  - Perforated ear drums
  - Negative middle-ear pressure
  - Otitis media
  - Otosclerosis
  - Negative pressure
  - Drug-induced cochlear hearing losses
  - Ménière's syndrome
  - Disease-induced cochlear hearing loss
  - Vascular cochlear hearing loss
  - Noise-induced hearing loss
  - Age-related hearing loss
  - Hearing loss due to presence of tumors
  - Tinnitus
  - Other pathological conditions of interest to the group

- ✔ Types of hearing loss
  - Conductive loss
  - Sensorineural hearing loss
  - Mixed hearing loss
  - Central processing difficulty

- ✔ How hearing losses are treated

- ✔ Interpretation of the audiogram
  - Decibels
  - Hertz
  - Audiometric symbols
  - Degree of hearing loss
  - Configuration of hearing losses

- ✔ The audiologic test battery and its purpose
  - Pure-tone thresholds
  - Speech discrimination testing
  - Immittance testing

- ✔ Qualifications, training, and the role of various hearing-care professionals
  - Audiologists
  - Otolaryngologists
  - Hearing aid dispensers

➤ Group Counseling Topics

- ✔ Explanation of patients' audiograms

- ✔ Discussion of familiar-sounds audiogram and patients' experiences

- ✔ Demonstration tape of filtered speech for significant other

- ✔ Further discussion concerning pathological conditions of interest to the group

➤ Individual Counseling or Testing

- ✔ Further explanation of patients' audiograms

- ✔ Handicap profiles

- ✔ Patient training in manipulation of hearing aid, if needed.

SECTION 3: ASSISTIVE TECHNOLOGY

➤ Group Topics

- ✔ Situational limits of hearing aids
  - Noise
  - Distance listening
  - Signal-to-noise ratio
  - Reverberation

- ✔ Rationale and explanation of ALDs

- ✔ Types of assistive listening device technologies
  - Hard-wired systems
  - Loop systems
  - FM systems
  - Infrared systems

- ✔ Demonstrations of assistive devices, including discussion of advantages, disadvantages, and costs

- Large-area systems
- Interpersonal communication devices
- Telephone devices
- Television and radio devices
- Alerting devices

✔ How to obtain or order assistive devices

✔ Availability of ALDs in the community

✔ Implications of the Americans with Disabilities Act

➢ Individual Counseling or Testing

✔ Listening questionnaire

✔ Recommendations about purchase or trial use of assistive technology

✔ Practice with use of the devices

✔ Practice with use of hearing aid telephone coils for those who have them

SESSION 4: AUDITORY AND VISUAL NATURE OF SPEECH

➢ Group Topics

✔ Speech acoustics

✔ Effects of noise on speech perception (video-tape demonstration)

✔ Definition, demonstration, and discussion of the effect of reverberation on speech perception

✔ Visible aspects of speech perception

✔ Limitations on speechreading
- Low visibility sounds
- Homophenous sounds
- Speaker differences in sound production
- Rapidity of speech compared with ability of the eye to follow
- Coarticulation effects
- Environmental constraints

✔ Advantages of the audiovisual perception of speech (video-tape demonstration)

✔ Suggestions to optimize speechreading performance

✔ Listening versus hearing

➢ Group Counseling Topics

✔ Visual, auditory, and audio-visual tests of speech perception

✔ Group-administered speechreading tests using speakers who vary in their visual intelligibility

➢ Individual Counseling or Testing

✔ Visual screening

SESSION 5: COMMUNICATION STRATEGIES

➢ Group Topics

- ✔ Need and suggestions for manipulating acoustic, visual, and psychosocial environments
- ✔ Assertiveness training
- ✔ Coping strategies
- ✔ Suggestions for significant others to improve communication
- ✔ Stress management
- ✔ Advocacy
- ✔ Self Help for the Hard-of-Hearing (SHHH)
- ✔ Need for a sense of humor

➢ Group Counseling Topics

- ✔ How do group members contribute to their own communication problems?
- ✔ Group members' suggestions for tips on communicating more effectively
- ✔ Final questions and comments

➢ Individual Counseling or Testing

- ✔ Following up testing with handicap inventories or profiles
- ✔ Hearing Aid Program Satisfaction Questionnaire
- ✔ Final recommendations

GRADUATION

APPENDIX VIII-J

Specific Content Protocol for Adult Group Aural Rehabilitation Sessions[1]

SESSION 1:
- Audiogram of familiar sounds
- Understanding an audiogram
- Lifestyle affects on hearing loss
- Understanding speechreading and communication strategies

SESSION 2:
- Brief explanation of session one
- Understanding each individual's own audiogram
- Teaching communication strategies, including the communication event
- Social and emotional issues related to hearing loss
- Limitations regarding hearing and speechreading

SESSION 3:
- Review
- Role playing
- How to use your hearing better
- Handling frustration

SESSION 4:
- Role-play
- Home work
- Assistive listening devices

SESSION 5:
- Post-test
- Hearing handicap inventories
- Review of course and family support

---

[1] Adapted from "Facilitation of Aural Rehabilitation Programs in Geriatric Communities," by S. S. Krutt and J. Shea, 1998. Instructional Course presented at the Tenth Annual Convention of the American Academy of Audiology.

APPENDIX VIII-K

Hearing Aid Skills Checklist[1]

SHADY PINES NURSING HOME
"For their golden years..."

HEARING AID SKILLS CHECKLIST

QUESTION	Yes	No
➢ General health	☐	☐
➢ Is the hearing aid being worn?	☐	☐
➢ Is the hearing aid inserted into the ear correctly?	☐	☐
➢ Does the hearing aid have a good battery that is inserted correctly?	☐	☐
➢ Is the M-T-O switch set correctly?	☐	☐
➢ Is the volume control adjusted appropriately?	☐	☐
➢ Is the remote control used correctly?	☐	☐
➢ Is the hearing aid functioning properly?	☐	☐
➢ Can the patient remove the hearing aid with ease?	☐	☐
➢ Is the earmold and hearing aid clean?	☐	☐
➢ Can the patient use the aid properly on the telephone?	☐	☐

[1]Adapted from "Evaluating the Success of Hearing Aid Orientation Programs," by P. B. Kricos and S. L. Lesner, 1997. Instructional course presented at the Ninth Annual Convention of the American Academy of Audiology.

APPENDIX VIII-L

Group Interaction Checklist[1]

SHADY PINES NURSING HOME
"For their golden years..."

HEARING AID SKILLS CHECKLIST

QUESTION	Yes	No
➤ Is the audiologist doing no more than 30% of the talking, with 70% of the talking conducted by group participants?	☐	☐
➤ Are group members actively participating in sessions?	☐	☐
➤ Are families or other "significant others" actively participating in the program?	☐	☐
➤ Does participant make use of visual cues and watch the talker?	☐	☐
➤ Are participants using effective repair strategies?	☐	☐
➤ Are participants demonstrating assertiveness?	☐	☐
➤ Do participants offer suggestions to talkers in order to improve communication?	☐	☐
➤ Are participants comfortable with stating publicly that they are hearing impaired?	☐	☐
➤ Do group members show evidence of attempting to modify the environment to maximize communication?	☐	☐
➤ Do participants come to the hearing aid orientation group sessions wearing their hearing aids?	☐	☐
➤ Do participants make use of assistive technology?	☐	☐
➤ Are nonverbal signals displayed by participants indicative of comprehension of and interest in group topics?	☐	☐

[1]Adapted from "Evaluating the Success of Hearing Aid Orientation Programs," by P. B. Kricos and S. L. Lesner, 1997. Instructional course presented at the Ninth Annual Convention of the American Academy of Audiology.

APPENDIX VIII-M

Consumer Groups for Elderly Persons with Hearing Impairment[1]

SHADY PINES NURSING HOME
"For their golden years..."

CONSUMER GROUPS WITH PUBLIC INFORMATION SERVICES FOR ELDERLY PERSONS WITH HEARING IMPAIRMENT

Consumer Groups

Alexander Graham Bell Association for the Deaf
3417 Volta Place, NW
Washington, DC 20007-2778
(202) 337-5220

American Tinnitus Association
1618 SW 1st, #417
Portland, OR 97207
(503) 248-9985

Association for Late Deafened Adults (ALDA)
10310 Main Street, #274
Fairfax, VA 22030
TTY (404) 289-1596

Self Help for Hard-of-Hearing People (SHHH)
7910 Woodmont Ave., Suite 1200
Bethesda, MD 20814
(301) 657-2248

Public Information Sources

National Information Center on Deafness
Gallaudet University
800 Florida Ave, NE
Washington, DC 20002
(202) 651-5051

National Technical Institute for the Deaf
Resources Catalog
P.O. Box 9887
Rochester, NY 14623-0887

---

[1]Adapted from "Effective and Relevant Programming," by J. Abrahamson, 1995. In P. B. Kricos and S. L. Lesner (Eds.), *Hearing Care for the Older Adult: Audiologic Rehabilitation* (pp. 75–112). Boston: Butterworth-Heineman.

APPENDIX VIII-N

Documentation of ALD Selection Protocol[1]

SHADY PINES NURSING HOME
"For their golden years..."

ALD SELECTION PROTOCOL

Patient's Name:_____ Room No:_____ Date:_____

ALD Selected (Make, Model, & Serial No.):

Rationale for device:

Counseling provided:

Procedures for assessment:

Patient's response to device:

Prognosis for benefit:

Plan for monitoring and orientation:

Final disposition/reassessment plans:

---

[1] Adapted from *Preferred Practice Patterns for the Profession of Audiology*, 1997. Rockville, MD: American Speech-Language-Hearing Association.

APPENDIX VIII-O

ALD Fitting and Orientation Checklist[1]

SHADY PINES NURSING HOME
"For their golden years..."

ALD FITTING AND ORIENTATION CHECKLIST

TASK	Yes	No
Patient can:		
➢ install device	☐	☐
➢ turn device on and off	☐	☐
➢ change batteries	☐	☐
➢ clean and care for device	☐	☐
Patient can select appropriate coupling method for ear.	☐	☐
Patient understands principle of sound/source microphone proximity for proper operation.	☐	☐
Patient understands that device will only work when there is one sound source at a time.	☐	☐
Patient can explain:		
➢ presence of the device	☐	☐
➢ what it is	☐	☐
➢ what purpose it serves	☐	☐
➢ what speaker needs to do to use it	☐	☐
Patient has developed an inventory of situations to use the device.	☐	☐
Patient has selected situations to use the device.	☐	☐
Patient can troubleshoot potential problems with device including:		
➢ installation	☐	☐
➢ coupling	☐	☐
➢ operation	☐	☐

Notes:

[1] Adapted from "Assistive Technology: Too Legit to Quit," by C. Compton, D. Lewis, C. Palmer, and M. Thelen, 1994. Pittsburgh, PA: Support Syndicate for Audiology.

CHAPTER 9

Sustaining Stellar Support Programs: Outcome Measures

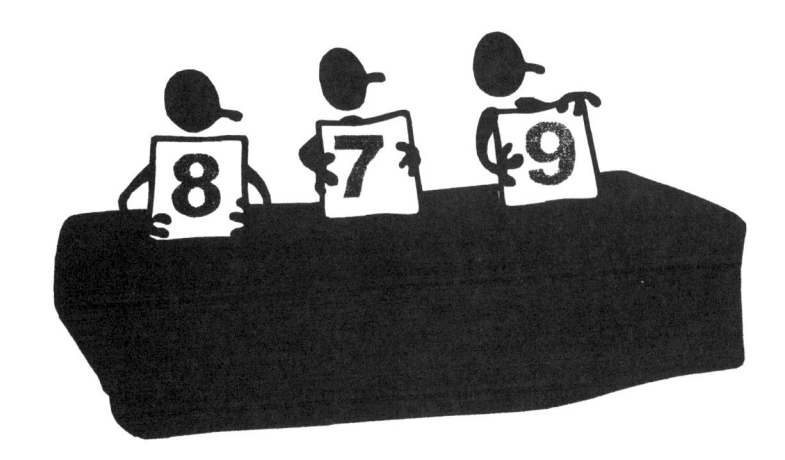

Figure 9–1. Outcomes measurement is critical for support program success.

INTRODUCTION

The United States health-care system is rapidly and dramatically undergoing changes that challenge practitioners to deliver quality health care at a reasonable price (Hicks, 1998). *Third-party payers expect coordinated services, facilities, and systems, as well as providers that are willing to be accountable and demonstrate quality* (Hicks, 1998). Donabedian (1980) believed that quality of care requires a unifying framework involving structure (e.g., providers of care, tools, resources, and organizational settings), process (e.g., activities that go on between and among health-care providers and patients), and outcomes (changes in patients' current and future health status that can be directly tied to prior audiologic care). Earlier chapters of this textbook have discussed support programs for patients with hearing impairment across service-delivery sites. Securing start-up funds to initiate these programs is only the first step in a continuous process of development, planning, and evaluation that is required for sustaining stellar support programs in a highly competitive health-care system. Not only must support programs be based on Continuous Quality Improvement (CQI) (Hosford-Dunn, Dunn, & Harford, 1995; Reisberg & Frattali, 1990; Walton, 1986), but their quality and quality improvement must be verified through outcomes measurement. Thus, managing audiologists must have some knowledge of outcomes measurement. The purpose of this chapter is to familiarize readers with the basics of outcomes measurement and to suggest sensitive measures for demonstrating the quality of support programs in specific service-delivery sites.

> **LEARNING OBJECTIVES**
>
> **This chapter will enable the reader to:**
>
> - Understand the terminology in outcomes measurement
> - Acknowledge the existence of various accrediting bodies and third-party payers who require outcomes measurement
> - Consider various types of outcome measures specific to service-delivery sites

TERMINOLOGY IN OUTCOMES MEASUREMENT

Frattali (1998) stated that outcomes are simply the result of intervention and can differ along several dimensions. One dimension can be defined by the agent (i.e., consumer of care) that can involves patients, their families, clinicians, teachers, employees, administrators, and so on. These types of outcome measurements can be (Frattali, 1998):

- clinically driven (e.g., ability to speechread),
- functional (e.g., ability to manipulate personal hearing aids independently, ability to use a remote control with a programmable hearing aid),
- administrative (e.g., patient referral rates, number of staff members satisfied with inservice program),
- financial (e.g., cost-effective care, average length of stay),
- social (e.g., employability, reduction of hearing handicap), and
- patient-defined (e.g., satisfaction of services provided, quality of life).

Another dimension relates to when outcomes occur (Frattali, 1998):

- *Immediate outcomes* provide information about the day-to-day benefits from treatment. A stroke patient's daily increase in independence with regard to hearing aid use is an example of immediate outcomes.
- *Instrumental outcomes* are those that activate the learning process. For example, once stroke patients have learned new motor skills to manage their hearing aids, they no longer need intervention and will continue to improve on their own.
- *Ultimate outcomes* are those that socially or ecologically validate our interventions. For example, interventions to promote independent hearing aid use validate the rehabilitation hospital's goal to return patients to home and work.

Immediate, instrumental, and ultimate outcomes occur at different times and influence each other. Figure 9–2 shows a model illustrating the interdependence of these time-based outcomes. The immediate outcomes from daily therapy, for example, will influence both the instrumental (i.e., what the patient learns) and the ultimate outcomes (i.e., social validation of intervention). The day-to-day accomplishments of the stroke patient in independently managing his or her hearing aids will determine if that patient can learn necessary skills to function at home and at work. Conversely, audiologists' ultimate outcomes for their support programs will influence the immediate and instrumental outcomes. A rehabilitation hospital's ultimate goal to move patients quickly through a continuum of intervention to home and to outpatient care influences immediate and instrumental outcomes of inpatient rehabilitation programs.

IMMEDIATE OUTCOMES
Day-to-day Progress

⇕

INSTRUMENTAL OUTCOMES
Activation of the Learning Process

⇕

ULTIMATE OUTCOMES
Social and Ecological Validation

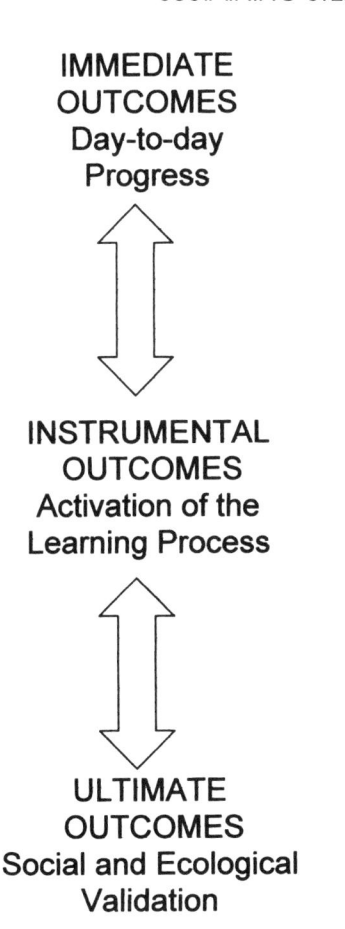

Figure 9-2. Interdependence of time-based outcomes.

Outcome measures are usually submitted to some type of analysis that can be classified into the following group designs (Fineberg, 1990; Frattali, 1998):

- *Experimental designs* are those that involve either a random or fully specified assignment to intervention and control groups (e.g., clinical trials).
- *Quasi-experimental designs* are those that involve nonrandom (and not fully specified) assignment to treatment and control groups (e.g., program evaluation and quality-improvement studies).
- *Nonexperimental designs* are those that involve no clear comparison groups (e.g., case reports, use of data registries, group judgments, and expert opinion).

Use of experimental and quasi-experimental designs requires some knowledge of research methodology and consideration of dependent, independent, and confounding variables. *Dependent variables* are those that are measured, such as outcome measures. *Independent variables* are those that are manipulated. *Confounding variables* are those that must be either controlled for or eliminated. In clinical trials, for example, researchers investigate the effectiveness of a particular treatment for patients that have some type of pathology. In addition to having a common pathology, patients must also have to satisfy other selection criteria to control for any confounding variables that may influence results. A researcher may choose to recruit patients under 40 years of age if the disease process is differentially affected by age, thereby confounding treatment effects. Patients satisfying selection criteria are randomly assigned to one of two groups: a control group and an experimental group. The independent variable in this case is treatment condition. Researchers must select a dependent variable or a sensitive measure that is both reliable and valid in measuring the condition of the patients' pathology. Recall that the *reliability* is the consistency of measurement. A reliable dependent variable is one that provides a consistent measure over time. *Validity*, on the other hand, is the truth in measurement. A valid dependent variable is one that measures what it claims to measure. A dependent variable can be reliable, but not valid. For a measure to be valid, it must also be reliable, however. Once a dependent variable has been selected, measures are obtained on both groups of patients pretreatment and post-treatment. Data are then submitted to statistical analyses to determine the existence of any significant difference between the two groups of patients that may infer the degree of effectiveness of the treatment protocol.

Audiologists wanting to quantify the quality of their support programs for patients with hearing impairment will rarely use the experimental or quasi-experimental designs. In most cases, audiologists will be using nonexperimental designs in assessing outcome measures from support programs. In addition, many clinicians do not have the academic training in research design or statistical procedures to carry out independent investigations. Audiologists should not feel that they are "off the hook" and do not have to be involved in the research process, however. They must consider the reliability and validity of both the clinical measures used in and the outcome measures selected for support programs. Some audiologists' lack of appropriate research training should not preclude them from participating in clinical research projects, provided that they seek the assistance of trained investigators within their own facility or at a local university who may wish to participate in applied research. Our profession is in need of experiments that support the notion that attending to patients' hearing health-care needs results in positive outcomes and enhances quality of life. In particular, efficacy studies supporting the notion that aural rehabilitation is a necessary, rather than elective, component of health care (Bridges & Bentler, 1998) can assist in convincing HMOs, third-party payers, and other parties to fund support programs for patients with hearing impairment across service-delivery sites.

CRITICAL AREAS OF OUTCOMES MEASUREMENT FOR SUPPORT PROGRAMS

As mentioned in Chapters 3 and 4 of this textbook, audiologists must diligently market support programs in order to secure necessary start-up funding. Once established, collection of appropriate outcome measures can assist audiologists in securing needed resources for sustaining support programs. Three important areas of outcome measurement for support programs are: (1) patient-communication function, (2) customer satisfaction, and (3) fiscal accountability. A common mistake made by audiologists in measuring changes in patient function is only to use discipline-specific measures, while failing to consider facility-wide measures that are important to administrators, third-party payers, and accrediting bodies. Audiologists must be able to visualize the "big picture" and to think like those administrators who control the purse strings. In an effort to receive an increase in next year's budget, for example, an audiologist could execute a small quasi-experimental study assessing the efficacy of support programs in reducing the amount of rehabilitation-hospital patients' hearing handicap. Audiologists may assign 10 patients with hearing impairment each to an experimental group and a control group. The experimental group would participate in the support program, while the control group would not. Audiologists may choose a discipline-specific pre- and post-treatment measure, such as the *Hearing Handicap Inventory for Adults—Screening* (HHIA-S) (Newman, Weinstein, Jacobson, & Hug, 1991) or *Hearing Handicap Inventory for the Elderly—Screening* (HHIE-S) (Ventry & Weinstein, 1982). Administrators may be impressed that participation in the support program results in a significant reduction in the degree of hearing handicap in the experimental group. Rehabilitation-hospital administrators would be even more impressed, however, if support programs made significant improvement in patients' functioning using measurements they considered important, such as the *Functional Independence Measure*, (FIM) (State University of New York at Buffalo, 1993; Clark-Lewis, 1997). The FIM is an outcome measure designed to measure the burden of care quantitatively so that it is understandable to third-party payers (Frattali, 1998). The FIM rates functional abilities on seven-point scales along various agendas, which tap several skills, such as communication. If audiologists can show administrators significant reductions in patients' hearing handicaps and simultaneous improvements in FIM scores, then the chances of securing ongoing funding of support programs are significantly enhanced.

Another important area for outcomes measurement is customer satisfaction of support programs. In health care, patients now have a major role in provider selection and, if dissatisfied, will choose other providers (Hicks, 1998). Indeed, today's health-care system has placed an unparalleled emphasis on meeting consumers' demands. Consequently, providers are held accountable to meet—or even exceed—consumer expectations (Rao, Blosser, & Huffman, 1998). Rao and Goldsmith (1991) identified seven factors to compel providers to adopt a satisfaction survey as part of outcomes measurement:

- standards of accreditation bodies (e.g., The Rehabilitation Accreditation Commission (CARF), the Joint Commission on Accreditation of Health Care Organizations (JCHAO), and so on),
- industry dictate (e.g., consumer lobby),
- components of risk management,
- components of institutional marketing programs,
- components of program/service evaluation,
- research on consumer needs/patient-care perspective, and
- components of quality-improvement process.

Audiologists must consider the various methods for measuring consumer satisfaction.

It is important to realize that the customer is not just the patient. It can mean the patients' friends, family, and even staff. The customer of support programs for children with hearing impairment in public schools, for example, can include the child, the parents, the classroom teacher, the speech-language pathologist, and so on. The success with which consumer satisfaction of support programs is measured depends on the audiologists' ability to answer the following questions (Leebov & Scott, 1994; Rao et al., 1998):

- What are the current customer-satisfaction assessment methods, both formal and informal? Can patient satisfaction regarding support programs be implemented into current methods? Or must audiologists devise their own methods?
- How effective are the current methods in improving customer satisfaction?
- How is the information shared with people who can use the feedback to improve service delivery?
- To improve assessment of customer satisfaction, do you focus on identifying priorities? Identifying customer groups? Identifying which methods work best?
- How effective are your methods in measuring customer satisfaction with specific aspects of support programs?
- Which aspects of the support program have the greatest impact on customer satisfaction?
- What are the critical control points in those aspects?
- What methods need to be devised to monitor these aspects so that you have the data to identify priorities and monitor support-program progress?

Audiologists should investigate the current methods of assessing customer satisfaction by asking their immediate supervisor about the outcomes measurement practices within the particular facility. Audiologists should not be complacent if told to relax and not worry about it. Just because the facility does not have a system in place or take the current system seriously does not mean that audiologists can afford to not measure customer satisfaction with support programs. Audiologists must realize that the fate of their support programs may be in their own hands. No support program can function on the principles of CQI without assessment of customer satisfaction. Without these data, it is impossible to identify program priorities and monitor support-program progress. Furthermore, these data are critical for support-program viability. Audiologists need accountability data to justify increases in necessary materials, allocation of human resources, and so on. Indeed, audiologists must take a proactive approach to outcomes measurement and devise their own methods of assessing customer satisfaction.

There are various methods for surveying customer satisfaction that vary according to format (i.e., multiple-choice formats, yes/no questions, rating scales, or open-ended questions), time frames (i.e., retropsective, concurrent, or prospective), frequency of use (i.e., continuous, monthly, quarterly, or intermittent/sporadic), subject sample (i.e., all discharged patients, all patients receiving X visits), administration (i.e., mail, telephone, manual distribution and immediate return, manual distribution and mail return, or face-to-face interview), patient tracking (anonymous, identified by name, coded, or identified by program), and responsibility for gathering data (i.e., administration, communications/media relations, outcomes management/program evaluation, consumer affairs, quality improvement, or separate clinical department) (Rao et al., 1998)

The questionnaire format should contain items that can provide numerical data that can *quantify* customer satisfaction. A questionnaire composed of yes/no questions provides little information as to the degree of patient satisfaction and limits ways to measure improvement in service delivery. Rating scales, on the other hand, can easily quantify patient satisfaction and can show improvement in customer satisfaction over time. In addition, the questionnaire should have at least one open-ended question to give customers the opportunity to provide suggestions or information that cannot be conveyed through closed-response items. The time frame for completing the questionnaire should always be retrospective (e.g., at the end of treatment or after a set period of time) and either continuously (e.g., as each patient is discharged) or annually administered (e.g., at the end of each school or fiscal year). Rehabilitation-hospital patients who have therapy all day may be too busy or tired to think about the adequacy of the support program, for example. These patients are best surveyed after discharge. In educational settings, however, support-program evaluation is best accomplished at the end of each school year.

The sample should include every customer participating in the support program for three reasons. First, audiologists should be concerned about the opinions of all support-program participants to establish priorities and target areas for improvement. Second, the larger the number of respondents, the more representative the sample. Third, the number of participants in the support program may be highly variable over time, and consistent feedback is required for CQI. The administration of the questionnaire should be manual distribution and immediate return for patients. All audiologists know that even patients with the best of intentions fail to fill out questionnaires and return them by mail. Thus, patients must be strongly encouraged to fill out the questionnaire before they leave the premises. Some off-site customers may require a mail-distribution and mail-return format if their schools are on the perimeter of a large, urban school district. Customer tracking of questionnaires should be anonymous. After all, most respondents will not provide their true impressions if their responses can be traced back to them. It does help to know of which customer group the respondent is a member, however. If customer satisfaction with support programs is low, it may help to know the specific origin of the dissatisfaction so that corrective measures can be put in place. Finally, an independent department should collect and analyze the data from the questionnaires to increase the credibility of customer-satisfaction ratings, although audiologists should provide input about how to analyze the data. Audiologists may wish to analyze customer-satisfaction ratings before and after major program modifications, for example.

OUTCOMES MEASUREMENT ACROSS SERVICE-DELIVERY SITES

Collecting appropriate outcome measures for support programs for patients with hearing impairment differs based on service-delivery site due to the different requirements of the associated accrediting bodies and to the nature of service provision.

Outcomes Measurement in Educational Settings

Outcomes measurement is becoming increasingly important in educational settings because public agencies must be accountable to taxpayers. Audiologists in educational settings must consider the long history of outcomes measurement in education (this topic is not covered in great detail here). Outcomes measurement in educational settings are governed by rules and regulations at the federal, state, and local levels. At the federal level, for example, the Individuals with Disabilities Education Act (IDEA) dictates that children who qualify are entitled to a free and appropriate public education and an Individualized Education Program or (IEP) that has both short-term and long-term goals related to student communication function. Unfortunately, few if any of those goals are related directly to the effectiveness of support programs for students with hearing impairment, although support programs may have an indirect impact on children's IEP goals. If audiologists provide excellent classroom support to teachers in self-contained classes for students with hearing impairment, then those children may have a greater likelihood of achieving their IEP goals. In this case, customer satisfaction may be a better indicator of support-program viability than other outcome measures.

Within educational settings, customers of support programs for students with hearing impairment include teachers (regular and special educators), other special-education providers (e.g., nurses, speech-language pathologists, and psychologists), administrators (principals, special-education coordinators, and supervisors), community agencies, community audiology and communication disorders clinics, physicians, parents, reimbursement and funding agencies, students, taxpayers, and the school board (Johnson, Benson, & Seaton, 1997; Rao et al., 1998). Possible areas of satisfaction to be measured differ according to who the customer is. Outcomes measurement should focus on teachers' satisfaction with the timeliness of attending to problems with auditory trainers, the scheduling of classroom visits, and personal interaction with the audiologist, for example. For administrators, measurement should include their satisfaction with the overall scheduling of services, the service-delivery model, the audiologist as a "team player," the timeliness of reports, and the overall competence and conduct of the audiologist (Rao et al., 1998). Unfortunately, using multiple questionnaires based on the existence of multiple-customer groups becomes cumbersome and complicated. Development of a generic customer-satisfaction questionnaire concerning program effectiveness is not only more feasible, but it will be more readily received, understood, and appreciated by the administration. An example of a generic customer-satisfaction questionnaire for this purpose appears in Appendix IX-A.

In addition to improvement in individual students' communication function and customer satisfaction, numerous other data can serve as outcome measures. The total numbers of activities for the year can be very impressive to administrators. Support-program viability can be bolstered by reporting the total number of classroom visits made by the audiologists, the total number of hearing aids and auditory trainers checked, the number of hearing aids and auditory trainers repaired on-site, the number of inservices given, and so on. Audiologists also need to report other indices of support-program quality, such as participants' rating of inservices, inservice-participant scores on quizzes, and so on. Other data, such as the average length of time needed to respond to reported problems or requests for assistance or information can be very powerful but require a highly organized and tenacious audiologist. Every consultation and every phone conversation with a concerned parent should be logged and considered as important data. *Documentation is the key!* In some cases, documentation can protect audiologists from unfair criticisms from vindictive individuals. Complaints to the district office of audiologists' neglect of reported problems can easily be quelled with accurate and thorough documentation. In addition, comparison of data collected from year-to-year can verify improvement in service delivery and can assist in verifying fiscal soundness of support programs.

Outcomes Measurement in Rehabilitation Hospitals and Long-term Residential Care Facilities for the Elderly

Although separate chapters are devoted to establishing support programs for patients with hearing impairment in rehabilitation hospitals and long-term residential care facilities for the elderly, these service-delivery sites are often accountable to the outcomes-measurement requirements of the same accrediting bodies that are leaders in quality assurance. Therefore, both sites are covered together here. The Rehabilitation Accreditation Commission, formerly the Commission on Accreditation of Rehabilitation Facilities (CARF), is a national, nonprofit organization founded in 1966. It is the preeminent standard-setting body that promotes the delivery of quality services to people with disabilities and those in need of rehabilitation (Hicks, 1998). The CARF has placed increased importance on outcomes-based program evaluation, outcome measures, and evidence of patient involvement in treatment planning (Gallagher, 1998). The CARF accreditation standards are "national consensus standards," meaning that a wide variety of individuals (e.g., providers, consumers, and so on) has a chance to provide input (Hicks, 1998). It is critical that audiologists provide input to those standards as well. Another major accrediting body is the Joint Commission on Accreditation of Healthcare Organizations (JCAHO), which was formed in 1951 as the Joint Commission on Accreditation of Hospitals by the American College of Physicians, the American Medical Association, the Canadian Medical Association, and the American Hospital Association (Gallagher, 1998). The JCAHO develops standards for hospitals, nonhospital-based psychiatric and substance-abuse organizations, long-term care organizations, home-care organizations, ambulatory-care organizations, pathology and clinical laboratory services, and healthcare networks (Hicks, 1998). Included in those standards are procedures for measuring quality of care and treatment outcomes (Gallagher, 1998). Although these outcome measures are not yet required for rehabilitation, efforts are currently underway by the American Speech-Language-Hearing Association to submit performance measures to JCAHO's National Library of Healthcare Indicators (Gallagher, 1998). There are other accrediting bodies that require outcomes measurement pertaining to service delivery in rehabilitation hospitals and nursing homes, but they are not discussed here.

Even though rehabilitation hospitals and nursing homes share several of the same accrediting agencies, their ultimate outcomes for patients are different. In rehabilitation hospitals, traumatically injured patients are admitted for a limited period of time with the ultimate outcome of returning to home and work. The rehabilitation-hospital patient population is transient with constant change and turnover. In this case, the focus of the support programs is to maximize patients' communication potential so that they may optimally benefit from their individual rehabilitation programs. Services include screening for hearing loss; audiologic evaluation; hearing aid evaluation, fitting, and delivery; use of assistive listening devices; and initial aural rehabilitation (i.e., communication tips). For many patients, their admission to the rehabilitation hospital may be their entry point into the continuum of hearing health-care that may end or extend to outpatient services after discharge. However, patients in long-term residential care facilities are admitted and may live the remaining years of their lives in the facility. Therefore, the patient population is more static, and the ultimate outcomes of the support program for nursing-home residents with hearing impairment are to:

- restore and maintain the highest possible level of patients' functional independence;
- preserve patient autonomy;
- maximize patients' quality of life, perceived well-being, and life satisfaction; and
- stabilize patients' chronic medical conditions (ASHA, 1997; Kane, Ouslander, & Abrass, 1989).

As mentioned earlier, ultimate outcomes influence all outcomes measurement, including assessing customer satisfaction. Thus, the method of assessing customer satisfaction may vary in some ways between these two service-delivery sites. In both settings, questionnaires are the best tool for surveying customer satisfaction. The questionnaires used in long-term residential care facilities may have to be printed in larger font, easily read by elderly patients, however. In addition, the method of administration may vary. For rehabilitation hospitals, manual distribution and immediate return is the best option for most patients. By contrast, some nursing-home residents may not have the stamina to fill out a questionnaire and may require a face-to-face interview. For both service-delivery sites, the survey should use rating scales, be retrospective, include all support-program participants, employ manual distribution and immediate return, and be anonymous but classified according to customer group. They should also be collected and analyzed by someone other than the audiologist. Examples of customer-satisfaction questionnaires for use in rehabilitation hospitals and nursing homes appear in Appendixes IX-B and IX-C, respectively.

As in educational settings, there are numerous types of data that can be used as outcome measures in rehabilitation hospitals and long-term residential care facilities for the elderly.

Examples include the number of patients screened; sensitivity and specificity of screening programs; the number of patients receiving audiologic evaluations, hearing aid evaluations, hearing aid fittings, and hearing aid deliveries; the number of hearing aids checked, number of aural rehabilitation sessions provided, number of inservices given, participants' ratings of inservices, and so on. Again, documentation is the key and is required for outcome measures for fiscal responsibility.

OUTCOME MEASURES FOR FISCAL RESPONSIBILITY

Outcome measures for fiscal responsibility vary according to service-delivery site. Similarly, methods of reimbursement are highly variable across and within service-delivery sites, between and among various aspects of audiologic service provision within support programs, and among patients making it difficult to discuss outcomes measurement using specific scenarios. One basic underlying principle of fiscal responsibility is that third-party payers expect more high-quality services at lower costs. Audiology networks, for example, expect providers to capitate the costs of audiologic services in exchange for a flat fee that covers the costs of patients' hearing aids. Similarly, administrators across service-delivery sites expect the benefits of support programs to far exceed their costs. Audiologists must be able to demonstrate fiscal responsibility to sustain stellar support programs. This is best accomplished through a careful comparison of actual program cost to their full market value. All program costs must be accounted for, ranging from the exact number of batteries distributed to the cost per hour for audiologic services. Audiologists should not be shy in assessing the full market value of the support program. One source of cost-efficiency for support programs lies in the use of multiskilling and the use of audiologic support personnel. For example, audiologists should charge the market price for daily hearing aid checks performed by trained audiologic support personnel even though the actual cost is low.

Fiscal soundness is determined by comparing the actual cost of the support program to its estimated full market value. Fiscally viable support programs are those in which full market value exceeds their actual costs. Both the agency and the managing audiologist should analyze the fiscal viability of support programs. Fiscal viability is particularly important to contract-for-service audiologists who must determine if managing support programs across service-delivery sites is lucrative to their private practices. This may be difficult because not only must the estimated full market value exceed actual program costs, but private-practice audiologists must also make a profit from these endeavors. They must consider how much profit could have been achieved through other services (e.g., in-office audiologic evaluations and hearing aid sales) that could have been provided during the time it took to plan, establish, oversee, and evaluate aural rehabilitation support programs. If these endeavors are not profitable, then audiologists should consider terminating this aspect of their practices. Audiologists who are employees of the agency need to be concerned about the fiscal soundess of the program, but their personal survival may not be tied to it. Fiscal soundness begins with obtaining initial funding sources for support programs. *Sustaining stellar support programs on a long-term basis, however, lies in our profession's ability to qualify aural rehabilitation services for reimbursement by third-party payers.* Chapter 10, "Aural Rehabilitation Programming in the Future," discusses these issues.

SUMMARY

This chapter discussed sustaining stellar support programs through the use of outcomes measurement. Outcomes measurement is a theme that can be found in every aspect of the U.S. health-care system. Audiologists must realize that outcomes measurement of support programs for patients with hearing impairment is their responsibility. This fact may be more elusive for audiologists who work for someone else than for audiologists who head their own practices. Different aspects of outcomes measurement were discussed here, such as types of outcomes, when outcomes occur, methods for measuring customer satisfaction, outcome measures across service-delivery sites, and fiscal soundness of support programs. Readers need to understand that outcomes measurement is required to sustain stellar support programs for patients with hearing impairment across service-delivery sites.

LEARNING ACTIVITIES

- Inventory and classify outcomes measurement in your university speech and hearing clinic or place of employment.
- Design and implement a patient-satisfaction questionnaire.

REFERENCES

American Speech-Language-Hearing Association. (1997, Spring). Guidelines for audiology service delivery in nursing homes. *Asha, 39*(Suppl. 17), 15–29.

Bridges, J. A., & Bentler, R. A. (1998). Relating hearing aid use to well-being among older adults. *The Hearing Journal, 51*(7), 39, 42–44.

Donabedian, A. (1980). *Explorations in quality assessment and monitoring. Volume 1: The definition of quality and approaches to its assessment.* Ann Arbor, MI: Health Administration Press.

Fineburg, H. V. (1990). The quest for causality in health services research. In L. Sechrest, E. Perrin, & J. Bunker (Eds.), *Conference proceedings: Strengthening causal interpretation of nonexperimental data* (pp. 215–220). Rockville, MD: U.S. Department of Health and Human Services, Public Health Service, and Agency for Health Care Policy and Research.

Frattali, C. M. (1998). Outcomes measurement: Definitions, dimensions, and perspectives. In C. Frattali (Ed.), *Measuring outcomes in speech-language pathology* (pp. 1–27). New York: Thieme.

Gallagher, T.M. (1998). National initiatives in outcomes measurment. In C. Frattali (Ed.), *Measuring outcomes in speech-language pathology* (pp. 527–557). New York: Thieme.

Hicks, P.L. (1998). Outcomes measurement requirements. In C. Frattali (Ed.), *Measuring outcomes in speech-language pathology* (pp. 28–49). New York: Thieme.

Hosford-Dunn, H., Dunn, D. R., & Harford, E.R. (1995). Audiology business and practice management. San Diego, CA: Singular Publishing Group.

Johnson, C. D., Benson, P. V., & Seaton, J. B. (1997). *Educational audiology handbook.* San Diego, CA: Singular Publishing Group.

Kane, R., Ouslander, J., & Abrass, I. (1994). *Essentials of clinical geriatrics* (2nd edition). New York: McGraw-Hill.

Leebov, W., & Scott, G. (1994). *Service quality improvement: The customer satisfaction strategy for health care.* Chicago: American Hospital Publishers Inc.

Newman, C. W., Weinstein, B. E., Jacobson, G. P., & Hug, G. A. (1991). Test-retest reliability of the Hearing Handicap Inventory for Adults. *Ear & Hearing, 12,* 355–357.

Rao, P. R., Blosser, J., & Huffman, N. P. (1998). Measuring consumer satisfaction. In C. Frattali (Ed.), *Measuring outcomes in speech-language pathology* (pp. 89–112). New York: Thieme.

Rao, P., & Goldsmith, T. (1991). How to keep your customer satisfied: Consumer satisfaction measure. Poster presented to the American Congress of Rehabilitation Medicine, Washington, DC.

Reisberg, M., & Frattali, C. (1990). Toward total quality management. *Quality Assurance Digest,* 1–5.

State University of New York at Buffalo, Research Foundation. (1993). *Guide for use of the uniform data set for medical rehabilitation: Functional independence measure.* Buffalo, NY: Author.

Ventry, I., & Weinstein, B. (1982). The hearing handicap inventory for the elderly. *Ear and Hearing, 3,* 128–134.

Walton, M. (1986). *The Deming management method.* New York: Pedigree/Putnam.

APPENDIX IX-A

Customer-Satisfaction Questionnaire for Educational Support Programs

ABC INDEPENDENT SCHOOL DISTRICT
"For their future..."

HEARING SUPPORT PROGRAM SATISFACTION QUESTIONNAIRE

READ each item carefully and CHECK THE BOX for the answer that best describes your opinion.

Please write any comments you may have on the back of this form. Thank you!

SA = Strongly Agree   MA = Moderately Agree   N = Neutral
MD = Moderately Disagree   SD = Strongly Disagree

ITEM	SA	MA	N	MD	SD
It is important that the children receive the highest quality hearing health-care services. Audiologist was:					
• skillful and knowledgeable.	☐	☐	☐	☐	☐
• well-prepared and organized.	☐	☐	☐	☐	☐
• prompt and attentive to children's needs.	☐	☐	☐	☐	☐
• prompt in responding to needs of teachers and other educational personnel.	☐	☐	☐	☐	☐
• courteous, respectful, and a "team player."	☐	☐	☐	☐	☐
• effective as an advocate for children's needs.	☐	☐	☐	☐	☐
Our children must have access to the highest quality amplification systems.					
• Hearing aids and personal FM systems were checked on a daily basis.	☐	☐	☐	☐	☐
• Accessories for these instruments were always available for replacement.	☐	☐	☐	☐	☐
• Loaner instruments were available for use.	☐	☐	☐	☐	☐
• Instruction for hearing aid care was provided to staff, parents, and children.	☐	☐	☐	☐	☐
• Assistive listening devices were available as needed.	☐	☐	☐	☐	☐
Educational personnel were prepared with the latest knowledge and skills to facilitate children's hearing health-care needs.					
• Timely, informative, and relevant inservices were provided on a regular basis.	☐	☐	☐	☐	☐
• Information was presented in a way that optimized learning.	☐	☐	☐	☐	☐
• Participants had adequate opportunity to practice new skills.	☐	☐	☐	☐	☐
Children's hearing health-care needs were met.					
• Communication between audiologist and educational personnel was effective.	☐	☐	☐	☐	☐
• Communication between audiologist and children's families was effective.	☐	☐	☐	☐	☐
• Classrooms and teaching styles were optimized for adequate listening.	☐	☐	☐	☐	☐
• Hearing Support Program is effective and well organized.	☐	☐	☐	☐	☐

APPENDIX IX-B

Customer-Satisfaction Questionnaire for Rehabilitation-Hospital Support Programs

XYZ REHABILITATION HOSPITAL
"On the road to your recovery..."

HEARING SUPPORT PROGRAM SATISFACTION QUESTIONNAIRE

READ each item carefully and CHECK THE BOX for the answer that best describes your opinion.

Please write any comments you may have on the back of this form. Thank you!

SA = Strongly Agree   MA = Moderately Agree   N = Neutral
MD = Moderately Disagree   SD = Strongly Disagree

ITEM	SA	MA	N	MD	SD
It was important that your communication was considered in your transition from acute care to our facility.					
• Nurse liaison was effective in communicating the importance of hearing to the rehabilitation process.	☐	☐	☐	☐	☐
• Nurse liaison reminded me to bring my hearing aids with me to the facility.	☐	☐	☐	☐	☐
Your hearing health-care needs were important to us.					
• Staff (e.g., secretaries, transporters, nurses, and so on) had effective communication skills.	☐	☐	☐	☐	☐
• All clinicians (e.g., occupational and physical therapists, and so on) were considerate of my hearing needs.	☐	☐	☐	☐	☐
• My family was included in the management of my hearing health-care needs.	☐	☐	☐	☐	☐
Our speech-language pathology and audiology staff is highly trained and knowledgeable in attending to patients' hearing health-care needs.					
• Audiologist was well prepared and organized.	☐	☐	☐	☐	☐
• Audiologist was experienced and knowledgeable.	☐	☐	☐	☐	☐
• The hearing health-care services were explained to me in ways I could understand.	☐	☐	☐	☐	☐
It was important that you were provided with efficient and comprehensive hearing health care.					
• My hearing loss was competently identified, diagnosed, and managed.	☐	☐	☐	☐	☐
• My hearing aids were checked daily.	☐	☐	☐	☐	☐
• Assistive listening devices were provided for my use as needed.	☐	☐	☐	☐	☐
• Useful communication tips were provided.	☐	☐	☐	☐	☐
• Overall, the Hearing Support Program enhanced my rehabilitation program.	☐	☐	☐	☐	☐

APPENDIX IX-C

Customer-Satisfaction Questionnaire for Support Programs in Nursing Homes

SHADY PINES NURSING HOME
"For their golden years..."

HEARING SUPPORT PROGRAM SATISFACTION QUESTIONNAIRE

READ each item carefully and CHECK THE BOX for the answer that best describes your opinion.

Please write any comments you may have on the back of this form. Thank you!
SA = Strongly Agree   MA = Moderately Agree   N = Neutral
MD = Moderately Disagree   SD = Strongly Disagree

ITEM	SA	MA	N	MD	SD
Your hearing health-care needs are important to us.					
• Staff (e.g., secretaries, transporters, nurses, and so on) have effective communication skills.	☐	☐	☐	☐	☐
• All clinicians are considerate of my hearing needs.	☐	☐	☐	☐	☐
• My family is included in the management of my hearing health-care needs.	☐	☐	☐	☐	☐
Our speech-language pathology and audiology staff is highly trained and knowledgeable in attending to patients' hearing health-care needs.					
• Audiologist is well prepared and organized.	☐	☐	☐	☐	☐
• Audiologist is experienced and knowledgeable.	☐	☐	☐	☐	☐
• The hearing health-care services are explained to me in ways I can understand.	☐	☐	☐	☐	☐
It is important that you are provided with efficient and comprehensive hearing health care.					
• My hearing loss was competently identified, diagnosed, and managed.	☐	☐	☐	☐	☐
• My hearing aids are checked daily.	☐	☐	☐	☐	☐
• My hearing aids are fixed promptly.	☐	☐	☐	☐	☐
• Assistive listening devices are provided for my use as needed.	☐	☐	☐	☐	☐
• Audiologist visits our facility frequently and reliably.	☐	☐	☐	☐	☐
• Useful communication tips were provided.	☐	☐	☐	☐	☐
• The Hearing Club is useful, fun, and informative.	☐	☐	☐	☐	☐
We respect and value your comments.					
• Overall, the Hearing Support Program enhances the quality of life at Shady Pines.	☐	☐	☐	☐	☐

CHAPTER 10

Aural Rehabilitation Programming in the Future

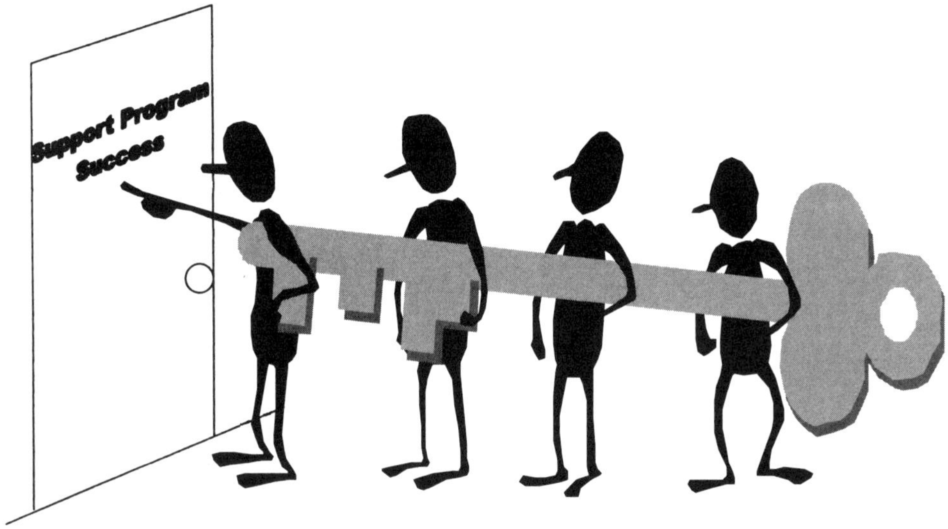

Figure 10-1. A team approach to aural rehabilitation is the key to support-program success.

INTRODUCTION

This textbook has discussed innovations in aural rehabilitation through the establishment of support programs for patients with hearing impairment in educational settings, rehabilitation hospitals, and long-term residential care facilities for the elderly. In each case, optimal delivery of aural rehabilitation services has numerous obstacles. A severe shortage of educational audiologists compromises comprehensive service provision in educational settings, for example. Similarly, most rehabilitation hospitals do not employ audiologists in inpatient treatment facilities, and many audiologists choose not to provide aural rehabilitation services in long-term residential care facilities for the elderly because of the unpleasant nature of the surroundings and limitations in reimbursement. Clearly, in these and other service-delivery sites, audiologists must devise innovative ways to provide aural rehabilitation services that are compatible with the increasing needs for health care in the United States for the year 2000 and beyond. Audiologists may be able to accomplish this goal through the establishment of stellar, cost-efficient aural rehabilitation support programs for patients with hearing impairment. Recall that in order to do so, however, they often must market and obtain start-up funds for such endeavors.

Our inclusion of two separate chapters in this book devoted exclusively to marketing and funding reflects our belief that the audiology profession has a long way to go in establishing the importance of comprehensive audiologic services, especially aural rehabilitation, for the health of our nation's citizens. Audiologists must realize that the entire profession must work toward this goal. Everyone must become involved. Audiologists cannot afford to think only about the profit margins of their own practices and leave the "dirty work" to their colleagues. Ultimately, the fate of the profession depends on everyone doing his or her part. The purpose of this chapter is to discuss the necessary steps that researchers, training programs, and individual practitioners can make to promote the importance of aural rehabilitation as a necessary component of health care.

LEARNING OBJECTIVES

This chapter will enable the reader to understand:

- Research needs in aural rehabilitation
- Aural rehabilitation needs in training programs
- Audiologists' promotion of aural rehabilitation

RESEARCH NEEDS IN AURAL REHABILITATION

Recently, interest has increased in the use of Quality of Life (QOL) assessments as indicators of outcome measures and as instruments for health policy decision making (Hnath-Chisholm, Reese, Ridge, & Abrams, 1998). QOL measures have been suggested for use in aural rehabilitation to increase the likelihood of these services being viewed as a necessity, rather than as an elective course of treatment for patients with hearing impairment.

Since the 1970s, some important research has assessed the impact of hearing on physical and psychosocial health. Table 10-1 summarizes the results of some studies in this area. Preliminary research toward this goal has shown that patients with hearing impairment have a higher incidence of health-related difficulties, such as heart arhythmias, ischemic heart disease, high blood pressure, and osteoarthritis (Crandell, 1998). Bess, Lichtenstein, Logan, Burger, and Nelson (1989) reported a significant direct, positive relationship between the degree of sensorineural hearing loss and the severity of functional health difficulties in 153 elderly listeners. Other studies have found similar relationships between patients' hearing status and health (e.g., Dye & Peak, 1983; Laforge, Spector, & Steinberg, 1991). Data are still needed, however, to support the notion that aural rehabilitation efforts do indeed improve the overall health status and QOL of patients with hearing impairment.

Crandell (1998) investigated the effects of hearing aid use on function-related disorders of elderly listeners with sensorineural hearing loss. Twenty elderly patients (8 males, 12 females), who ranged in age from 65 to 91 years of age and were new hearing aid wearers, served as subjects in the investigation. Two behaviorally based measures of sickness-related dysfunction were administered to these subjects on three occasions: (1) prehearing aid fitting, (2) 3 months post-hearing aid fitting, and (3) 6 months post-hearing aid fitting. Results indicated that hearing aid use over time reduced the amount of functional health deficits in elderly patients with sensorineural hearing loss. Similarly, Mulrow, Tuley, and Aguilar (1992) found that elderly male patients undergoing audiologic evaluations and a course of aural rehabilitation management at a Veterans Administration Hospital demonstrated improvements in their QOL 1 year after being fitted with hearing aids. However, in both investigations, the subject samples were limited, and there were no attempts at selecting subjects randomly or including control groups for comparison (Bridges & Bentler, 1998). Therefore, Bridges and Bentler investigated the overall well-being of elderly individuals, in general and then in the following subgroups, who: (1) reported no hearing impairment; (2) reported hearing impairment; (3) did not wear hearing aids; (4) wore hearing aids, but without much success; and (5) wore hearing aids and reported success. The investigators distributed 257 questionnaires through inclusion of the instrument in a monthly newsletter of a local area agency. Of the 251

Table 10-1. Investigations assessing the impact of hearing on physical and psychological health.

Year & Author	Purpose	Methods	Results	Conclusions
1979, Oyer & Oyer	To discuss the aging process and problems caused by hearing loss	Literature review	Hearing aids, aural rehabilitation, and counseling can reduce negative effects of hearing loss on physical and psychosocial health.	More research is needed investigating the impact of hearing on physical and psychological health.
1980, Thomas & Herbst	To investigate effects of acquired deafness on mental health, personal well-being, social, and family life	Administered two questionnaires to 212 subjects (ages 16–64), hearing aid users and a control group of 410 people matched on several factors	Respondents with hearing loss had greater incidence of negative psychological conditions (anxiety, depression, unhappiness, loneliness, and dissatisfaction with life) and health problems than those with normal hearing.	Hearing loss has a negative impact on general health and well-being. Patients with hearing loss should benefit from long-term aural rehabilitation.
1982, Harless & McConnell	To determine: (1) any differences in self-concepts between hearing aid users and nonusers, and (2) role of improved communication skills on self-concept	Administered a self-concept scale and speech intelligibility questionnaire to 68 patients (>60 years old) referred by physicians for audiologic evaluation and divided into two groups: (1) hearing aid users, and (2) non-hearing-aid users	Hearing aid users had a more defined self-concept, were more sure of themselves, and had higher communication function than nonusers.	Hearing aid use and other factors are significant in elderly patients' self-concept and communication function.
1982, Weinstein & Ventry	To assess: (1) the relationship between social isolation and hearing loss, and (2) the hypothesis that greater hearing loss contributes to greater social isolation	Administered hearing evaluation and two psychological function questionnaires to 80 male veterans (between 65 and 88 years old) meeting specific criteria	Respondents with greater hearing loss had greater isolation and hearing handicap than those with less hearing loss.	Hearing loss in the elderly is directly related to social isolation (greater hearing loss → greater social isolation) and indirectly related to communicative skills (greater hearing loss → poorer communication skills).
1983, Dye & Peak	To determine if hearing loss has a variable effect on psychological function and if any effects can be reversed with amplification	Administered a battery of tests pre- and 6 weeks post-hearing aid fitting to 58 male veterans (>45 years old) divided into two groups (more	Respondents with more severe hearing losses showed more dysfunction (less alert, poorer memory, less able to learn new information, more	Hearing loss has a variable effect on psychological function that can be partially remedied through the use of amplification.

continued

Table 10-1. *continued*

Year & Author	Purpose	Methods	Results	Conclusions
		severe vs. less severe hearing loss) matched for illnesses, general health, and severity of hearing loss.	paranoid, more depressed, and less able to cope) than those with less severe hearing loss. Both groups showed improvements 6 weeks post-hearing aid fitting, however.	
1989, Bess, Lichtenstein, Logan, Berger, & Nelson	To determine if sensorineural hearing loss has an adverse effect on the day-to-day functioning of elderly persons	Administered hearing tests, visions tests, and two questionnaires (sickness impact and mental status) to 153 veterans (65 years old and older) in relatively good health (ambulatory, no upper-respiratory disease or strokes) referred by local internists	Respondents with greater hearing loss had higher scores on the sickness-impact questionnaire (more physical and psychological handicap).	Sensorineural hearing loss is strongly associated with increased psychosocial dysfunction in elderly persons.
1990, Mulrow, Aguilar, Endicott, Tuley, Velez, Charlip, Rhodes, Hill, & DeNino	To determine if: (1) hearing loss affects elderly persons' quality of life and (2) if wearing amplification can improve these individuals' quality of life.	Administered five questionnaires, three times (initially, at 6 weeks, and then 4 months later) to 194 elderly persons randomly assigned to two groups: (1) fitted with one hearing aid on the poorer ear and (2) placed on a hearing aid waiting list	The hearing aid user group showed reduction of self-reported hearing handicap and communication difficulty and increases in mental status after 6 weeks, but not after 4 months. The waiting-list group did not show any improvement.	Hearing aid use can make some positive changes in the social, emotional, and communication dysfunction caused by hearing loss.
1990, Mulrow, Aguilar, Endicott, Valez, Tuley, Charlip, & Hill	To determine if: (1) elderly persons with hearing loss have more dysfunction than peers without hearing loss, (2) how much dysfunction is associated with hearing loss, and (3) which quality-of-life measures are most valid with this population	Administered five standardized questionnaires and hearing screenings to 204 non-hearing aid user veterans (64 years and older) with no severely disabling diseases	Respondents with hearing loss were older, less educated, had greater hearing handicap, and were less likely to have hypertension, diabetes, or congestive heart failure than peers with relatively normal hearing. No association between hearing loss and dementia or depression and hearing loss.	Elderly persons with hearing loss had more hearing handicap than their peers with relatively normal hearing.
1991, Bess, Lichtenstein, & Logan	To assess the associations	Administered hearing screenings,	Elderly persons with hearing loss had a	The relationship between hearing

Year & Author	Purpose	Methods	Results	Conclusions
	between hearing loss and scores ontests of disability and global function	vision screenings, and three questionnaires to 153 patients (65 years and older) referred by local internists	higher sickness-impact score and hearing handicap than their peers without hearing loss. Sickness-impact scores were more affected by PTA1 (500, 1000, and 2000 Hz), while hearing handicap correlated better with PTA2 (1000, 2000, and 4000 Hz).	handicap and hearing loss is complex and highly individualistic from patient-to-patient.
1992, Mulrow, Tuley, & Aguilar	To assess the long-term benefits of hearing aids for elderly patients with hearing loss	122 non-hearing-aid user veterans (64 years and older) with hearing losses greater than 40 dB and no severely disabling disease were fit monaurally with in-the-ear hearing aids; received a 45-minute fitting and orientation session; and were administered five standardized questionnaires at the hearing aid fitting and 4 months, 8 months, and 12 months post-hearing aid fitting	Respondents showed improvements in quality of life from baseline to 4 months, but none thereafter.	Hearing aid use can improve the quality of life for elderly persons with hearing loss.
1993, Carabellese, Appollonio, Rozzini, Bianchetti, Frisoni, Frattola, & Trabucchi	To assess the relationship between hearing aid and vision impairments and quality-of-life measures	Interviewed and administered four standardized questionnaires to 1192 inhabitants (between 70 to 75 years old) of a small town in Italy, who were divided into four groups: (1) Normal hearing and normal vision, (2) Normal hearing and impaired vision, (3) Impaired hearing and normal vision, and (4) Impaired hearing and impaired vision	Interviewees with a single deficit reported depression, poor self-sufficiency, and minimal social relations. In addition, those with double deficits reported lower mental status.	Presence of sensory deficit is associated with reduced quality of life. Impaired hearing has more of an affect on self-sufficiency, while impaired vision has more of an effect on depression and social relationships.

Source: Adapted from "Impact of Hearing on Physical and Psychological Health," by Hearing Industries Association and Beltone Electronics, 1998. *The Hearing Review, 5*(11), 26–30.

respondents, 77 males (30.7%) and 174 females (80.5%) responded to *The Geriatric Depression Scale* (GDS) (Yesavage, Brink, Rose, et al., 1983) and the *Satisfaction with Life Scale* (SWLS) (Diener, Emmons, Larsen, & Griffin, 1985). The GDS is a 30-item self-assessment measure of depression. The SWLS is a five-item self-assessment of life satisfaction. Subjects who reported no hearing impairment indicated significantly less depression than those who reported a hearing impairment. Subjects with a hearing impairment who no longer wore hearing aids reported less life satisfaction and significantly higher depression than the successful hearing aid users. In addition, successful hearing aid users reported significantly higher ratings in satisfaction with life than current, unsuccessful hearing aid users. The results of this study strengthen the association of increased hearing function and enhanced perception of well being.

The results of these studies have two major implications for aural rehabilitation. First, *hearing health-care professionals should consider including improved functional health status and overall QOL as measures of hearing aid benefit* (Bridges & Bentler, 1998; Crandell, 1998). Second, *these results may contribute to third-party payers' viewing hearing aids as necessary, rather than elective, components of health care for patients with hearing impairment* (Bridges & Bentler, 1998). Fortunately, as discussed in Chapter 1, increasing numbers of managed-care organizations (MCOs) are offering hearing plans that provide for the purchase of hearing aids for their enrollees. Audiologic evaluations and aural rehabilitation services, however, are too often expected to be capitated, or covered under the cost of the hearing aids. Clearly, our profession has a long way to go in convincing third-party payers about the value of aural rehabilitation services beyond the purchase of hearing aids. Further research that demonstrates improvements of patients' functional health status, QOL, and other outcomes measures are required before MCOs will cover the costs of comprehensive aural rehabilitation services.

Chapter 9 discussed the use of outcomes measurement in sustaining stellar support programs for patients with hearing impairment across service-delivery sites. Recall that the type of outcome measure used can vary across these sites. Efficacy data for support programs can include other outcome measures beside patients' functional health status and overall QOL. Students' academic achievement scores can be used as efficacy data for support programs in educational settings, for example. School administrators would be more likely to fund aural rehabilitation support programs if they contributed to significant improvement in the achievement scores of students with hearing impairment. Similarly, patients' average length of stay may be an important outcome measure relevant to support programs for rehabilitation hospitals. Health administrators probably would provide the necessary resources for a program that cuts health-care costs by reducing patients' length of stay. Research investigations are needed to show these trends on the national level. Unfortunately, many audiologists lack the time, means, and training to undertake these types of research endeavors single-handedly. Few audiologists consider research their primary job responsibility, and those who do are rarely involved with the investigation of applied research questions. Our training programs need to prepare tomorrow's professionals with the skills needed to conduct efficacy studies that validate patient benefit through comprehensive aural rehabilitation services. The future of the profession depends on it.

The increased focus on the audiology doctorate (Au.D.) over the traditional research and teaching Ph.D. places further limitations on the numbers of clinical researchers to conduct aural rehabilitation efficacy studies for two reasons. First, students are electing to pursue Au.D. degrees, rather than Ph.D. degrees. Second, most Au.D. curricula require little, if any, research experience from students. We believe that Au.D. training programs are ideal settings in which to foster the skills necessary to undertake these investigations. Training of research skills enhances both students' academic and clinical preparation. Certainly, teaching basic research skills in Au.D. curricula would benefit students, training programs, the profession, and ultimately the patients we serve. We believe that training programs can make a huge impact in this area.

AURAL REHABILITATION NEEDS IN TRAINING PROGRAMS

Throughout this textbook, we have mentioned critical areas of instruction for our training programs so that future professionals will be able to devise innovative aural rehabilitation service-delivery models that are compatible with the realities of the U.S. health-care system. Students must be knowledgeable about current health-care policies in the managed-care arena and their impact on the practice of audiology. We have advocated that training programs begin including this type of information in their curricula to prepare students to meet the challenges of managed care. Many university faculty members are often inexperienced in the basics of managing a successful private practice in today's health-care arena. Most faculty were trained and later taught in traditional academic teaching and research institutions that did not recognize, permit, or reward participation in "real world" clinical pursuits. Institutions from this academic model generally have no means to evaluate or reward faculty for these endeavors. Few faculty members establish private practices, and therefore few have to deal with the harsh realities of practicing in the "real world." For this reason, training programs tend to teach students "pie-in-the-sky" aural rehabilitation service-delivery models that exist in a vacuum and may not be fiscally viable. This text is perhaps the only book on aural rehabilitation that begins with a chapter on managed care. Our basic premise is that to be useful aural rehabilitation service-delivery models must always be designed within a realistic context. Consequently, we believe that training programs should educate our future professionals in the same way.

Many audiologists fear the new hearing networks that are growing throughout the country (e.g., HEARx, Helix Hearing Care, Newport Audiology Centers, Sonus, and so on). These fears may be rooted in ignorance. Some audiologists would rather "stick their heads in the sand" and not worry about it; others may choose to work for someone else rather than be the masters of their destiny through ownership of sole-proprietor practices. Because professional delivery of services is evolving in our profession, training programs must teach future practitioners the topography of the marketplace and the implications of these large, multi-office organizations. Future practitioners should make career decisions based on their knowledge of the facts, not out of ignorance or fear. *Knowledge is power!* Young professionals should feel confident in their ability to make a living whether they choose an academic, teaching-and-research career or pursue a more professional direction; whether they choose to work for someone else, for themselves, or to affiliate with a hearing network.

Managed care has had profound effects (both positive and negative) on the U.S. health-care system. Students must realize that managed care can offer some benefits to the profession as discussed in Chapter 1 (e.g., case-management approach, guaranteed referral base, multidisciplinary approach, multiskilling and the use of support personnel, outcomes measurement, steady cash flow, stimulation of business, and unification of practice patterns). Furthermore, training programs must emphasize how the benefits of managed care can improve provision of audiologic services across service-delivery sites. For example, Chapter 2 discussed the premise of using multiskilling in the development of support programs for persons with hearing impairment. A model was presented to illustrate how the use of innovative procedures utilizing multiskilled audiologic support personnel is governed by our code of ethics, federal laws, state laws, facility regulations and standards, scope of practice, preferred practice patterns, position statements, and practice guidelines. Furthermore, managed-care principles can be used in any area of specialization within the profession.

Our training programs should provide opportunities for specialization. Sole-proprietor practices can compete with these hearing networks by carving out their own niches in serving specific populations (e.g., infants, children, baby boomers, or geriatrics) or by emphasizing particular areas of expertise (e.g., tinnitus evaluation and treatment, evoked response audiometry, otoacoustic emissions, vestibular system assessment, and so on) (Danhauer, 1998). In the future, private-practice audiologists may find it lucrative to offer aural rehabilitation services through support programs for patients with hearing impairment across service-delivery sites. Instructors in training programs must acquire a better understanding of the unique clinical aspects of our profession and, in so doing, realize that they need to modify existing programs to include teaching of basic marketing skills and the fostering of resourcefulness in their students. Chapter 3 provided basic knowledge on defining and marketing aural rehabilitation support programs, and Chapter 4 discussed resourceful ways of finding initial start-up funds. Students must do more than just read about these aspects of audiologic practices in textbooks, however. They need to observe successful practitioners in the field as part of their academic preparations so they can "hit the ground running" when they graduate and assume professional roles as service providers. Therefore, training programs should encourage, support, and reward their faculty for professional and clinical endeavors and for forming partnerships with the private practitioners and equipment manufacturers. Such activities provide students with the necessary "real world" experience to reach more of the population with hearing impairment.

AUDIOLOGISTS' PROMOTION OF AURAL REHABILITATION

Individual practitioners can have a major impact on promoting the importance of aural rehabilitation services. *The challenge for audiologists is to provide quality aural rehabilitation services across service-delivery sites in spite of the changing health-care climate, personnel shortages, public-policy initiatives, economic considerations, and nonexistence of provider reimbursements* (ASHA, 1997). Audiologists must be aware of the need for strategic advocacy with legislators and for marketing services to health-care providers and MCOs to ensure that persons with hearing impairment will have access to quality aural rehabilitation of their disorders (Hallowell, 1996). Chapter 1 discussed the importance of audiologists assuming a proactive approach to managed care in three realms: (1) personal, (2) professional, and (3) clinical practice.

On a personal level, audiologists should learn as much about managed care as possible through books, Internet resources, local MCOs, and their professional organizations. Professionally, audiologists should consider affiliating with provider networks to be able to enact necessary changes from within the organization. As part of the system, audiologists can assist hearing networks in writing hearing plans that include reimbursement for aural rehabilitation service provision. Affiliated audiologists may be able to negotiate with their hearing networks to approach rehabilitation hospitals and long-term residential care facilities for the elderly about providing the cost of hearing plans as part of their patients' fees, for example. Both hearing aids and the costs of aural rehabilitation support programs could be funded using reasonable and mutually beneficial fee structures. Audiologists can enlist patients and their families to lobby legislators about the need for hearing healthcare coverage for all citizens, and for hearing networks, and insurance companies to provide aural rehabilitation services to their members.

Recent national efforts in achieving Universal Infant Hearing Screening show how effective coalitions of audiologists (clinicians and researchers), equipment manufacturers, hearing networks, patients, and their families can be in affecting legislation (Arehart, 1999). This is achieved by creating an awareness of and demonstrating the need for screening programs, and then implementing them. If we can do this for infant hearing screening, we can do the same for aural rehabilitation programs. After all, screening and diagnostic programs will do little good if we fail to treat those individuals who are identified and subsequently diagnosed with hearing impairment. Perhaps the time is right to start promoting aural rehabilitation programs that will treat those identified by the new screening programs. The fact that these screening programs must be financed once they are mandated bodes well for the future of aural rehabilitation programs. This means that someone finally will pay for our services, and thus more value will be placed on them. In that respect, the future looks much brighter for aural rehabilitation.

Clinically, audiologists must operationally define aural rehabilitation protocols that result in positive patient outcomes in the most cost-efficient manner possible (Frattali, 1991; Goldberg, 1996). The importance of consumer satisfaction on sustaining stellar support programs through the documentation of outcomes measurement was emphasized in Chapter 9. *Services provided without documentation have no chance for coverage by third-party payers* (Frattali, 1991; Goldberg, 1996).

Unfortunately, until aural rehabilitation services are considered necessary rather than elective health care, audiologists must play the role of fundraiser for patients who cannot afford to purchase the help they need. Chapter 4 suggested that audiologists use "strategic philanthropy" in locating sources of funding for the initiation of support programs across service-delivery sites (Chartrand, 1998). At first glance, these endeavors may appear to be a drain on time and resources, but audiologists can build a bridge of trust, recognition, and acceptance, however, with the largely untapped and distrustful segment of the population with hearing impairment (Chartrand, 1998), as well as with other hearing health-care professionals. Often, audiologists must form alliances with local service organizations and national philanthropic hearing-health networks to secure funding. *Audiologists must work as part of a team to establish support programs and meet the needs of indigent patients.*

Throughout this textbook, the importance of teamwork has been emphasized in meeting patients' hearing health-care needs through aural rehabilitation support programs across service-delivery sites. Chapter 2 introduced an innovative transdisciplinary approach to team building (ASHA, 1996) that involves breaking down boundaries between professional disciplines, which has the promise of being a more cost-efficient method of providing aural rehabilitation. *Audiologists must take leadership in managing support programs aimed at satisfying patients' hearing health-care needs.* Patient satisfaction begins with a vision of quality care and service. Audiologists must share this vision with team members. It is a process as much as an attitude, so it must be well planned, continually monitored, and frequently measured (Bronkesh, 1998). Chapter 3 discussed how support programs must undergo a continual process of development, planning, and evaluation (Johnson, Benson, & Seaton, 1997) as part of Continuous Quality Improvement (CQI) (Hosford-Dunn, Dunn, & Harford, 1995; Reisberg & Frattali, 1990; Walton, 1986).

Audiologists must show leadership toward these efforts whether in a hospital setting, private practice, or a hearing network. Leadership means daring to be different and to go out on a limb. It is required when attempting to establish support programs for patients with hearing impairment that may be viewed with skepticism by colleagues and facility administrators. Leaders can see relationships between and among practitioners from different disciplines in organizing cost-effective team approaches to aural rehabilitation through the use of multiskilling and support personnel. *Audiologists' greatest challenge in this role is to form a team from a group of individuals who may have little in common with each other except the desire and charge to help people with health problems.* Bronkesh (1998) presented Mark Kelly's (i.e., author *The Adventure of a Self-Managing Team*) characteristics of an effective team:

- Clearly defined goals and expectations
- Clearly established roles and responsibilities
- Well-documented guidelines and ground rules
- Open communication in an atmosphere of trust and respect
- Continuous learning and training in appropriate skills
- Patience and support by management
- Rewards tied to results
- A desire to improve and innovate

In this textbook, we have discussed how to accomplish all of these things. Above all, Bronkesh (1998) *advised audiologists not to be afraid to lead their team, no matter where they might be in the practice hierarchy.* Audiologists must be reminded that teams, like support programs, do not blossom overnight. Rather, they grow and mature together when given plenty of coaching, nurturing, and leadership (Bronkesh, 1998).

SUMMARY

This chapter concludes our discussion of innovations in aural rehabilitation through the establishment of stellar support programs for patients with hearing impairment. These ideas are considered within the context of specific service-delivery sites and in view of the current realities (e.g., managed care) of the U.S. health-care system. It is hoped that this textbook has served as a guidebook for students and professionals in managing multiskilled professionals and support personnel in aural rehabilitation support programs. For each service-delivery site, clinical management and managed-care principles are integrated for contextual relevance and for direct application of knowledge. Now it is up to us all, as audiologists to develop and sustain these programs for persons with hearing impairment and their families and friends. We hope this book facilitates that effort.

LEARNING ACTIVITIES

- List 10 qualities of a good leader.
- Discuss the current efforts of the American Speech-Language-Hearing Association and the American Academy of Audiology in enhancing the viability of aural rehabilitation services to third-party payers.
- List the 10 most important things learned from this textbook.

REFERENCES

American Speech-Language-Hearing Association. (1996). *Curriculum guide to managed care.* Rockville, MD: American Speech-Language-Hearing Association.

American Speech-Language-Hearing Association. (1997, Spring). Guidelines for audiology service delivery in nursing homes. *Asha, 39*(Suppl. 17), 15–19.

Arehart, K. H. (1998). Marion Downs National Center for Infant Hearing. *Audiology Today, 10*(Special Edition), 12–14.

Bess, F. H., Lichtenstein, M. J., & Logan, S. A. (1991). Making hearing impairment functionally relevant: Linkages with hearing disability and handicap. Acta *Otolaryngologica, 476*(Suppl), 226–231.

Bess, F., Lichtenstein, M., Logan, S., Burger, M., & Nelson, E. (1989). Hearing impairment as a determinant of function in the elderly. *Journal of the American Geriatrics Society, 37,* 123–128.

Bridges, J. A., & Bentler, R. A. (1998). Relating hearing aid use to well-being among older adults. *The Hearing Journal, 51*(7), 39, 42–44.

Bronkesh, S. J. (1998). Improving patient satisfaction: Leadership. *Audiology Today, 10*(4), 24.

Carabellese, C., Appollonio, I., Rozzini, R., Bianchetti, A., Frisoni, G. B., Frattola, L., & Trabucchi, M. (1993). Sensory impairment and quality of life in a community elderly population. *Journal of the American Geriatrics Society, 41,* 401–407.

Chartrand, M. S. (1998). Growing your practice/business with strategic philanthropy. *The Hearing Review, 5*(7), 35–36.

Crandell, C. C. (1998). Hearing aids and functional health status. *Audiology Today, 10*(4), 20–21, 23.

Danhauer, J. (1998). Who are those major multi-office audiology groups moving in on us, and—Is this town big enough for the both of us? *Audiology Today, 10*(2), 47–51.

Diener, E., Emmons, R. A., Larsen, R. J., & Griffin, S. (1985). The Satisfaction with Life Scale. *Journal of Personality Assessment, 49,* 71–75.

Dye, C., & Peak, M. (1983). Influence of amplification on the psychological functioning of older adults with neurosensory hearing loss. *Journal of the American Academy of Rehabilitative Audiology, 16,* 210–220.

Frattali, C. (1991). From quality assurance to total quality management. *American Journal of Audiology: A Journal of Clinical Practice, 1*(1), 41–47.

Goldberg, B. (1996). Imagining tomorrow: What's ahead for our professions? *Asha, 38*(3), 22–23, 25–28.

Hallowell, B. (1996). *Measuring educational outcomes.* Paper presented at the Annual Conference of the Council of Graduate Programs in Communication Sciences and Disorders, San Diego, CA.

Harless, E., & McConnell, F. (1982). Effect of hearing aid use on self-concept in older persons. *Journal of Speech and Hearing Disorders, 47,* 305–309.

Hearing Industries Association & Beltone Electronics. (1998). Impact of hearing on physical and psychosocial health. *The Hearing Review, 5*(11), 26–30.

Hnath-Chisholm, T., Reese, J., Ridge, R., & Abrams, H. (1998, November). *Quality of life outcomes for aural rehabilitation.* Miniseminar presented at the Annual Convention of the American Speech-Language-Hearing Association, San Antonio, TX.

Hosford-Dunn, H., Dunn, D. R., & Harford, E. R. (1995). *Audiology business and practice management.* San Diego, CA: Singular Publishing Group.

Johnson, C. D., Benson, P. V., & Seaton, J. B. (1997). *Educational audiology handbook.* San Diego, CA: Singular Publishing Group.

LaForge, R., Spector, W., & Sternberg, J. (1991). The relationship of vision and hearing impairment to one-year mortality and functional decline. *Journal of Aging and Health, 4*(1), 126–148.

Mulrow, C. D., Aguilar, C., Endicott, J. E., Tuley, M.R., Velez, R., Charlip, W. S., Rhodes, M. C., Hill, J. A, & DeNino, A. (1990). Quality of life changes and hearing impairment. *Annals of Internal Medicine, 3,* 188–194.

Mulrow, C. D., Aguilar, C., Endicott, J. E., Valez, R., Tuley, M. R., Charlip, W. S., & Hill, J. A. (1990). Association between hearing impairment and quality of life of elderly individuals. *Journal of the American Geriatric Society, 38,* 45–50.

Mulrow, C. D., Tuley, M. R., & Aguilar, C. (1992). Sustained benefits of hearing aids. *Journal of Speech and Hearing Research, 35,* 1402–1405.

Oyer, H. J., & Oyer, E. J. (1979). Social consequences of hearing loss for the elderly. *Allied Health and Behavioral Sciences, 2*(2), 123–138.

Reisberg, M., & Frattali, C. (1990). Toward total quality management. *Quality Assurance Digest,* 1–5.

Thomas, A., & Herbst, K. G. (1980). Social and psychological implications of acquired deafness for adults of employment age. *British Journal of Audiology, 14,* 76–85.

Walton, M. (1986). *The Deming management method.* New York: Pedigree Putnam.

Weinstein, B., & Ventry, I. (1982). Hearing impairment and social isolation in the elderly. *Journal of Speech and Hearing Research, 25,* 593–599.

Yesavage, J. A., Brink, T. L., Rose, T. L., et al. (1983). Development and validation of a Geriatric Depression Screening Scale: A preliminary report. *Journal of Psychiatric Research, 17*(1), 37–49.

Index

A

Abbreviated Profile of Hearing Aid Benefit (APHAB), 216–217, 283, 285
Academy of Dispensing Audiologists, 20
Acoustics, classroom, 164
ADA. *See* Americans with Disabilities Act
Adult learning experiences, meaningful, 74–76
Advantages and disadvantages of managed care
 for health-care providers, 3–5
 for patients, 3–5
Advantages of multiskilling, adapted, 18
Aging, aspects of, 265–267
ALDs. *See* Assistive listening devices
Alzheimer's disease and elderly populations, 266
American Academy of Audiology (AAA), 20
American Association of Preferred Provider Organizations (AAPPO), 7
American Dietetic Association, 17
American Managed Care and Review Association (AMCRA), 7
American Nurses Association, 17
American Physical Therapy Association, 17
American Speech-Language-Hearing Association (ASHA)
 Ad Hoc Committee on Multiskilling, 19
 ASHA-PAC, 23
 position statement and guidelines of consensus panel on support personnel in audiology, 27–29 (*app*)
 position statement on multiskilled personnel, 26 (*app*)
 position on use of support personnel, 16
 preferred practice pattern for ALD selection, 295–296
Americans with Disabilities Act (ADA), 21, 293, 294
 instructor's overhead, 86–98 (*app*)
 resources for high school seniors with hearing impairment and their families, 205 (*app*)

Amplification device support programs, 154–161
 children's role in serving as amplification device support personnel, 160
 establishing need for, 155–156
 monitoring program setup, 156–160
  devising program logistics, 159–160
  inventory of amplification devices, 156–157
  obtaining informed consent, 157
  obtaining necessary equipment and materials, 158–159
  selection of model or multiskilling and training support personnel, 157–158
APHAB. *See* Abbreviated Profile of Hearing Aid Benefit
Assessment
 of marketing plan, 42
 resources for CAPD, 163
Assisted-living residence checklist, 304–305 (*app*)
Assistive listening devices (ALDs), 52, 136
 fitting and orientation checklist, 330 (*app*)
 manufacturers, 63 (*app*)
 program and communication accessibility, 220–222
 selection, preferred-practice pattern for, 295–296
Association of Higher Education on Disabilities, 170
Audience, determining market, 38–39
Audiologic evaluation, appropriate, 274–275
 suggestions for modifications for elderly patients, 275
Audiologic service-delivery model in rehabilitation hospital, typical, 209–210
Audiologic support personnel, preparedness of related professionals to serve, 66–68
Audiologists
 allowances afforded by good networks, 7
 assisting students in transition, 173–175
 programs for students with disabilities, 175–176

Audiologists *(continued)*
  promotion of aural rehabilitation, 352–353
  relationship of to service-delivery sites and patients, 53–54
  shortage of, 148
Audiology program, full-service for elderly in long-term care facilities, 272–273
Audiometric and receptive communication screening, 273
Audiometric data from communication assessment, 286
AUDIOSCAN, 158
Aural rehabilitation services
  group programs, 291–292
  implications for, 6–7
  individual support programs, 292
  programming, future of, 345–353
  short-term, 222
  team concepts in, 16–17
Automatic gain control (AGC) hearing aid systems for elderly, 282

B

Baby boomer generation
  aging of, 264–265
  increased life expectancy of, 268–269
Basics of OAE screening program, 231–239 *(app)*
Batteries for hearing aids, 67, 132
Behavioral objectives for rehabilitation-hospital staff inservice, 71
  equipment needed to accomplish, 72
  example topics for informational and skill-based formats, 72
Behind-the-ear hearing aids, 170, 171
Benefit administrators, evaluating health plans by, 6
Business and Professional Women's Clubs International, 56, 62

C

CAPD. *See* Central auditory processing disorders
Central auditory processing disorders (CAPD) service delivery, support programs in
  challenges facing CAPD service-delivery support programs, 167
  implementation of management goals, 163–167
  resources for CAPD assessment, 163
  screening procedures, 162
  training and educating key individuals, 161–162
Central Oklahoma Association for the Deaf and Hearing-Impaired (COAD-HI), 57
Cerumen management, 273–274
Challenges facing CAPD service-delivery support programs, 167
Checklist of holistic factors in planning aural rehabilitation, 318 *(app)*
Children's role in serving as amplification device support personnel, 160
Chronic health problems in elderly, 266–267
CICs. *See* Completely-in-the-canal hearing aids
Civitan International, 56, 60
Classroom amplification device inventory sheet, 181 *(app)*
Clear speech, handout on, 262 *(app)*
Client-Oriented Scale of Improvement (COSI), 285
Clinical practice, proactive approach to, 9
Clinical researchers, limitations on numbers of, 350
Cochlear implants, 52
  understanding, 137–148
Collateral multiskilling, 17
Collateral-subordinate multiskilling, 17
Communication
  aids and services, examples of, 223
  and the ADA, 84–87
  barriers, 124–127
  as critical element in rehabilitation hospital, 207–208
  model for informal support programs, 155, 156
  with someone with hearing loss, inservice on how, 120–128 *(app)*
Communication disorders in elderly, incidence of, 267
Communication network for support programs in long-term residential care facilities for elderly, 288, 289
Communication/environment assessment and planning guide, 273, 311–316 *(app)*
Completely-in-the-canal (CICs) hearing aids, 170, 171
  for elderly, 276–281
    decision chart for assessment of, 277–278
  styles, 276–281
Compression limiting hearing aid systems for elderly, 282
Consumer groups for elderly persons with hearing impairment, 328 *(app)*
Continuity of management of patients' hearing health–care needs, 213
Continuous Quality Improvement (CQI), 42–43, 70

Continuum of housing for elderly, 301–303 (app)
Costs
  for audiologic support personnel, 57–58
  for materials, 58
  patient-related, 55–57
Counseling support programs, 167–170
CQI. See Continuous quality improvement
Cross-training, 26
Customer-satisfaction questionnaire
  for educational support programs, 341 (app)
  for rehabilitation-hospital support program, 342 (app)
  for support programs in nursing homes, 343 (app)

D

Daily log of hearing aid use for patients requiring assistance, 254 (app)
Dementia, characteristics of elderly residents with, 293
Diagnostic hearing evaluation, 274–276
Dietetics, 17
Digital hearing aids, 286–287
Disabilities, students with
  postsecondary students
    laws and related organizations regarding, 170
    programs for, 170–173
Disability and hearing loss, effects of, 210–212
Disadvantages and advantages of managed care
  for health-care providers, 3–5
  of multiskilling, 18
  for patients, 3–5
Distortion product otoacoustic emissions (DPOAE), 214–215
Documentation of aid selection protocol, 329 (app)

E

Ear, and hearing loss, instructor overheads, 111–117
Educational Audiology Association (EAA), 20
Educational setttings establishing support program in
  amplification device support programs, 154–160
    children's role in serving as amplification device support personnel, 160
    establishing need for, 155–156
    monitoring program setup, 156–160
  audiologists, shortage of, 148
  current, realities in, 152–154
  counseling support programs, 167–170
  informal support programs, 152–156
  learning activities, 176
  learning objectives, 150
  legislation on public education and, 148–152
  realities in educational settings, current, 152–154
  summary, 177
  support programs in central auditory processing disorders (CAPD) service delivery, 161–167
    challenges facing CAPD service-delivery support programs, 167
    implementation of management goals, 163–167
    resources for CAPD assessment, 163
    screening procedures, 162
    training and educating key individuals, 161–162
  support programs in postsecondary educational institutions, 170–176
    audiologist's role in assisting students in transition, 173–175
    audiologist's role in programs for students with disabilities, 175–176
    laws and related organizations regarding postsecondary students with disabilities, 170
    programs for postsecondary students with disabilities, 170–173
Educational support programs, customer-satisfaction questionnaire for, 341 (app)
Elderly, establishing support programs for in long-term residential care facilities
  aspects of aging, 265–267
  establishment of, 263–264, 270–273
  facility services, 293–296
    inservice training for staff, 293–294
    other facility services, 294–296
  housing, important considerations of, 269–270
  learning activities, 297
  learning objectives, 265
  obstacles for audiologic service delivery, 267–269
  patient services, 273–292
    audiometric and receptive communication screening, 273
    cerumen management, 273–274
    diagnostic hearing evaluation, 274–276
    group and individual aural rehabilitation services, 291–292

Elderly, establishing support programs for in long-term residential care facilities *(continued)*
    hearing aid evaluation and fitting program, 276–286
        hearing aid features, 283–287
        hearing aid monitoring and maintenance, 288–289
    residents of long-term care facilities, 56
    special services, 296
    summary, 296–297
Equipment and materials, obtaining, 158–159
Evaluation for hearing aid, 216–219

F

Facility Communication Accessibility Checklist, 221, 255 *(app)*
Facility services for elderly in long-term residential care
    inservice training for staff, 293–294
    other facility services, 294–296
Failed hearing screenings, audiologic evaluations for patients with, 214
Family resource centers, at schools, 170–172
Feasibility study, worksheet for, 46–47
Field of Dreams, 51
Fiscal responsibility, outcome measures for, 338–339
Fisher's Auditory Problems Checklist, 166
Fitting program for hearing aids, 216–219, 276–286
FM systems, guidelines for fitting and monitoring, 155
Formats, inservice, 70–74
    example topics for informational and skill-based, 72
    types of, 65–66, 70–74
Free and appropriate education (FAPE), 55
Full level of assistance, 219
Functional listening evaluation, 191–194 *(app)*
Funding
    for support program, securing, 51–52
    sources for support programs, 55–59
Fundraising. *See* Sources for support program
Future of aural rehabilitation programming
    audiologists' promotion of aural rehabilitation, 352–353
    innovations, 345–346
    learning activities, 353
    learning objectives, 346
    research needs in aural rehabilitation, 346–350
    summary, 353
    training program needs, 350–352

G

Geriatric Depression Scale (GDS), 350
Getting elderly patients ready for hearing aids, 319 *(app)*
Group aural rehabilitation
    services, 291–292
    sessions, room arrangements for, 290, 291
Group interaction checklist, 327 *(app)*
Guidelines
    for Audiology Services in the Schools, 150, 152
    for fitting and monitoring FM systems, 155, 164

H

Handout on clear speech, 260 *(app)*
Handouts for hearing aid delivery, 244–245 *(app)*
Healthcare, current climate of
    advantages and disadvantages of managed care, 3–5
    history, 1–2
    learning activities, 10
    learning objectives, 2
    managed care, overview, 2–3
        principles of, 2–3
        types of organizations, 3
    managed care and practice of audiology, 5–7
        hearing plans, 5–6
        implications for aural rehabilitation, 6–7
    proactive approach to managed care, 7–9
        clinical practice, 9
        personal level, 7
        professional level, 7–9
    summary, 9–10
Health Maintenance Organizations (HMOs), 3, 5–6
HealthClub, 173
HealthSouth model, 208–209
    inpatient rehabilitation programs, 210
    outpatient programs at inpatient facilities, 211
HEAR NOW, 57
Hearing, assessing impact of on physical and psychological health, investigations assessing, 347–349
Hearing aid
    check sheet, 184 *(app)*, 253 *(app)*
    evaluation and fitting program, 216–219
    fitting protocol, 217
    fitting shopping list, 243 *(app)*
    monitoring program, 219–220
    skills checklist, 326 *(app)*

Hearing aids in residential care facilities
  evaluation and fitting program, 276–287
  getting elderly patient ready for, 319 (app)
  monitoring and maintenance, 288–289
Hearing handicap inventory
  for adults—screening, 241 (app)
  for elderly—screening, 240 (app)
Hearing Handicap Inventory for the Elderly (HHIE), 215–216, 273, 334
  screening version, 215, 216
Hearing impairments, support programs for patients with, 213–222
Hearing loss
  confirmed, audiologic evaluation for patients with, 214
  and disability, effects of, 210–212
  and its effect on communication, 105–108
  and its effect on communication, inservice on, 102–119 (app)
  on education, impact of, 109–110
Hearing plans, 5–6
Hearing screening
  form, 239 (app)
  programs, effective, 213–216
High school seniors with hearing impairment
  ADA resources for, 205
  letters to, 206
High-performance compression circuitry hearing aids
  of other features, 283–286
  selection of, 281–283
  styles, CICs, 276–281
HMO. *See* Health Maintenance Organization
Holistic factors in planning aural rehabilitation, checklist of, 318 (app)
Hospitals, rehabilitation. *See* Rehabilitation hospitals
Housing of elderly, important considerations, 269–270
Human resources, 57–58

I

IDEA. *See* Individuals with Disabilities Education Act
Implants, 52
Independent level of assistance, 219
Individual aural rehabilitation services, 292
Individual Practice Association (IPA), 3
Individuals with Disabilities Education Act (IDEA), 21, 151
  amendment of, 175
Inefficient health care system, 1
Informal support programs, 152–156

Informed-consent form, 182–183
  consent, obtaining, 157
  for participation in support program, 255 (app)
Insertion and removal of hearing aid from ear, 133
Inservice for the Americans with Disabilities Act (1990), 82–102 (app)
Inservice on understanding cochlear implants, their care, and their use, 135–146 (app)
Inservice on understanding hearing aids, their care, and their use, 129–136 (app)
Inservice participant evaluation form, 81 (app)
Inservice programs, creating effective
  complete, 69–70
  components of, 69–70
  creating meaningful adult learning experiences, 74–76
  learning activities, 76
  learning objectives, 66
  preparedness of related professionals to serve as audiologic support personnel, 66–68
  selection of appropriate model of multiskilling, 68–69
  summary, 76
  types of, format, 65–66, 70–74
Inventory of amplification devices, 156–157

J

Joint Commission on Accreditation of Healthcare Organizations (JCAHO), 21, 334, 337
  National Library of Healthcare Indicators, 337

K

K-amp systems
  for elderly, 282
  processing, 218
Kiwanis International, 56, 60

L

Laws and related organizations regarding postsecondary students with disabilities, 170
Learning activities
  for educational support programs, 176
  fund raising, 59

Learning activities (continued)
  future, 353
  inservice programs, 76
  for long-term residential care facilities, 297
  managed care, 10
  for multiskilling, 24
  support programs, 43
  sustaining stellar support programs, 339
Learning objectives
  for educational support programs, 150
  fund raising, 52
  future, 346
  inservice programs, 66
  for long-term residential care facilities, 265
  managed care, 2
  multiskilling, 16
  rehabilitation hospital, 208
  support programs, 34
  sustaining stellar support systems, 332
Least restrictive environment (LRE), 55
Legislation on public education, 148–152
Letter of introduction to local service clubs and organizations, 61 (app)
Letter of request for consignment assistive listening devices, 64 (app)
Letter to administrators documenting inservice activity, 78–79 (app)
Letter to classroom teachers, 180 (app)
Letter to high school seniors with hearing impairment and their families, 206 (app)
Letter to patient and family regarding hearing screening results, 242 (app)
Letter to parents regarding support group, 202 (app)
Letter to request funding from local service clubs and organizations, 62 (app)
Lion's Clubs International, 56, 60
Listening questionnaire, 256–259 (app)
Long-term residential care facilities for elderly, establishing support programs for
  aspects of aging, 265–267
  continuum of housing, important considerations, 269–270
  establishment of, 263–264, 270–273
  facility services, 293–296
    inservice training for staff, 293–294
    other facility services, 294–296
  learning activities, 297
  learning objectives, 265
  obstacles for audiologic service delivery, 267–269
  patient services, 273–293
    audiometric and receptive communication screening, 273
    cerumen management, 273–274
    diagnostic hearing evaluation, 274–276
    group and individual aural rehabilitation services, 291–292
    hearing aid evaluation and fitting program, 276–286
    hearing aid monitoring and maintenance, 288–289
  special services, 296
  summary, 296–297

M

Maintenance and monitoring of hearing aids, 288–289
Managed health care
  advantages and disadvantages of, 3–5
  effects of on U.S. healthcare system, 351
  overview, 2–3
    principles of, 2–3
    types of organizations, 3
  and practice of audiology, 5–7
    hearing plans, 5–6
    implications for aural rehabilitation, 6–7
  proactive approach to, 7–9
    clinical practice, 9
    personal level, 7
    professional level, 7–9
Managed indemnity insurance programs, 3
Managed-care organizations (MCOs), 1, 3–9
Management goals for CAPD, implementation of, 163–167
Management of patients' hearing health-care needs, continuity of, 213
Manufacturers
  for assistive listening device, 63
  of OAE equipment, 229
Market penetration, 51–52
Market position and strategy, 40–42
  determining, 41
  developing timeline, 42
  selecting marketing tools, 42
Marketing
  audiologic services, 8
  effectiveness log, 49 (app)
  ideas for support programs, innovative, easy-to-do, 48 (app)
  positioning and strategy, 40–42
  resources, 45 (app)
  support programs
    assessment of plan, 42
    continuous quality improvement (CQI), 42–43
    preliminary work, 38–40
Masking level difference (MLD) testing, 163

Materials for families of children with hearing loss, 203–204 (app)
MCO. See Managed care organizations
Medicare
　and elderly, 268
　funds for, 56
Military Audiology Association (MAA), 20
Minimum Data Set for Nursing Home Resident Assessment and Care Screening (MDS), 273
Misconceptions of educational personnel about CAPD, 190 (app)
Model of multiskilling
　and training support personnel, selection of, 157–158
　selection of appropriate, 68–69
Model on multiskilling, 21–23
Monitoring amplification devices program setup
　devising program logistics, 159–160
　inventory of amplification devices, 156–157
　obtaining informed consent, 157
　obtaining necessary equipment and materials, 158–159
　selection of model or multiskilling and training support personnel, 157–158
Monitoring and maintenance of hearing aids, 288–289
Monitoring program for hearing aid, 219–220
Most comfortable listening level (MCL), 218
Multichannel compression systems, for elderly, 283
Multidimensional model of regulatory influences on practice of audiology, 22
Multimemory hearing aids for elderly, decision chart for considering, 284–286
Multiple-microphone technology (MMT), 286
Multiskilled personnel
　position statement on, 26
　resources on use of, 30–31
Multiskilling,
　multiskilling, 17–19
　　advantages, 18
　　disadvantages, 18
　resources on use of, 30–31
　selection of appropriate model of, 68–69
　use of support personnel, overview
　　learning activities, 24
　　learning objectives, 16
　　model, 21–23
　　summary, 23
　　support personnel, use of
　　　in audiology, 20
　　　history, 19–20
　　team concepts in aural rehabilitation, 16–17
　　technology, high cost of, 15–16
Myths associated with aging, 265–266

N

National Acoustics Lab—Revised (NAL-R), 218
National Hearing Conservation Association (NHCA), 20
National Philanthropic Hearing Health Networks, 52
Networks of HMOs, 3
　allowances afforded audiologists by, 7
Noise, definition, 163
Notification of patient participation in hearing support program, 226–227 (app)
Nurses' attitudes towards hearing aid wearers, 67–68
Nursing, 17
Nursing home checklist, 306–308 (app)
Nursing homes. See also Long-term residential care facilities for elderly
　support program, customer-satisfaction questionnaire for, 343 (app)

O

Obstacles for audiologic service delivery, 267–269
Occupational therapy, 17
Omnibus Budget Reconciliation, 273
Organizations for managed care
　types of, 3
　useful, 12
Otoacoustic emissions, 213–215
　equipment manufacturers, 215
　fact sheet, 228 (app)
　screening programs, 214
　test equipment manufacturers, 229 (app)
Outcome measures for fiscal responsibility, 338–339
Outcomes measurement across service-delivery sites, 336–338
　in educational settings, 336–337
　in rehabilitation hospitals and long-term residential care facilities for elderly, 337–338

P

Parents
　of children with CAPD, suggestions for, 195–199 (app)
　of children with hearing impairments
　　letter and informed consent for, 182–183 (app)
　　support group, 169

Partial level of assistance, 219
Participants in hearing aid monitoring inservice, 79 (app)
Patient services for long-term residential care facilities
　audiometric and receptive communication screening, 273
　cerumen management, 273–274
　diagnostic hearing evaluation, 274–276
　group and individual aural rehabilitation services, 291–292
　　group aural rehabilitation programs, 291–292
　　individual aural rehabilitation support programs, 292
　hearing aid evaluation and fitting program, 276–286
　　high-performance hearing aid styles, CICs, 276–281
　　selection of high-performance compression circuitry, 281–283
　　selection of other high-performance hearing aid features, 283–286
　hearing aid monitoring and maintenance, 288–289
Patient with confirmed hearing loss, audiologic evaluations for, 214
Patient's hearing aid status list, 251 (app)
　chart note, 252 (app)
Patient-related costs, 55–57
Patients and service-delivery sites, audiologists relationship to, 53–54
Personal FM system, 165
　check sheet, 186 (app)
Personal level, proactive approach to, 7
Philanthropy, strategic, 52–53
Physical and psychological health, investigations assessing impact of hearing on, 347–349
Physical therapy, 17
Pilot International, 56, 60
Placement in nursing home, negative effects of, 267
Position Statement and Guidelines of the Consensus Panel on Support Personnel in Audiology, AAA, 66, 158 (app)
Positive aspects of managed care, 3–4
Postsecondary educational institutions, support programs in
　audiologist's role in assisting students in transition, 173–175
　audiologist's role in programs for students with disabilities, 175–176
　laws and related organizations regarding students with disabilities, 170
　programs for students with disabilities, 170–173

Practice guidelines from American Speech-Language-Hearing Association pertaining to educational audiology, 150
Preferred provider organizations (PPOs), 3
Preliminary work, 38–40
　defining marketing goals and objectives, 38
　determine marketing audience, 38–39
　execute market research, 39–40
　identifying marketing tools, 40
Principles of managed care, eight basic, 2–3
Private practice, impact of on support programs, 34
Proactive approach to managed care, steps to, 8
Professional acoustic modification of classrooms, expense of, 163–164
Professional level, proactive approach to, 7–9
Professionals involved in support programs for CAPD service delivery, 162
Program for Students with Disabilities (PSD), 173
Program logistics, devising, 159–160
Proactive approach to managed care, 7–9
　clinical practice, 9
　personal level, 7
　professional level, 7–9
Protocol for children's educational program on hearing loss, 188–189 (app)
Provider networks, 33
Psychological health, investigations assessing impact of hearing on, 347–349
Public education, legislation on, 148–152
Publications for ASHA, relevant, 12–13 (app)
Publications on marketing, 44
　from ASHA, 44

Q

Quality of Life (QOL) assessments, 346, 350
Questionnaire format, use of to quantify customer satsifaction, 335, 341–343
Quiz, inservice
　on ADA, 101–102 (app)
　on communication tips, 128 (app)
　on hearing loss and its effect on communication, 118–119 (app)
　on understanding hearing aids, their care and use, 136 (app)
Quota International, 56, 60

R

Real-ear insertion responses (REIRs), 218
Receptive and audiometric communication screening, 273

Rehabilitation Accreditation Commission (CARF), 334
Rehabilitation Act and Americans with Disabilities Act (ADA), 170, 175
Rehabilitation hospital, establishing support programs in
  communication as critical element in, 207–208
  effects of disability and hearing loss, 210–212
  learning objectives, 208
  rehabilitation industry in next millennium, HealthSouth model, 208–209
  summary, 222
  support programs for patients with hearing impairment, 215–220
    assistive listening device program and communication accessibility, 220–222
    complete audiologic evaluations for patients with confirmed hearing loss and failed hearing screenings, 214
    continuity of management of patients' hearing health-care needs, 213
    effective hearing screening programs, 213–216
    hearing aid evaluation and fitting program, 216–219
    hearing aid monitoring program, 219–220
    short-term aural rehabilitation, 222
  typical audiologic service delivery model in, 209–210
Rehabilitation-hospital patients, funds for, 56
Rehabilitation-hospital staff member's attitudes towards patients wearing hearing aids, 68
Rehabilitation-hospital support program, customer-satisfaction questionnaire for, 342 (app)
Repair of children's hearing aids, obtaining funds for, 55
Research needs in aural rehabilitation, 346–350
Residential care facilities. See Long-term residential care facilities for elderly
Residents' rights in nursing homes, 270
Resources
  for CAPD assessment, 163
  on managed care and related profession issues, 12–13 (app)
  needed, 53–55
  use of multiskilling and support personnel, 30–31 (app)
Responsibilities of educational audiologists, 153
Rotary International, 56, 60

S

Sample case history intake form, 310 (app)
Sample items for resident assessment instrument, communication/hearing patterns, 317 (app)
Sample letter to nursing-home residents and their families, 309 (app)
Satisfaction with Life Scale, 350
Scope of Practice in Audiology, ASHA, 21–22
Screening Instrument for Targeting Educational Risk (SIFTER), 166
Screening procedures, CAPD, 162
Screening program for OAE, basics, 230–238
Self-contained FM systems, 164
Sequencing of motor skills for hearing aid use and manipulation, 246–247 (app)
Sertoma International, 56, 60
Service clubs and organizations, 60 (app)
Service-delivery sites, 53
  and patients, audiologist's relationship to, 53–54
Short-term aural rehabilitation, 222
Siblings of children with hearing impairment, suggestions for, 200–201
Silence, 149, 150
Single-channel hearing aid systems, for elderly, 282
Social assessment domain, for elderly patients, 283
Sound-field amplification system
  check sheet, 187
  efficacy of using, 167
  FM classroom, 165
Sources, finding for support programs
  factors related to, 53–55
    audiologist's relationship to service-delivery sites and patients, 53–54
    resources needed, 54–55
    service-delivery sites, 53
    status of support programs, 53
  funding sources for support programs, 55–59
    human resources, 57–58
    materials, 58–59
    patient–related costs, 55–57
  learning activities, 59
  learning objectives, 52
  market penetration, 51–52
  strategic philanthropy, 52–53
  summary, 59
Special services for long-term residential care facilities, 296
Specific content protocol for adult group aural rehabilitation sessions, 320–324, 325 (app)

Speechreading materials, 261–262 (app)
Staff inservice participation documentation form, 80 (app)
Start-up funds, securing, 53
Stellar support programs, sustaining, outcome measures
   changes in U.S. health-care system, 331–332
   critical areas of outcomes measurement for, 331–336
   learning activities, 339
   learning objectives, 332
   outcomes measurement across service-delivery sites, 336–338
     in educational settings, 336–387
     in rehabilitation hospitals and long-term residential care facilities for elderly, 337–338
   outcome measures for fiscal responsibility, 338–339
   summary, 339
   terminology in, 332–334
Strategic philanthropy, 52–53
Stroke, therapy for patient with, 212
Students in transition, audiologists role in, 173–175
Students with disabilities
   audiologist's role in programs for, 175–176
   postsecondary
     laws and related organizations regarding, 170
     programs for, 170–173
Subordinate multiskilling, 17
Suggestions for parents, teachers, and other persons close to children with CAPD, 195–199 (app)
Suggestions regarding siblings of children with hearing impairment, 200–201 (app)
Supervised-use level of assistance, 219
Support personnel in audiology
   panel on, 27–29
   resources on use of, 30–31
   use of in audiology, 20
     history, 19–20
     implementation, 20
Support personnel training, 65
Support programs, defining and marketing
   defining, 34–37
   impacts of on private practice, 34
   learning activities, 43
   learning objectives, 34
   marketing support programs, 37–43
     assessment of marketing plan, 42
     continuous quality improvement (CQI), 42–43
     market position and strategy, 40–42
     preliminary work, 38–40
   networks, 33
   summary, 43
Support programs for patients with hearing impairment, 213–220
   assistive listening device program and communication accessibility, 220–222
   complete audiologic evaluations for patients with confirmed hearing loss and failed hearing screenings, 214
   continuity of management of patients' hearing health-care needs, 213
   effective hearing screening programs, 213–216
   hearing aid evaluation and fitting program, 216–219
   hearing aid monitoring program, 219–220
   short-term aural rehabilitation, 222
   status, 53
Syllabic compression hearing aid systems for elderly, 282

T

TASK MASTERS, 173
Teachers of children with CAPD, suggestions for, 195–199 (app)
Team concepts in aural rehabilitation, 16–17
Technology, high cost of, 15–16
Telecommunication devices for the deaf (TDD), 220
Telephone, use of by individuals with hearing impairment, 58
Time-based outcomes, interdependence of, 333
Training program needs for aural rehabilitation, 350–352
Training and educating key individuals, for CAPD, 161–162
Training programs for MCOs, 8
Transient-evoked otoacoustic emissions (TEOAE), 214–215
Troubleshooting hearing aids, 134

U

U.S. health-care system, changes in, 331–332
Understanding Hearing Aids, their Care and Use, 292 (app)
Undetected or unmanaged hearing loss, 212
Universal Infant Hearing Screening, achieving, 352
Utah Assistive Technology (AT) Project, 58
Utilizing stations, inservice, 73

V

Visualization and imagery task for CIC insertion, 248–250 (*app*)
Visualization of Input/Output Locator Algorithm (VIOLA), 218

W

Web sites
   on managed care, useful, 12
   on marketing, useful, 45
Wide dynamic range compression (WDRC), 282
Worksheet for feasibility study, 46–47 (*app*)